HERE'S WHAT READERS HAV
THE 8-WEEK CHOLESTEROL C

"On April 10, my physician told m⌐ ⌐ ⌐⌐ cholesterol. It was 319 VDL and 83 HDL and a triglyceride level of 93. . . . I found your book about a month ago. . . . I was tested on May 23 and my cholesterol level was *142.* Can you believe that? I was so happy. . . . I thank you for writing a readable, informative and practical book."

—Frieda A. Jenkins
Miller Woods, Illinois

"You have done a tremendous amount of good for me!!! . . . My cholesterol went from 225 to 162. I am deeply grateful to you for facilitating my path."

—Ian Brown, M.D.
Beverly Hills, California

"For the modest investment . . . in the purchase of your book, and having followed the game plan religiously (almost), I have apparently reduced my cholesterol level from an all-high 308 to 188 . . . and in six weeks!"

—J. Keith Shackelton
Rancho Palos Verdes, California

"My reading was 263 in April. The countdown finally came two weeks ago and I am on top of the world. Thanks to you, my high-density cholesterol rose to a ratio of 4 to 1. I feel as though a thousand tons have been lifted from my shoulders and I can't thank you enough."

—Barbara Mraz
Strongsville, Ohio

"From a cholesterol level of 289 to . . . 174. . . . Both my doctor and I were amazed! In his words, 'Truly remarkable!' Also, as you said, along came the weight loss; from 201 to, at the moment, 180 pounds, and I still seem to be losing."

—P. Del Giudice
Convent Station, New Jersey

"Received your book on May 9 for my [61st] birthday. . . . April cholesterol reading—310 . . . July 17 cholesterol reading—141. This was a 54½ percent reduction!!! . . . Thanks again from the bottom of my heart!"

—Adam J. Herman
Cumberland Center, Maine

"I have been on your program for three months and my cholesterol level has dropped by 32 percent. It is now down to 202 and it has always been at 300. . . . I thank you very much for permitting me to reach the numbers that I never thought were possible."

—Robert E. Kushell
Glen Cove, New York

"Thank you so much—for helping me lower my cholesterol."

—Virginia Picard
Lawrence, Massachusetts

"I have read and followed Robert Kowalski's book. . . . My cholesterol dropped from 284 to 182 in eight weeks. At 5'8" tall, my weight decreased from 168 to 150–155 pounds and has remained stable."

—Robert W. Marling
Libertyville, Illinois

"Thank you very much for your book which has proved to be a real blessing for me. In mid-April, one day before starting your program, my cholesterol was 250 and my HDL was 42, a ratio of about 6. Three days ago my readings were: cholesterol 204, HDL 73, a ratio of 2.8. . . . Again, thank you so very much for your book. I feel certain it has added to my lifespan."

—Fred P. Kreis, Jr.
Treasure Island, Florida

"I recently completed your eight-week cholesterol cure and am pleased to report that it *works*. My cholesterol count dropped 54 points."

—M.C. Ellis
Birmingham, Alabama

"I have faithfully followed your advice. In exactly *three weeks* my total cholesterol dropped 40 points. . . . The greatest news for me, however, is the *improvement* of total, HDL, LDL and ratio. . . . Ratio from 6.2 to 3.6. . . . I am really thrilled. . . . The diet is *not* difficult—it makes sense and it *WORKS!* . . . I just want to share my exciting news with you and to *thank you* so much. . . . I am recommending your book to everyone! . . . I feel wonderful."

—M. Yvonne Thomas
Hillsboro Beach, Florida

"Since the first time I was aware of what my cholesterol level was it has averaged about 360. . . . In eight weeks my cholesterol was down by 140 points! . . . I tell everyone about your book. I told my doctor he should read it and he should prescribe it to all his patients. . . . You did a magnificent job. . . . I call it my Health Bible! It's worth its weight in gold."

—Sybil B. Ibey
Enfield, New Hampshire

"I picked up your book when I recently had my cholesterol tested and found that at the ripe age of 30 my total cholesterol was a whopping 261. . . . My latest tests showed my level to be 161—an astonishing decline of approximately 36 percent in just seven weeks. . . . Your book is an important contribution to this nation's health. Thanks for writing it."

—Charles R. Cross
Seattle, Washington

"I am a 49-year-old female and on June 3 my cholesterol level was 276. Last week, July 23, . . . mine tested 204! I had only been on your 'eight-week' cure for two weeks. . . . I am a believer!"

—Sue Genter
Bradenton, Florida

"I became aware of my high cholesterol [286] about five or six years ago and . . . I tried to do something about it. I tried it all: lecithin, fish oil, linseed oil, vitamin C, etc., and all in combination with a low-fat diet. . . . An attempt at cholestyramine was a disaster. . . . Needless to say, none of the above worked—my cholesterol remained in the two hundreds. So it was with some skepticism that I read your book. But I'm certainly glad I did. . . . I started your program in late May and in early August . . . the results were great. Cholesterol was 181, down from the most recent test of 250. HDL was 48—up from 37 and a total cholesterol-HDL ratio of 3.8. LDL was 92 and triglycerides 203—down from 236. Needless to say, I'm grateful for your program."

—Bill Manor
Wyandotte, Michigan

"I bought your book, read it thoroughly, and took the eight-week cholesterol cure. The results were beyond my expectation. In eight weeks my cholesterol dropped from 277 mg to 155 mg (44 percent). My weight went from 173 to 155 pounds . . . and I'm able to maintain this weight and still enjoy eating. I highly recommend your book to all my friends and workers. Keep up the good work—you have changed my life and hopefully my longevity."

—Ralph E. Dinsman
Las Vegas, Nevada

"I read your book with interest and . . . I followed your recommendations. . . . My blood cholesterol dropped from 288 to 150 in seven weeks. When I told my cardiologist this, his response understandably was 'unbelievable. I never heard of anything like that. How did you say you did it?' . . . You have made a marvelous contribution to your fellow man. I sincerely appreciate what you have done."

—David B. Boller
Los Angeles, California

"My husband has tried it all for 15 years, has been on the Pritikin diet . . . after trying the American Heart Association diet—a flop! Pritikin helped, but after hearing you on the radio a few months ago he bought your book and he started on the program right away. . . . It has helped! . . . He . . . has his cholesterol well under 200. It has been as low as 125. Thanks for your research and book and newsletter! It is the best help we have found, so far."

—Ramona Taylor
Tucson, Arizona

"My results were wildly dramatic: my cholesterol level dropped from 293 to 101! I told everyone I know about *The 8-Week Cholesterol Cure*. My doctor now gives copies of the book to his patients. And, for the first time in my life, I do not have digestive problems. . . . I think your book is terrific: intelligent, honest, appropriately personal and extremely helpful."

—Michael Padnos
Cambridge, Massachusetts

"I have followed the regimen that you suggested for three months now—all with good results. My total cholesterol was 265 and now it is 183."

—Josephine Dinsmore
Lake Charles, Louisiana

"In 1978 I had bypass surgery because of severe artery problems. I could not lower my cholesterol levels to any significant degree. . . . On March 7, 1987, I read your book. . . . I had a blood test on May 5 and the results were dramatic: 245 down to 165. . . . To say that I am pleased is a vast understatement. I for once feel that I am in some control of my own health and life. Thanks for opening my eyes to what I consider may well be a lifesaver. Also, for giving me hope again."

—George D. White
Oceanside, California

"I was doing really great after my triple bypass, but my cholesterol at 250 for my age and situation was too high. . . . A few days later I came across your book. . . . Today, I completed the eight-week course (less two days) and took a quickie serum: cholesterol test at a medical fair. . . . I held my breath as the machine kicked out 184—down 66 points."

—Earl E. Lane
Alexandria, Virginia

"A couple of months ago I purchased your book. . . . Thank you for writing it! Who knows, your book may have saved my life. For me your method worked, no doubt about it! Today my level is a healthy 182, that's a 30 percent drop in only 8 weeks."

—Bob Payne
Incline Village, Nevada

"7/11—bought your book. . . . 286 cholesterol: LDL 207, HDL 58, triglycerides 106. . . . 7/27—total cholesterol 189! LDL 103, HDL 70, triglycerides 81. Is this some sort of a record?"

—Barbara Vance, R.N.
Seattle, Washington

"Curiously, over the past couple of years [my cholesterol level] has risen although I've been on a strict low-fat diet for years. Now for the interesting news—immediately after reading your book I started eating three oat bran muffins a day. . . . I did have my cholesterol checked this past Monday and just got the results—a dramatic 35-point drop *in less than two weeks*. . . . A million thanks for your book."

—Tony DiMarco
Los Angeles, California

Also by Robert E. Kowalski

Cholesterol & Children: Giving Your Children
a Future Free of Heart Disease

The 8-Week Cholesterol Cure Cookbook

8 Steps to a Healthy Heart

The Revolutionary Cholesterol Breakthrough

The Type II Diabetes Diet Book

Robert E. Kowalski

THE 8-WEEK CHOLESTEROL CURE

How to Lower Your Blood Cholesterol by Up to 40 Percent Without Drugs or Deprivation

Foreword by
Albert A. Kattus, M.D.

Revised Edition

HarperLargePrint

An Imprint of HarperCollins*Publishers*

A hardcover edition of this book
was published by Harper & Row Publishers.
A revised trade paperback edition
was published in 1990 by Perennial Library.
A rack-sized paperback edition
was published in 1999 by HarperPaperbacks.

HarperCollins books may be purchased for educational,
business, or sales promotional use.
For information please write: Special Markets Department,
HarperCollins Publishers, Inc., 10 East 53rd Street,
New York, NY 10022.

FIRST LARGE PRINT EDITION

Library of Congress Cataloging-in-Publication Data
has been applied for.

ISBN 0-06-095574-0

00 01 02 03 04 ❖/RRD 10 9 8 7 6 5 4 3 2 1

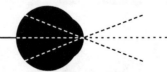

This Large Print Book carries the
Seal of Approval of N.A.V.H.

I dedicate this book to my father with loving memories of the past, and to my children, Ross and Jenny, with the joys and memories of the present and future.

Acknowledgments

Full acknowledgment of all those who contributed to the development of this book would be impossible, as they include my educators and mentors through the years, the doctors and nurses who helped me stay around in this world to write it, and all those whose lives have touched mine in ways reflected throughout these pages. I'm particularly grateful, however, to the late Dr. Albert A. Kattus, both for his medical ministrations and his personal support and confidence in the research documenting the basic premise of this book. My thanks also to the nurses at the Santa Monica Hospital Medical Center who contributed their time to our research project. I also deeply appreciate the confidence of all those involved in the process of bringing the manuscript dream to the published reality.

Contents

Tables

The Diet-Heart Newsletter

Reading this book will bring you up to date on the latest information about how the foods we eat affect our risk of heart disease and what we can do to reduce that risk. But this is an ever-expanding area of research and developments. To keep you abreast of current happenings in the field, I have developed *The Diet-Heart Newsletter.*

In fact, much of the new information in this updated edition of *The 8-Week Cholesterol Cure* was first brought to readers of the previously published hardcover edition by way of the *Newsletter.*

This quarterly publication summarizes current articles in the medical literature, ideas that often are not available to the public. You'll receive insights from medical meetings and seminars not typically reported to the public. You'll get newly developed recipes and dietary suggestions about new products. There is also a regular question-answer forum in which you can participate.

For a sample of *The Diet-Heart Newsletter* and subscription information send a stamped, self-addressed business-size (large) envelope to:

The Diet-Heart Newsletter
Post Office Box 2039
Venice, CA 90294

Foreword
by Albert A. Kattus, M.D.

Former Director, Cardiac Rehabilitation
Santa Monica Hospital Medical Center
Santa Monica, California

Honorary Professor of Medicine
University of California School of Medicine
Los Angeles, California
Deceased

In the last century the concept of preventive medicine had its first big triumph when the ravages of bacterial infective disease began to come under control. Pasteur taught how to destroy the germs of tuberculosis and typhoid fever and other diarrheal organisms in the milk supply. Pure water and uncontaminated foods, vaccination, and, at length, antibiotics brought many of the great scourges of the world under control, with the saving of innumerable lives.

The big recent triumph of disease control is highlighted by the mortality statistics of cardiovascular disease over the years from 1950 to 1980. The mortality rate due to diseases of the heart and blood vessels has fallen 40 percent in the United States over the past thirty

years. Whereas infectious disease was the leading cause of death in the first half of our century, the leading cause of death in the second
half of the century have been arteriosclerotic
diseases of the heart, brain, and other vital organs.

The fact that the mortality of these diseases
has been reduced by 40 percent, however,
does not mean that this epidemic is now under
control. The fact is that cardiovascular disease
(clogging of the arteries of the heart and other
vital organs) is still the leading cause of death
in our time. Thus, in order to complete the
victory over this disease, it is necessary that the
entire population of the country cooperate to
develop lifestyles that will minimize the likelihood of progression of the interior chemistry
that results in clogging of the arteries of the
body.

How did it happen that the mortality rates
fell by 40 percent in the years from 1950 to
1980? The key to understanding that big drop
is found in an analysis of what happened during those years. At the peak of the mortality
rate for heart disease, the Second World War
was just over. Americans were looking for a
better break. Veterans were getting benefits:
education, cheap mortgages, good health
care, and so forth. But a surprising number
were having heart attacks, and many who had

avoided bullets, shrapnel, and grenades were now falling victim to heart disease.

At about that time, the federal government took partial responsibility for the nation's health by establishing the National Institutes of Health, which is involved with pure food and drugs, vaccination, and pure water. Now that it was clear that heart and blood-vessel diseases were killing more Americans than any other disease, it didn't take long before the National Heart Institute was born. This organization developed and financed research programs on campuses, in university medical school laboratories, and in major nonuniversity medical centers.

At about the same time, the American Heart Association began to promote heart disease research by funding investigators, some of them eminent scientists and others promising young researchers and teachers, from private donations.

Thus a strong surge of scientific investigation began regarding the basic causes of heart disease and what might be done to reduce the terrible toll, much of it among young persons in the prime of life. Some of the fruits of the effort were the development of coronary care units, the heart-lung pump for open-heart surgery, cardiopulmonary resuscitation, drugs for controlling lethal abnormalities of the heart rhythm which often lead to cardiac arrest and sudden death and electronic heart pacemakers to keep the heart from beating too slowly. Many lives were saved among those presenting with heart disease. Mortality from heart attack (myocardial infarction) was significantly reduced. But the cost was enormous and the underlying disease of the arteries was still there, likely to strike at another time. No cures could be claimed. The magic Drano for cleaning out the arteries was not discovered.

The basic need was understanding the chemical mechanism resulting in the deposit of atherosclerotic plaque that clogs the arteries and leads to stroke and heart attacks. The idea is that if the mechanism is known and understood it may become possible to prevent the disease process before it has a chance to start. It may be much easier on the patient to avoid the disease that could kill him and it is likely to be much less expensive to prevent the disease rather than to treat it after it has done severe damage to health and longevity.

The research of the years of the fifties and sixties provided the information that paved the way to preventive cardiology. Discovery of the three major risk factors that are the most reliable predictors of coronary heart disease provided the clues to prevention. These factors are high blood pressure, cigarette smoking, and elevated blood levels of cholesterol. When these characteristics are present in an individual, that person has ten times greater risk of having coronary heart disease than those in whom the factors are absent.

Epidemiologists have studied the statistics of the falling rate of heart disease and have reached the conclusion that the remarkable reduction of heart-disease death cannot be due to better doctoring by the physicians who treat the disease after it is diagnosed. The answer is that the adoption of a more healthful lifestyle has taken place in a large segment of the population. The public has learned about the risk factors and has taken it upon itself to find out how it can help itself to a heart-disease-free future.

We know that in the years from 1963 to 1977 tobacco use fell by 30 percent and 40 million Americans stopped smoking. In recent years, consumption of animal fats and oils has dropped by 47 percent and butterfat intake has gone down by 33 percent. These data indicate that the public is taking action to improve health habits and has succeeded to a remarkable extent.

Smoking can be stopped by an act of the will. Nothing complex there: either you do it or you don't.

Blood-pressure control may depend on

maintaining appropriate body weight, avoiding too much sodium, and, if necessary, use of medicines which can lower the pressure.

Control of the blood cholesterol is the most complicated problem. Each person's own body chemistry determines how much cholesterol that body will make. We know that some people can lower the cholesterol manufactured and the amount in the blood just by cutting down the amount of fat they eat. However, some people have high levels even though they eat almost no fat. Some people respond well to certain medicines for cholesterol reduction and some do not. The problem is to be sure that the cholesterol which is so important in forming the blockage material in the arteries can be brought to a low enough level in the blood to assure that it won't deposit in the arteries and yet will be present in enough quantity to fulfill the basic jobs that it has to do, that is, to help build the membranes that form the walls of the body cells and to aid in the synthesis of a number of the body hormones vital for human function. Previous efforts have been largely unsuccessful.

Mr. Kowalski has provided the information needed for lowering one's cholesterol. It is a "how-to" book. How to find the foods that are least likely to bring about a cholesterol excess. How to avoid the foods that are most likely to yield a cholesterol excess. How to use special foods with special properties for lowering cholesterol. How to use the vitamins that tend to lower cholesterol.

This is a comprehensive work on how to deal with the chemistry of cholesterol so that it will enhance good health and avoid the diseases that are caused by clogged-up arteries.

Adherence to the program described in this book has resulted in lowering the serum cholesterol in a series of volunteer test subjects. Surprisingly these subjects also had the additional bonus of a significant rise in the level of high density lipoprotein, a protective component of cholesterol further lowering the risk of coronary artery obstructive disease.

I have watched the program evolve and I have seen the gratifying reduction in heart disease risk of most of the volunteer participants in the research. The results have indicated that the consumption of a low-fat diet, along with oat bran and niacin (one of the B-complex vitamins) is both safe and effective. I believe that this program will become a useful method for self-control of the serum cholesterol level, thus further reducing the risk of coronary heart disease by preventive measures.

Introduction to the Completely Revised Edition

On Monday, October 5, 1987, six months after the publication date of this book, the federal government and more than twenty health organizations declared war on cholesterol and heart disease. In a much publicized press conference, they issued the nation's first detailed guidelines for both physicians and the public.

They unequivocally stated that serum cholesterol levels should never exceed 200 mg/dl, regardless of age or sex. That's considerably lower than the previously accepted levels—and in keeping with the recommendations I had published in my book.

A major thrust to bring information regarding the identification and treatment of elevated cholesterol levels to both the public and physicians was initiated in the press and elsewhere. Diet, the authorities said, was the first order of business for those whose levels were above the cutoff point. And, if necessary, drugs could be used to bring this risk factor under control. Interestingly, in the many reports following that noteworthy press conference, the use of oat bran and niacin was mentioned as an excellent way to reduce cholesterol levels. In other words, the concepts first described in this book received widespread endorsement.

The response to the publication of *The 8-Week Cholesterol Cure* has been spectacular. Whenever I appeared on a television or radio interview show to which viewers or listeners could phone in questions and comments, the lines were jammed. Time and time again producers and hosts told me that no interview had ever evoked so many calls. When Dr. Art Ulene featured the book and its program on the *Today Show* on NBC-TV and invited viewers to write in for a printed summary of the report, NBC received 25,000 requests, setting a record at the network. Extra staff had to be hired to respond to those requests.

The public obviously had been waiting for practical information on how to deal with this major risk factor in the disease that results in the deaths of half of all Americans. The recommendations issued in the past had not been satisfactory; that fact was driven home in the thousands of letters I've received since the book's publication.

So many of my readers have told me that they never expected to be faced with a cholesterol problem because they had been following the advice they'd been given about cutting back on fats and cholesterol in the diet. They were shocked when their test results came back showing elevated cholesterol levels. And they were horrified when, all too often, their physicians were not aware that such levels were extremely dangerous. But they were as pleased as could be when, after following the simple recommendations in this book, their cholesterol levels fell to completely safe levels, thus totally eliminating this major risk factor for heart disease.

But it wasn't only the public who was reading the book; happily, the medical community has also responded very favorably. Most physicians and other health professionals have welcomed the book as a major step forward in our battle against heart disease. Many have written to tell me how they are using the book and its program both for themselves and for their patients. For some physicians, this was a way to work more effectively with their patients; they could prescribe reading the book, and then continue to monitor progress and answer questions regarding their patients' specific needs.

Of course, there have been some authorities who are not in complete agreement with the book's advice. Some have been concerned about my recommendations regarding the use of the vitamin niacin to lower cholesterol levels. The concern as stated was that men and women would take large doses without medical supervision, even though I had written—and even printed in italics—that such supervision was best. You'll read more about that in the completely updated chapter on niacin. But here again I'll state that no one should undertake a cholesterol-lowering program on his or her own. If nothing else, one needs to have blood tests done in order to determine cholesterol levels before and after following the program and annually thereafter. That's true even for those *not* using niacin.

A vast number of developments have occurred since the first publication of *The 8-Week Cholesterol Cure*. I've subsequently brought all this information together in this edition.

To date, many of my readers have been women. While most of the research in this area has focused entirely on men, coronary heart disease is far from just a man's disease. Since the first publication of this book, an article published in the *New England Journal of Medicine* cast new light on the relation of menopause to the risk of coronary heart disease. The number of women suffering heart attacks is growing, and the same risks that affect men must be considered for women, especially after menopause.

This completely revised edition of *The 8-Week Cholesterol Cure* contains four new chapters not published previously. I discuss the special considerations of women, children, and the elderly in detail. You'll learn all the most recent information on how HDL cholesterol can protect against heart disease, and, conversely, how low levels of that "good" cholesterol can be an independent risk factor for heart disease. You'll have all your questions answered about fats and oils, including fish oils.

When I first began writing about cholesterol and heart disease for this book in 1985, the only way to learn your cholesterol level was to go to your doctor or to a laboratory. Today there are a number of options. These are described and evaluated in Chapter 3.

At the beginning, I must admit that I believed lowering my own cholesterol levels would, at best, slow down the progress of heart disease. Today we know that modifying the risk factors of heart disease can completely halt the progress of the disease and in some cases can even reverse it. I'm a living example of just how well the program can work. And I can now give you definitive proof, in clinical studies and by way of my own angiogram, that heart disease can be defeated once and for all. Chapter 16, "Yes, You Can Reverse Heart

Disease," should be the best news you read on health and how you can save your own life, and the lives of those you love.

Finally, while I believe the program detailed in this book offers the most effective approach possible for most people, I recognize that all of us are as different on the inside as we are on the outside. Some people will require the most aggressive treatment available, in the form of prescription drugs. Ultimately everyone's cholesterol levels should be well below 200 mg/dl; for many this will require significant reduction in order to eliminate this critical risk factor. Since, for a very few individuals, prescription drugs do become necessary, then that option must be considered. And to provide the information you need to discuss this area intelligently with your physician, I've provided a complete chapter dealing with those drugs.

Similarly, I've brought other parts of the book up to date regarding new research developments, foods that have been found to lower cholesterol levels, new products that have reached the market, and a number of other details that have recently come to light. Many readers are already aware of those developments, since they have become subscribers to the *Diet-Heart Newsletter* I began publishing in order to keep readers up-to-date. For further details on how you, too, can stay in the mainstream, be sure to see the information on the newsletter preceding the foreword.

In a study conducted by Louis Harris and Associates for the Bristol-Myers Company in 1987, more than 200 scientists and physicians were asked what the number-one health problem in the United States and other Western countries will be in the year 2000. They immediately answered cardiovascular disease. While they were optimistic about future developments in medicine and surgery, those authorities recognized that men and women need to be educated and need to make some lifestyle changes in order to reduce their own risks of heart disease.

Here are the 1989 facts, direct from the data files at the American Heart Association: Heart attack is the leading cause of death in America, killing nearly one of every two Americans. This year as many as 1.5 million men and women in the U.S. will have heart attacks, and more than 500,000 of them will die. Nearly 66 million Americans have one or more forms of heart or blood-vessel disease. It's an equal-opportunity killer, claiming the lives of men and women, black and white, young and old.

To a very large extent, your health is in your own hands. You have a role in your own destiny. You're taking the right step by reading this book. And I sincerely hope you'll follow the program, thus significantly reducing the risk of developing heart disease. You *can* beat the odds!

Introduction:
The Program's Promise

By starting to read this book you've already taken the first step toward vastly improved health and vitality. The rewards to be gained by following the Ultimate Lifestyle Program outlined here are tremendous. Consider these promises:

- You'll be able to control your weight without feeling at all deprived.
- You'll eliminate a major heart disease risk factor from your life. Your cholesterol level will plunge dramatically, without drugs or deprivation diets.
- You'll vastly improve your chances for living a long, long life. The Fountain of Youth is a fantasy. This promise is a reality.

Probably the most astounding thing about this program is how really easy it is to follow. This is the program that says "yes, yes, yes" instead of "no, no, no." You can eat to your heart's content, knowing that you won't gain weight. Yes, you can go to restaurants. Yes, you can enjoy really taste-tempting foods. Yes, you can involve your entire family and all your friends—who wants to live like a monk, watching the world go by?

You'll look great and feel great. Think of how long you've wanted to lose those extra pounds. Now you can do so with confidence. And you'll have a vitality and exuberance you never knew possible. You'll wake up in the morning ready to face the day and all its challenges.

Remember Ponce de León and his search for that elusive Fountain of Youth? Practically everyone would like to live to a ripe old age. Biology books say the human lifespan should be one hundred years. The Bible states that the life of man is "three score and ten," but many men and women never reach that promised seventy. Yet science has methods to offer to achieve longevity, and you *can* use them.

No one can promise you won't be hit by a truck tomorrow. Or be struck dead by lightning. But you *can* cut the risk of heart disease and other life-shortening diseases. That's a promise. The chapters to come explain how you can eat to live, following this Ultimate Program for Cholesterol Control and Longevity.

As Mr. Spock says on *Star Trek*, "Live long and prosper."

Looking for the Silver Lining—a Personal Introduction

At forty-one years of age I'd already had one heart attack and two coronary bypass surgeries. I had been denying my problem for years, but suddenly came to the realization that something had to be done to improve my chances of survival. I began a search for alternative approaches and therapies that finally led me to the formulation of a complete, thoroughly enjoyable lifestyle, which I'm quite sure will help me live for decades to come, deriving full pleasure from all that life has to offer. Simply enough, I've found the silver lining in the black cloud, and I want to share it with you.

I sincerely hope that you'll follow the suggestions this program offers so that you can reap its benefits. Before going on to describe the program and how it can turn your life around for the better, I'd like to introduce myself and tell you *my* story in a bit more detail.

For the past several years I've specialized in writing about medicine. At Iowa State University I received my B.S. and M.S. degrees in Science Journalism, with additional study in medical physiology. During the next few years I had the opportunity to work in the pharmaceutical industry, with a medical association, and in the food industry. Finally in 1980 I became a freelance medical writer.

But during the time when I was writing about health, my own was deteriorating. Fast.

Heart disease was rampant in my family. My father died of a coronary attack in 1969. And, when I was only twenty-nine, a free blood analysis at a medical convention revealed that my cholesterol level was 250 milligrams per deciliter. The national adult average is about 210, and experts were starting to say at that time that even 200 milligrams was too high. But I ignored the findings.

Then in 1978, on Memorial Day, I had a myocardial infarction. A heart attack. Subsequent testing showed badly clogged coronary arteries, and it was time for my first coronary artery bypass surgery. A triple.

Still I denied the problem. I told friends that all was well, and that my "new pipes" were as clean as a baby's. I did very little to stop or slow the progress of the disease that had led to the clogging in the first place.

Sure, the doctors told me to cut down on fats and cholesterol. But when I did so, following the American Heart Association's guidelines at the time, my cholesterol level changed very little. Besides, I kept telling myself, the whole idea of cholesterol and its effect on heart disease was still "controversial." So I stopped having my blood tested and passed the next six years in ignorant bliss.

Then came the shocker.

After my annual treadmill stress-test examination, a cardiologist told me that the results were not encouraging. How could that be? I asked. I had been regularly swimming a mile of laps in the pool, usually three to five times a week. My weight was completely in control. I wasn't smoking cigarettes. Still, the doctor suggested another angiogram.

Like the guy who closes the barn door after the proverbial horse has run off, I suddenly became very diet conscious. Maybe there *was* something to the idea after all. And my cholesterol level was now 284 milligrams. Not good.

I went on a very strict fat- and cholesterol-lowered diet for the next two months. The American Heart Association would have been proud of me. But, after I had cut out all egg yolks, all red meat, practically all cheese (and all the other foods I loved), the tests showed my cholesterol level had dropped only 13 points. Discouraging, to say the least.

Then came the finishing note: the angiogram showed the need for another coronary bypass, this time a quadruple. The surgeon agreed with the need, but wasn't encouraging. He told me the mortality rate for "re-dos" was 5 to 6 percent. I went home and cried like a baby.

I had so much to live for! I adored my very young children; Jenny was three and Ross was six at the time. They needed me! Never before had I wanted so badly to live.

Well, the surgery went particularly well. I wasn't one of the mortality statistics. In fact, the experience wasn't nearly as bad as the first. My recovery was spectacular, and within a couple of weeks I was back at the typewriter.

But this time I decided, in effect, enough was enough. *Something* had to be done about the cholesterol problem. I was absolutely determined that this was one risk factor that I would get rid of. But how?

Diet hadn't done the job in the past, and my readings in the medical literature bore out the conclusion that some people—like me—just couldn't properly metabolize cholesterol. Even with just a bit in the diet, it seemed, the blood levels would be high.

There seemed to be only two alternatives, and neither was terribly appealing.

First there was the Pritikin Program. I had read Nathan Pritikin's books and heard about the good results some adherents had while scrupulously following this strict regimen. While I have a great deal of respect for this approach and its founder, for me this seemed like a life of deprivation.

I loved eating in restaurants, and Pritikin said to avoid eating out. I loved a wide variety of foods, and he said to stick almost exclusively with steamed rice and vegetables. Here's what Pritikin says in his chapter titled "Hanging in While Dining Out." It's on page 196 in the paperback edition: "Dietary sabotage away from home is impossible to avoid, but it can be countered successfully. Confronted with this kind of terrorism, many people simply give up. . . . Don't get into the habit of eating out too often. It can get wearying to make a production of ordering your foods in the enemy camp."

When I read this I was really discouraged. One of the true pleasures of my life has always been experiencing delicious foods in a variety of restaurants all over the country. But I was willing to give it all up if that's what it took to get my cholesterol down and give myself a fighting chance.

The other alternative was one of the cholesterol-lowering drugs. They *had* been demonstrated to be effective. But think of what they do to your life. First, the cost is out of sight. A month's supply of cholestyramine, one of the most prescribed drugs in this category, runs over $100. I could think of lots of ways to spend that $1,200 a year more pleasantly. Second, you not only have to buy the drug, you have to take it. Now, I was never a very good medicine taker, even as a child. I'm probably worse now. But this drug sounded like something out of a horror script. It comes in little packets, looking like gritty sand. You stir the granules into a glass of juice or water and gulp it all down before the mixture settles out. Four times a day. But that's just the beginning. Reading about the adverse reactions listed in the *Physicians' Desk Reference*, I learned that the most common problem is constipation. But one can also develop "abdominal discomfort . . . flatulence, nausea, vomiting, diarrhea, heartburn, anorexia, indigestive feeling and steatorrhea." That last one means your bowel movements may have the consistency of grease, since the drug acts by binding fats coming through the digestive tract. Not a very appealing alternative at all.

But what else could I do?

Because of the nature of my work as a medical writer, I had ready access to the medical literature. Never was I more motivated to "do my homework." And I was well rewarded. There was a viable alternative after all. People have elevated, high-risk cholesterol levels for three reasons. First, their diets contain too much fat and cholesterol, which their bodies are unable to properly handle. Second, they do not excrete sufficient amounts of cholesterol through bile acids in the colon. Third, they produce a large amount of cholesterol in their livers. Put the three together, and the cholesterol count soars. It seemed logical, then, to consider all three aspects of the problem.

You've probably heard that sometimes "the whole is greater than the sum of its parts." Well, I read about three quite different approaches to lowering cholesterol, all of which had been demonstrated to be somewhat effective, but none of which did the trick completely. My hypothesis was that if I put the three together they would work synergistically to achieve the total effect I was hoping for.

Bingo!

From a dangerously high serum cholesterol level of 284 (that's milligrams per deciliter, the designation typically used in medicine) my rate went to a comfortably safe 169! In just eight weeks. My doctors and nurses were amazed and delighted. Results like these had never before been achieved in such a short time, especially without drugs or an extremely restricted diet. The magic I'd been looking for seemed to be within my grasp: the combination of a common breakfast cereal, over-the-counter vitamins, and a reasonable and healthful diet, along with a program of exercise. Best of all, there was no reason why everyone in the world couldn't share the benefits. No impossible-to-follow dietary restrictions. No unpleasant drugs to take. No superhuman athletic demands.

Next, working with my cardiologist, I put the concept to a test to see if other men and women could benefit to the same degree. They did. The results of that study are in another chapter, and they are quite dramatic.

Needless to say, I was ecstatic over my own results. Now that my cholesterol level was only 169, one of the major risk factors had been removed, I could stop worrying about my arteries clogging up so quickly again.

But there were other rewards I hadn't even counted on. I had lost about twelve pounds during and after my surgery, which I expected would come right back when I started to follow a normal eating pattern and my appetite returned.

My appetite did return, and I did start eating a great deal of food every day. But I did not gain the weight back. So I started to eat even more. *Still* no weight gain. On top of everything else, it appeared that my program had a special weight-control bonus.

Digging further into the medical literature, I found out there was a scientific explanation

for all this. Part of the program calls for including oat bran in one's diet in the form of
muffins and cooked into other foods. Not
only does this cereal whisk fats and cholesterol
through the digestive system, but it also creates tremendous feelings of fullness—not the
bloated feeling some fad diet drugs give, but a
nice satisfied feeling. You just don't feel hungry between meals. You have no desire for
snacks. Scientists call this "satiety." I call it
wonderful.

But there's still more good news. With my
old eating habits, I had used Alka-Seltzer
antacid formula pretty often to relieve indigestion and heartburn. With my new program, I
could throw those antacids in the trash, or
save them for friends who hadn't seen the
light yet.

Speaking of friends, we all know how people feel sorry for those on diets. It seems dieters have no fun at all; they must feel
deprived and hungry all the time. But my
friends, even those who didn't have to worry
about their weight, were eager to try my program, asking for recipes and sampling my
muffins. I'm a walking testament to how *good*
a person can feel!

Finally, a word about longevity. To tell the
truth, I had never thought much about the
long-term future. My father and many in my

family died young, and I had assumed that I had inherited that legacy. Now my cholesterol level is way down, my blood pressure is a low-normal, my weight is completely under control, and I'm looking forward to a long life.

This program does more than just protect against heart disease. In the coming chapters, I'll tell you what medical authorities have learned about longevity and how the program puts you ahead of the game.

Read the book, follow its recommendations, and start on your way to a long, healthy life. Nothing like this program has ever been offered to the public before. Since it is truly new and revolutionary, I'd love to hear about your own results. I'd greatly appreciate your taking a few moments to tell me a bit about yourself and how the program has worked for you.

In the meantime, good luck and good health!

1

Cholesterol:
No More Controversy

Ironically, cholesterol has affected my own life over and over again during the past twenty years.

I first heard of cholesterol in college, when the professor simply described the substance as he would any other chemical covered in the course. Cholesterol, he said then and it remains true today, is an organic chemical compound in the family of alcohols. It looks and feels like soft wax. Cholesterol is just one of a whole group of compounds in the body known as sterols, all of which are essential to life. Cholesterol enters the body through the foods, specifically the animal foods, we eat. It is also manufactured by the body in the liver. On the other hand, if the body didn't have enough cholesterol to form vital hormones and metabolic products, we would not be able to survive. On the other hand, if the body has too much cholesterol, the excess begins to line the arteries, leading to atherosclerosis.

A long time ago, scientists noticed that in cultures where very little saturated fat and cholesterol were consumed, there was a parallel lessening of heart disease. But did the eating of cholesterol *lead* to the heart disease, or was it just another of the many aspects of the modern lifestyle that could be blamed? Thus began the controversy, the so-called diet/heart debate that raged for many years.

On a holiday when I was home from college, my father mentioned that his doctor had noticed that his cholesterol level was elevated, and had advised staying away from certain foods that had a lot of cholesterol. Of course, not much was known about dietary modification back in 1965. Dad and I had a number of discussions about cholesterol. I pointed out that Eskimos eat a lot of blubber and they don't get heart disease. There just was no proof about the whole thing. Just to be on the safe side, Dad avoided oysters, then thought to be high in cholesterol, when we ate out in restaurants. He ate fish because he actually preferred seafood over steaks. But, without much guidance, he still ate a lot of cheese and drank whole milk, and his cholesterol level was affected not a bit. One day in 1969 I got a phone call that Dad had died, at age fifty-seven, of a massive coronary.

Should I blame cholesterol? Well, Dad also had very high blood pressure. He was under a great deal of stress the year he died. And there was a family history of heart disease. Actually,

I thought it was too bad that he had missed out on the oysters.

Two years later, while working for a medical association in Chicago, I attended a medical meeting where a new computerized blood-analyzing device was being unveiled. All of us attending the meeting got free blood tests, and I learned from mine that while everything was in the "normal" range my cholesterol level was a bit high. One of the doctors at the association said that 250 milligrams was too high for someone only twenty-nine years old.

I shrugged it off and went on with my normal, all-American eating habits. There was no proof, I reasoned, that changing my diet would lower my cholesterol level.

My career path led, in 1973, to a job as a science writer at the National Dairy Council. Over the next seven years I became Director of communications, managing a great number of projects designed to improve the public's nutrition in general, and to increase the consumption of dairy products in particular by stressing their high calcium content.

During that seven-year period of time I read extensively about the cholesterol issue and met most of the scientists conducting research on the topic. Of course a great deal of my time was spent defending dairy foods against those who brought up the cholesterol problem. Even though I knew I had an elevated cholesterol level myself, I still felt there was no proof that diet could affect cholesterol levels, no reason to recommend altering the eating patterns of the entire nation. It was a "controversy." There was room for "debate."

A number of research studies during those years swayed many individuals, including me, to believe that altering the diet was not the proper course of action to reduce cholesterol levels. First, those who did change their eating habits found that their cholesterol levels did not decrease significantly. Second, the "average" cholesterol level in adult men was in the low to middle range of 200 to 250 milligrams per 100 cubic centimeters of blood. If that was average, therefore "normal," why try to change anything? Third, studies showed that people with low levels of cholesterol did not increase those levels when fed an extra-large load of cholesterol. Even the American Medical Association, after reviewing these data, concluded that there was no reason to give a blanket prescription of dietary modification to the general public. Many other medical and scientific organizations agreed.

Then, in 1978, at the age of just thirty-five years, I had that heart attack. After I recovered from the attack, the doctors recommended a triple coronary artery bypass; three of the arteries supplying blood to the heart were blocked and needed to be bypassed with bits of vein taken from my legs.

Yes, they took samples of my blood. Yes, the cholesterol levels were elevated. But even after the surgery I didn't really alter my diet. You might ask why.

The answer is very simple, or at least it appeared simple to me at the time. When I did try to alter my diet somewhat by cutting back on butter, whole milk, steaks, and the like, the results were so minimal that I concluded that I was just one of those unlucky people who didn't respond to dietary modification. This was the cholesterol level my body had "chosen" to maintain no matter how much or how little cholesterol I ate. Besides, the surgery had "cleaned up" my system and I was as good as new. So I thought. Six years later, I had my second bypass operation, this time a quadruple. I was only forty-one years old. Not a very good record, and not a very good omen for the future.

It was time for a re-examination of the situation. Diet still did not seem to be the answer in my own case. Just before the surgery my cholesterol level tested out to 284 milligrams. By rather strict dieting over the next two months I was able to achieve only a drop to 271. During that time, I drank only skim milk, ate no butter or red meat, and forgot the egg entirely.

Still, the evidence that cholesterol levels in the blood are a major risk factor in heart disease was building up faster than ever before. In 1984 even *Time* magazine ran a cover story on cholesterol, picturing a typical breakfast plate of eggs and bacon forming a frowning face. No more controversy, the article read. Cholesterol must be reduced to decrease the risk of heart disease. A crucial piece of data had been delivered in the scientific community after years of study. There was no longer any question about it: lowering cholesterol significantly reduced the incidence of heart disease.

For me, this began, rather belatedly, a comprehensive review of the medical and scientific literature dealing with cholesterol, heart disease, and what could be done. What I read led to an awakening, albeit a rude one. I'd like to share with you the most important data and recommendations I found in the vast library of available literature. I think you'll agree when you read the data that some action should be taken about cholesterol—and that the approach needed has not been available before. A new, safe, effective, and not unpleasant method of cholesterol reduction is needed. But first a brief explanation of terms.

CHOLESTEROL AND LIPID TERMINOLOGY

Actually, cholesterol is just one of a number of fats, also called lipids, found in the blood. Some of those fats are harmful when levels rise too high. Other lipids, the neutral sterols, are chemically related to cholesterol but have no detrimental effects. Finally, cholesterol itself is a broad term referring to a number of fractions.

The term we hear most often, *cholesterol,* usually refers to *total cholesterol,* the total amount of all cholesterol in the blood. The amounts are measured in milligrams per deciliter, abbreviated as mg/dl or mg/dL. This is the number most people and most physicians talk about when trying to "keep the cholesterol down."

A number of years ago, researchers found that the total cholesterol in the blood could be broken down into a number of fractions, determined by the *lipoproteins,* which carry cholesterol: low-density lipoprotein cholesterol (LDL), very-low-density lipoprotein cholesterol (VLDL), and high-density lipoprotein cholesterol (HDL).

Low-density lipoprotein cholesterol (LDL) is generally regarded as the real culprit in coronary heart disease.[1] LDL carries cholesterol

[1]Notes will be found beginning page 607.

through the blood and deposits it in the arteries in a concretion of calcium, fibers, and other substances collectively referred to as plaque. The formation of such plaque is called atheroma, and the disease is atherosclerosis. It is this atherosclerosis that we commonly call heart disease. Actually, the heart usually is healthy, but the arteries are blocked. So a more proper term is coronary heart disease, with the word *coronary* referring to the coronary arteries supplying the heart with blood. The higher the level of LDL in the blood, the greater the risk of heart disease occurring.

Very-low-density lipoprotein cholesterol (VLDL) is the substance used by the liver to manufacture LDL. Scientists refer to VLDL as a precursor of LDL. In other words, the higher the level of VLDL, the more LDL can be produced by the liver.

High-density lipoprotein chloesterol (HDL) is the protective fraction of cholesterol. HDL actually acts to draw cholesterol away from the linings of arteries. The higher the HDL level, the more protection against heart disease. The ratio between total cholesterol and HDL cholesterol, or between LDL cholesterol and HDL cholesterol, is extremely important. The higher the ratio, the greater the risk of heart disease, since there is far more LDL trying to line the arteries than there is

HDL trying to keep the cholesterol away from the arteries.

How does HDL exert its protective effect? Investigators at the University of Alabama have suggested an explanation. Dr. Byung Hong Chung and his associates think HDL protects blood-vessel walls against toxic remnant particles of fats that are broken down by enzymes in the bloodstream after a meal. Damage to blood-vessel walls by these blood-fat remnants may be at least as important in the development of atherosclerosis as the cholesterol deposited in those walls by LDL.

Others believe that HDL works by way of removing fat and cholesterol from the blood vessels and carrying them back to the liver, where they are readied for elimination from the body through the gastrointestinal system.

In either case, we know that cholesterol does its damage by clogging the arteries. That probably happens when some microscopic damage occurs in the vessel wall, and cholesterol along with other materials such as fibrinogen—a factor in blood clotting—and white blood cells and calcium are used to repair the damage. Thus we want to keep cholesterol out of the walls of those arteries.

Blood tests prescribed by doctors will usually include information about levels of *triglycerides*. These fats in the blood have quite a different pattern from that of cholesterol. Some people may have normal levels of cholesterol but very high levels of triglycerides, and vice versa. Scientists generally agree that there is, however, an association between elevated triglycerides and elevated cholesterol. Lowering triglycerides can help bring down cholesterol as well.

In total, then, it's best to have low levels of total cholesterol, LDL cholesterol, VLDL cholesterol, and triglycerides, as well as low cholesterol ratios, while keeping a high level of the protective HDL.

Diet and Coronary Heart Disease

The first indications ever put down on paper that diet might be linked to heart disease, as well as to other diseases, came from observations of the eating habits of a wide variety of populations. Comparisons were made, for example, between Japanese men living in Japan and relatives who had come to the United States. More than thirty such studies have been done over the years, and the conclusions remain the same each time. Those groups consuming less saturated fat and cholesterol have less coronary heart disease.[2]

Parenthetically, it's also worth mentioning

that similar studies were performed in terms of sodium consumption. Again the results are conclusive. The more salt and other forms of sodium in the diet, the higher the incidence of hypertension, high blood pressure.[1]

Certainly other factors must also be considered, as practically nothing in science and medicine is perfectly cut and dried. For example, in a study done with accountants, cholesterol levels rose tremendously during the stressful months just before the April 15 filing of income-tax returns. Those cholesterol levels drop back down after the due date passes. Thus stress has a great deal to do with cholesterol levels. In fact, Dr. Meyer Friedman first postulated that the Type A—or high-strung, anxious—individual is more prone to heart disease and elevated cholesterol levels than is the more relaxed Type B person. Friedman and his partner, Dr. Ray Rosenman, in their book *Type A Behavior and Your Heart*,[3] recommend finding ways of changing behavior—of avoiding anger and time-driven stress factors—in order to reduce cholesterol levels.

It is also known that certain individuals have a definite genetic predisposition to elevated lipid levels of all sorts. Simply enough, this appears to be a genetic metabolic disability to handle dietary fats and cholesterol. Even in animal studies, some are able to consume large amounts of cholesterol with no problem, while others need just a trace in their diets to cause havoc. The bottom line seems to be that many people, *but not all,* have the cholesterol problem. Some people, despite a diet filled with sinful goodies, nonetheless maintain low cholesterol levels. My brother Tom, for example, is one of those lucky ones. Tom eats everything he wants, with no regard to anything but taste. He watches calories only to stay fashionably slender. Tom loves eating in fine restaurants, and views the baked potato as a vehicle for butter and sour cream. Double portions, at that. Yet every time he has a blood test the results show that his cholesterol level is actually on the low side!

This is the same guy I grew up with. My mother fed us the same foods. We've had practically parallel lives. Yet his system handles dietary fats perfectly while mine goes wild. No one ever said life was fair.

Anyway, back to the literature.

In studies at the University of Illinois and elsewhere pigs were fed a variety of diets. Pigs are used because their vascular systems are very similar to those of human beings. The pig's aorta, the large artery coming out of the heart, is practically the same as ours. No doubt about it, diet can alter the accumulation of the so-called atherosclerotic plaque that lines the aorta and other arteries. Pigs with a predisposition to a high cholesterol diet will clog up their arteries rather quickly. Many studies have shown this to be true.

Certain groups of people, even those living in the affluent United States, have a very low level of heart disease. And the diet is involved. Such a group is the Seventh Day Adventists, whose lives are built around a vegetarian diet.[4] But even those data are not clear. Yes, they have little heart disease. Yes, they avoid meat. But they follow what is known as a lacto-ovo vegetarian diet, which includes lots of cheese and eggs almost every day. Yet the egg and cheese are where a large amount of dietary cholesterol is found. It appears, to me at least, that some other factors are operating for the Seventh Day Adventists. Probably this comes down, once again, to simple genetics. They tend to be a rather closed group of people, with individuals marrying within their religion. Perhaps the trait of handling dietary fats properly has been handed down through the generations. On the other hand, if a Seventh Day Adventist were to have a genetic problem, reducing saturated fat and cholesterol by avoiding red meats would be important.

It is such conflicting and confusing data and information that have developed the controversy over the years. But, as we're about to see, that discussion is really moot for those who *do* tend to develop high cholesterol levels.

Does any controversy still exist regarding diet and heart disease? To answer that question, Dr. Kaare Norum of the University of Norway in Oslo sent a questionnaire to more than two hundred of the leading authorities all over the world. These were the men and women doing the cutting-edge research dealing with dietary fat and coronary heart disease. He asked them whether they believed there is a connection between diet and the development of coronary heart disease. Ninety-seven percent said yes. Asked whether they thought there is a connection between diet and blood cholesterol level, 98 percent said yes. And when asked whether there is a connection between plasma cholesterol and the development of coronary heart disease, 98 percent again said yes. The conclusion anyone can reach is that there is no more controversy.

A survey conducted by the Food and Drug Administration in 1984 indicated that cholesterol and salt are the two top health threats as perceived by the American public. The Roper Organization survey found that 65 percent of those contacted considered cholesterol a significant health concern. That number was 10 percent higher than the year before.

The month before the 1984 survey was published, the National Institutes of Health strongly advised Americans to reduce dietary fat and cholesterol because of their direct link with the rate of heart attacks. The government panel reported that 60 percent of all Americans have high cholesterol levels and should make significant efforts to reduce the fat and cholesterol content of their diet.

The problem has always been, however, that while the link between the cholesterol levels in the blood and heart attacks has been well established, the connection to the diet has been less clear. In other words, while it may be true that reducing cholesterol levels in the blood will reduce the threat of heart disease, will a reduction in dietary fat and cholesterol lower that threat? The hang-up has been that, for the most part, attempts to reduce fat and cholesterol in the diet have not shown tremendous success in lowering cholesterol in the blood. Actually, early intervention studies looked only at the amount of cholesterol, not the fat, in the diet. Later, both fat and cholesterol were viewed together as responsible for raising serum cholesterol levels. And, as time went on, it was found that saturated fat has more impact on serum cholesterol than does cholesterol itself.

A major four-year study by the National Institutes of Health—the Multiple Risk Factor Intervention Trial (MR FIT)—was conducted primarily to zero in on nutrition intervention for individuals at high risk of heart disease.[5] Cholesterol levels of those persons in the study were 220 mg/dl or higher. The "mg/dl" stands for milligrams of cholesterol per deciliter of blood; previously the designation was milligrams per cubic centimeter. The diet suggested to the men in the study contained 300 milligrams or less of cholesterol, with 35 percent of calories as fat.

How successful was the test? At the end of the first year there was an overall decrease of only 6 to 7 percent from initial cholesterol levels. For those who did particularly well, also losing weight during the year, there were reductions up to 10 percent. After four years, the MR FIT program achieved an average cholesterol reduction of 6.7 percent.

Clearly this level of success is just not enough. For those men and women at risk, with, say, cholesterol levels of 250 mg/dl or higher, even a full 10 percent drop is not sufficient.

Another study was published, also in 1984, by the National Heart, Lung, and Blood Institute. This was the result of the Lipid Research Clinics Coronary Primary Prevention Trial.[6] In that particular investigation, scien-

tists tried to determine whether lowering cholesterol levels could actually reduce the incidence of coronary heart disease.

Recognizing that diet alone probably
would not bring cholesterol levels down
significantly, the researchers decided to increase the likelihood of success by adding a
cholesterol-lowering drug to the program.
The drug was cholestyramine, frequently prescribed by doctors to bring down dangerously
high cholesterol levels.

This drug lowers cholesterol levels by binding fats in the intestine, causing them to be excreted in the feces. To be effective, the drug
often must be taken three to four times a day.
It comes in packets of granules which can be
mixed with water or fruit juice. Taking the
drug is rather unpleasant, and not everyone is
willing to stick with it.

Subjects in the study were asked to follow a
modified diet with reduced fat and cholesterol. They received either the drug or a
placebo. No one knew which.

Results were published in the *Journal of the
American Medical Association.* Altered diet
alone produced a 3.4 percent decrease in cholesterol levels. Altered diet along with
cholestyramine brought the decrease to 14
percent during the first year. Not surprisingly,
the placebo had little if any effect. Over the

succeeding years of the study, the cholesterol levels slowly rose back up, for a total decrease of only 6.5 percent. Compliance was a problem.

However, some of the subjects did stick with the program. They achieved significant lowering of their cholesterol levels over the eight-year period of time. And their risk of coronary heart disease dropped proportionately.

Medical authorities believe that while the total level of cholesterol is an important indicator of risk, an even more precise measurement is the LDL cholesterol levels.

Within the cholestyramine-treated group, patients experienced a 22.3 mg/dl drop in LDL cholesterol levels. This was associated with a 17.2 percent reduction in the actual incidence of coronary heart disease.

In other words, those individuals who were able to significantly reduce cholesterol levels experienced far less heart disease. Conversely, those who did not drop their cholesterol levels during that eight-year period had far more heart disease.

Moreover, the authors of the published study state that for subjects taking the full amount of cholestyramine LDL cholesterol levels fell by 35 percent. Total cholesterol levels dropped 25 percent. This much of a reduction, they say, would reduce the incidence of coronary heart disease by 49 percent. Consider the incredible implications of that statement: **The risk of coronary heart disease is cut in half by lowering LDL cholesterol levels 35 percent!**

Another way of looking at these data was discussed by a panel of the National Institutes of Health. Those experts said unequivocally that **each 1 percent reduction in blood cholesterol levels produces a 2 percent reduction in coronary heart disease.** For example, a 5 percent reduction in total blood cholesterol should reduce disease rates by 10 percent. Combinations of diet, drugs, and reduction of other risk factors can reduce disease by up to 50 percent, they said. Feeling strongly about their findings, the NIH set out to convey this information to physicians, to educate them as to the value of cholesterol reduction for their patients.

But, once again, we're faced with the dilemma of just how to achieve that 35 percent LDL reduction. The study's authors point out that it can be done with diet and drugs. But is this reasonable to expect for the entire American population? Millions of people are at risk from heart disease, but it's highly unlikely that these millions would or could take the drugs used in the study.

An alternative might be strict dietary restriction. Nathan Pritikin has published a number of books detailing his approach to dietary control of cholesterol.[7] It is an effective program. To reduce cholesterol significantly with the Pritikin Program, fat and protein are each kept to only 10 percent of total calories. Compare this with even the recommendations given by the American Heart Association of limiting fat to 30 percent, or even 20 percent. Meat, fish, and poultry combined must not add up to more than one pound per week. The result is practically a vegetarian diet. Again, not many individuals could comply with this program—especially for the rest of their lives.

These were the choices available to me when I determined that it was essential to reduce my own cholesterol levels. Neither the radical dietary program nor the drugs seemed appealing. That's why I developed the program by which I lowered my own levels by not just 30 percent, or even 35 percent, but a full 40 percent.

Now that you've seen how effective cholesterol lowering can be in reducing the incidence of heart disease, and knowing that there is a safe, effective way to do so pleasantly, let's learn a bit more about cholesterol chemistry. You've probably heard the terms and names

before, but it's good to have a firm understanding so that you can take better control
over your own life.

How Much Is Too Much?

Until fairly recently, the majority of physicians
were not concerned if one's cholesterol level
fell into the normal/average range for adult
American men and women. The problem with
being "average," however, seems to be that
most Americans—including many children—
have levels much too high. The "normal" level
may not be a safe level. This is especially true
when comparing those levels with profiles of
other ethnic groups. The conclusions are clear
from dozens of studies: those cultural groups
with lowest levels of cholesterol have the lowest incidence of heart disease.

The attitudes and opinions of physicians as
to how high is too high began to change in
1983 with the publication of an article by Drs.
Basil Rifkind and Pesach Segal in the *Journal
of the American Medical Association*.[8] In the
study reported, plasma cholesterol and triglyceride levels were established for more than sixty
thousand participants in ten separate American
populations. New definitions were set for those
who are *hyperlipidemic* (with elevated fats in

the blood in general) and *hypercholesterolemic* (with elevated cholesterol levels).

The tables toward the end of this chapter, from Drs. Rifkind and Segal's paper, give breakdowns of cholesterol levels for men, women, and children. As an example, in Table 1, only 5 percent of the population of males have a cholesterol level of 150 mg/dl or lower in the age group forty to forty-four years. Conversely, looking at the 75th percentile, 25 percent of the same population have a level of 230 mg/dl or more. The average level for this group is 205 mg/dl. More and more authorities today are recognizing that safe levels are much, much lower than what has been accepted for the past twenty years, and intervention of one sort or another is called for whenever the level exceeds 200 mg/dl. Thus the *average* adult male, and many other Americans of both sexes and in all age groups, need to do something to reduce elevated cholesterol levels.

As the average cholesterol level rises above 200 mg/dl, the incidence of coronary heart disease increases proportionately. Thus, the Council on Scientific Affairs of the American Medical Association concludes, "average total plasma cholesterol levels of 180 to 200 mg/dL in adult populations seem to be associated with a low incidence of both cardiovascular and other diseases and probably should be considered optimal."

Medical and scientific authorities finally came to a national consensus in 1987 with the issuance of the first guidelines for cholesterol. The maximum acceptable serum cholesterol level, the government-sponsored panel declared, is 200 mg/dl, regardless of age or sex. That, of course, is a far cry from what physicians had believed to be "normal."

The panel members said they hoped that cholesterol levels would be more strictly controlled, thus greatly reducing a major risk factor in heart disease. They pointed to a parallel situation in 1970, when physicians were told that all patients should be examined for hypertension and that elevated blood pressure should be aggressively treated to eliminate or reduce that heart disease risk. Some optimistically voiced the feeling that in years to come the risk of cholesterol would also be cut back tremendously.

Yet even the 200 mg/dl maximum cited by the panel may not be low enough. An eminent cholesterol researcher, Dr. Jeremiah Stamler, published unequivocal proof of the value of lowering cholesterol levels even further. His article in the *Journal of the American Medical Association* reported the latest findings of the MR FIT (Multiple Risk Factor Intervention

Trials) program, discussed earlier, in which 356,222 men aged thirty-five to fifty-seven were screened for heart disease risk.[9] In the years since the program's first screening in 1973, death rates have been compared. The findings concerning cholesterol are striking.

Dr. Stamler states clearly that "the relationship between serum cholesterol and CHD is *not* a threshold one, with increased risk confined to the highest quintiles, but rather is a continuously graded one that powerfully affects risk for the great majority of middle-aged American men." He has concluded that even levels of 200 mg/dl are not low enough. Deaths from heart disease, he says, are "attributable to serum cholesterol levels equal to or greater than 180 mg/dl." Dr. Stamler recommends getting cholesterol levels as low as possible.

Of course, in looking at the total lipid levels and their effect on heart disease, we cannot lose track of the importance of the protective levels of HDL. But, rapidly accumulating evidence strongly points to low HDL cholesterol levels as an independent risk factor, and many within the medical community have already called for revisions of the 1987 government-issued guidelines on cholesterol, since they ignore this essential aspect of heart disease. It appears that high levels of HDL protect against heart disease, and that even for those with seemingly desirable total cholesterol levels, low HDL counts can lead to blockage of the coronary arteries. For men, HDL levels ideally are at least 40; for women, HDLs should be at least 45.

Speaking at the American Heart Association meeting in Washington, D.C., in November, 1988, Dr. Robert Wones of the University of Cincinnati explained that while public cholesterol screenings have become increasingly popular, such tests which reveal only total cholesterol miss those individuals at risk owing to low levels of HDL cholesterol. The testings can also mislabel those with high total cholesterol levels as being at risk when in truth they are protected by high HDL counts.

Dr. Wones pointed out that errors in testing owing to HDL levels are more likely in women than in men, since women tend to have higher HDL counts. Testing errors are infrequent in those with cholesterol levels in excess of 240 mg/dl. Conversely, women with total cholesterol levels of 200 to 239 are likely to be protected by their HDL elevations. The only way to be sure, in any case, is with a complete cholesterol analysis.

In one study, the vast majority of men with coronary heart disease had total cholesterol/HDL level ratios of six-to-one or

more.[10] Researchers at Laval University in
Quebec looked at lipid levels in 2555 French-
Canadian men aged 45 to 75 years. They
found that low levels of HDL cholesterol were
the most-prevalent factor associated with both
angina and heart attacks.

HDL cholesterol, in fact, may be a more
important consideration, in many cases, than
even total cholesterol or LDL cholesterol.
Studying this issue at the University of California at Berkeley, researchers concluded that
increased LDLs and decreased HDLs are both
associated with a higher incidence of heart disease. But the importance of LDL levels was
reduced when HDL was taken into consideration; that is to say, HDL was more predictive
of heart disease than LDL.

Even individual physicians have begun to
take special notice of HDL levels in their patients. One such doctor, W. E. Freeman, Jr.,
M.D., of Bowling Green, Ohio, wrote to the
publication *Medical World News* in December
1987 to report that in his experience with
more than 7000 patients, their HDL readings
were more important to him than total cholesterol. Using total cholesterol readings
alone, he pointed out in his letter, many patients would be missed in terms of recognizing
them as candidates for future heart disease
owing to their low HDL counts.

In fact, for some time doctors have wondered why a large number of heart-attack patients have shown completely normal cholesterol levels. Two very recent studies have shown that the culprit probably is low HDL levels.

Dr. G. S. Ginsburg of Beth Israel Hospital in Boston reported his findings at the 1988 AHA meeting. In his study, a total of 1748 patients had a cholesterol measurement and 1445 had their HDLs measured as well. Of these, 1381 had both total and HDL cholesterol measured during the first forty-eight hours after admission to the hospital following heart attack. Forty percent had total cholesterol of less than 200 mg/dl. The patients' average cholesterol level was 214; that's not very high when you consider that 211 is the average in the U.S. population. Of that 40 percent, 549 patients in all, 344 had coronary heart disease. Most of them were male. And 74 percent of those with heart disease had HDLs of less than 40.

In part two of his study, Dr. Ginsburg and his associates selected patients who had undergone coronary angiography (a procedure in which a catheter is inserted through an artery into the heart so the interior of the coronary arteries can be inspected directly). Of 1428 patients, 1208 tested positive for heart disease.

Of those patients with coronary heart disease, 659 had HDL and total cholesterol tested. Thirty-two percent, 213 patients, had total cholesterol readings under 200. Patients with CHD had an average HDL cholesterol level of less than 40. Those without the disease were above 40. That comes to about four to five milligrams lower HDL for those with the disease. Just a little bit can mean a lot when it comes to HDLs.

Speaking at the same meeting, Dr. Michael Miller of Johns Hopkins stated that more than 20 percent of those with CHD have cholesterol levels in the desirable range. Over a three-year period of time, 1000 patients underwent coronary angiography at Johns Hopkins; two-thirds of those were male. They excluded 138 patients who had had recent heart attacks. Another 65 were excluded because of drugs given. Of the 797 remaining patients who were analyzed, 288 had a cholesterol level of 200 mg/dl or less. Those patients became the study group. Most had CHD, and 194 were male. Two-thirds of patients had HDLs under 40, and four out of five had HDLs under 45. Dr. Miller feels confident that low HDLs represent an independent risk of heart disease.

Conversely, researchers in Helsinki, Finland, have shown that elevated levels of

HDLs can offer protection against heart disease. The Helsinki Heart Study was a five-year project involving 4081 men with abnormally high cholesterol levels but no symptoms of heart disease. One group received the drug gemfibrozil while another got a placebo. Gemfibrozil reduces triglycerides significantly, lowers LDL cholesterol a bit, and raises HDL cholesterol somewhat. Those getting the drug showed an 11 percent drop in LDL with an 11 percent rise in HDL. By the end of the five years, those taking gemfibrozil showed a reduction of 34 percent in heart disease in terms of heart attacks and deaths. The authors, writing in the *Journal of the American Medical Association* in August 1988, concluded that both elevating HDL and lowering LDL cholesterol levels are effective in the primary prevention of coronary heart disease.

Interesting, also, is the case of those fortunate individuals whose total cholesterol level is very low. Dr. William Connor of the University of Oregon studied the Tarahumara Indians, who live a truly primitive life in the mountains of Mexico. Their diet is spare and contains very few animal foods. They exercise extensively, often playing a game of kicking a ball while racing on foot for up to twenty-four hours at a time without stopping. Taking blood samples, Dr. Connor and his group found cholesterol levels in the 120s and 130s. HDL levels were also very low. But there was no trace of heart disease in the entire population. Dr. Connor concludes that when the total cholesterol level falls to very low values, the importance of the protective HDL becomes less significant.

We're beginning to see the benefits not only of testing for HDL levels but also of doing something about improving those numbers. During the 1988 AHA meeting, Dr. Meir Stampfer of Harvard Medical School presented a report on an on-going study with 22,071 male physicians in the U.S. In this study, doctors have agreed to take aspirin and beta carotene to determine the respective roles of those two substances in protecting against heart attacks and cancer. Blood was collected from 70 percent of all participants, when they were free of heart-disease symptoms and cancer at the beginning of the study. Blood from 97 men who had subsequent heart attacks were analyzed, along with samples from 97 men who did not have heart attacks. The best predictor of heart disease, when comparing those blood samples, was HDL cholesterol level. Dr. Stampfer concluded that "A 1 mg/dl increase in HDL corresponded to a 7% decrease in risk, even after adjustment for other lipids and apoproteins and other risk factors."

The immediate implication of this information about HDL cholesterol levels is that you shouldn't rely entirely on tests that measure only total cholesterol. The best bet is to ask your doctor to refer you to a good laboratory where you can learn about your HDLs as well as your LDLs and triglycerides. Then you can discuss the best approaches to control with your physician.

The goal is to have a ratio of total cholesterol to HDL cholesterol below 4.5. The ratio can be affected by either raising the HDL or lowering the LDL. The latter is more practical. The 4.5 ratio is the level associated with the standard risk of women, who have far less heart disease than men. Even better is a ratio of 3.5, which is associated with half the standard risk for men.[11]

Here are some examples of total cholesterol/HDL ratios:

$$\frac{200 \text{ mg/dl total cholesterol}}{50 \text{ mg/dl HDL cholesterol}} = 4.0 \text{ ratio}$$

$$\frac{175 \text{ mg/dl total cholesterol}}{55 \text{ mg/dl HDL cholesterol}} = 3.0 \text{ ratio}$$

$$\frac{250 \text{ mg/dl total cholesterol}}{40 \text{ mg/dl HDL cholesterol}} = 6.0 \text{ ratio}$$

$$\frac{210 \text{ mg/dl total cholesterol}}{60 \text{ mg/dl HDL cholesterol}} = 3.5 \text{ ratio}$$

No one should be satisfied until the total cholesterol is less than 200 or at least until the ratio is less than 4.5.

We do not have definitive evidence that aggressively trying to elevate HDL cholesterol levels will have as dramatic an effect on reducing the incidence of heart disease and death as we've seen in lowering total cholesterol. Remember, though, that for many years scientists pointed to the correlation between high cholesterol levels and heart disease. It took literally decades for the medical mainstream to have the ironclad proof that allowed them finally to embrace the idea that all men and women should lower their cholesterol levels to 200 mg/dl or lower. It will probably take a few more years for the majority in medicine to recognize the benefits of bringing cholesterol levels down dramatically in order to stop completely the progress of the disease or even to reverse it as I've discussed in Chapter 16. And no doubt it would take many years of research to provide the documentation needed to convince the medical community that changing HDL levels unequivocally can provide protection from heart disease.

The question remains as to whether you

want to wait until that unequivocal proof is delivered. I don't.

WHERE TO BEGIN

Where do we begin, then, in lowering total cholesterol and LDL cholesterol, and increasing HDL cholesterol?

The recommendation from all authorities is to begin with diet. According to the Council on Scientific Affairs of the American Medical Association, "There is good reason to believe that the average cholesterol levels in persons in the United States may be higher than optimal due in part to the typical United States diet."[12]

Adults in primitive and Oriental societies have an average total cholesterol level between 150 and 200 mg/dl. Remember that total cholesterol levels between 140 and 180 mg/dl are consistently found to be related to the lowest rates of atherosclerosis and coronary heart disease.[12]

The American Heart Association has recommended three phases of dietary modification. Each is increasingly restricted, with increased expectations for success.

In Phase I, the diet would include no more than 300 milligrams of cholesterol daily. There should be a fat intake of not more than 30 percent of total calories, with 10 percent each from saturated, polyunsaturated, and mono-unsaturated fats and oils. This approach will usually reduce cholesterol levels by 10 to 15 percent in normal individuals.

In Phase II, fat and cholesterol intake should not exceed 30 percent of calories and 250 milligrams per day, respectively. Finally, in Phase III, the restricted diet would contain only 20 to 25 percent of calories as fat, with less than 10 percent coming from animal sources. Cholesterol intake should be kept under 100 milligrams daily.

In 1986 the American Heart Association refined and clarified its position on cholesterol intake for the general population. While 300 milligrams remained the daily limit, the AHA recommended a maximum of 100 milligrams per 1000 calories consumed daily. So 300 milligrams would be the limit for someone eating 3000 calories; someone consuming 2000 calories should limit cholesterol to only 200 milligrams.

This would obviously necessitate a proportionate drop in recommendations for Phases II and III, although those recommendations have not yet been formulated. Interestingly, however, the AHA seems awkwardly unable to face the increasing evidence that the 20 percent-of-calories level of fat intake is best for everyone and that this goal *can* be achieved. An AHA principal spokesperson and policy formulator told me it could take years for the general population to lower intake to Phase I. Those with insight will make the changes much, much sooner.

The place to begin, it seems logical to assume, is with Phase I. This is the same approach advocated by many health and medical authorities. The U.S. Department of Agriculture and the U.S. Department of Health, Education and Welfare jointly published the official "Dietary Guidelines for Americans" in 1980.[13] That report suggests eating a wide variety of foods, avoiding too much fat, saturated fat, and cholesterol, eating foods with adequate starch and fiber, and avoiding too much sugar and sodium. That seems like good advice everyone can live with without feeling like a martyr. Then, as needed, fat intake can be further reduced.

To achieve the desirable 4.5 or lower total cholesterol to HDL cholesterol ratio, decreasing LDLs and lowering total cholesterol is the most effective route, but there are ways to alter HDL levels favorably.

A diet low in fats and cholesterol, reduced in total calories, and including a moderate amount of alcohol[14] produces increases in HDL levels.

The next thing to do is to quit smoking cigarettes. Every single study done shows that smokers have consistently lower HDL levels than nonsmokers. While you're at it, stay away from smokers as much as possible. It appears that even passive smoking by way of other persons' smoldering cigarettes can drop the HDL numbers. Sadly, children of smokers have lower HDL counts than do those in homes with nonsmoking parents.

If you're overweight, try to bring your weight down to normal. Looking at data from the Multiple Risk Factor Intervention Trial, researchers have reported that weight loss results in both a decrease in LDL and an increase in HDL—by as much as 5 milligrams, which can be enough to protect against heart attack.

If you routinely supplement your diet with vitamins and minerals, check to see whether the dosage for zinc is above 50 milligrams. Dosages higher than that can lower HDL levels. Few people do take large doses of zinc on a routine basis, but zinc lozenges are sometimes recommended for treatment of colds and the flu, and those large doses could do some damage. You should be aware that once HDL levels go down, it's difficult to get them back up, so I would urge you not ever to take large doses of zinc for any reason.

Virtually every study has shown that moderate alcohol intake is associated with elevated HDL levels. Some have even postulated that this may be the reason we see moderate drinkers enjoying longer lives than teetotalers. Moderate drinking has been defined as one or two drinks daily, taken as wine, beer, or mixed drinks.

On the other hand, it has been questioned whether the effect alcohol has on HDLs is truly beneficial, depending on the type of HDL particle involved. Researchers at the Veterans Administration Medical Center in Wood, Wisconsin, have looked into this issue. The concern was whether alcohol elevates the truly protective subfraction of HDL, the HDL_2. Previous reports indicated alcohol may only raise the HDL_3, thought to be not as protective. But the Wisconsin study shows that both HDL_2 and HDL_3 rise with the intake of alcohol in moderate amounts.

No one, including myself, believes that current nondrinkers should be encouraged to start imbibing in order to increase their HDL levels. The potential harm of alcohol consumption, including accidents, must be taken into consideration. But for those who currently enjoy a cocktail before dinner or a glass or two of wine or beer during the meal, there's no reason not to continue the pleasant ritual.

Exercise also has a beneficial effect on HDL levels. Researchers at the National Defense University in Washington, D.C., examined the relationship between miles run per week and HDL levels in 1020 healthy males with an average age of 43 years. They found that optimal changes in lipid levels occur when a person runs an average of sixteen miles a week; that is, LDL levels go down a bit, and HDL levels rise. That comes out to be about three miles a day, five days a week, which is not terribly much if you're a runner. Running more than that didn't further improve HDL levels. On the other hand, running less than nine miles weekly produced no beneficial effects in terms of HDLs. Walking is just as good.

Looking at the improvements in lipid profiles of those involved with a cardiac rehabilitation program, researchers in West Virginia found that exercising three times weekly for three months resulted in an increase of 7.5 percent in HDLs, with a rise from an average of 41.6 mg/dl to 44.3 mg/dl. The patients exercised at 70 to 80 percent of their maximum heart rate.

More of the benefits of exercise can be seen in Chapter 9. Some research indicates even moderate exercise has good effects on HDLs.

Early research done with cholesterol-lowering diets showed that increasing the amount of polyunsaturated fats could significantly drop total cholesterol levels. Many advocated significant increases in consumption of cooking oils rich in polyunsaturated fatty acids, such as corn oil and safflower oil. Now we know that, while total cholesterol levels do drop with this approach, so do HDL numbers. Today there's agreement that monounsaturated fats are the better way to go. When used to replace saturated fats in the diet, monounsaturated fats such as olive oil can lower total cholesterol while preserving HDLs. You can read more about that in Chapter 7.

We also now know that very-low-fat diets can significantly lower the levels of the protective HDLs. The benefit of total cholesterol reduction may be completely offset by concomitant drops in HDLs. That's often the case when following such regimens as the Pritikin Program. Very seldom does one achieve such dramatic reduction in total cholesterol, down to, say, 130 to 140 mg/dl, that the need for HDLs diminishes. Most followers of such programs see only moderate cholesterol reduction, accompanied by drops in HDL. That's why I recommended a more moderate approach, along with the increased consumption of foods that will selectively lower LDLs while sparing HDLs entirely.

There are two approaches you can discuss

with your physician beyond the obvious measures of quitting smoking, controlling weight, and exercise in order to raise HDLs. One is the use of the drug gemfibrozil, which we've seen from the Helsinki study was effective. I've provided some details about that drug in Chapter 15. The other possibility is the use of niacin, an integral part of my overall program for those who can tolerate it. You can read more about that in Chapter 6.

For many individuals, diet alone can reduce a moderately elevated total cholesterol level of, say, 210 or 215 down to less than 200. This, as we'll see, is made even easier now with the addition of oat bran to the diet, as fully described in Chapter 5, "Getting the Scoop on Oat Bran."

SELECTING A SOUND DIET

The problem for most people trying to do something to change a lifetime of dietary habits is thinking, "What do I have to give up?" Instead, the proper approach should be "What are the thousands of delicious foods I should pick?"

First of all, what is the purpose of eating? Basically, we should eat to live. Too many have learned to live to eat. It's time to get back to basics.

The purpose of a good diet is to provide all the nutrients we need to live a hearty, robust life. Those nutrients help us maintain and, in the case of children, grow our bodies.

While the plan has been criticized from time to time for being too simplistic, the basic four-food-group approach remains an excellent guideline for selecting foods. This plan calls for a wide variety of foods.

Adults need a minimum of two servings from the meat and dairy groups and four servings each from the fruit-vegetable and grain groups. Is this plan possible and practical for a calorie-and-cholesterol-conscious person? It definitely is if one remembers the advice to consume a *wide variety* of foods from these groups. And the plan comes to life when one stresses the importance of the latter two groups of foods. Stress the word *minimum* in the four servings.

In order to get all the protein needed, two servings from the meat group are completely sufficient. Some prefer to call this the protein group, since it also includes protein sources such as poultry, fish, and beans.

Is there anything wrong with beef? Or with any of the other red meats? Absolutely not, if eaten in moderation. But what constitutes a "serving" of meat? It's not a sixteen-ounce steak! A serving of meat should be no more than four ounces. And it's really not asking that much to trim the excess fat from the edges.

But there's more to the meat group than just red meat. Actually relying on just one type of food becomes boring. Don't forget poultry and seafood. Practically every great chef in the world prides himself on thinking of fantastic ways to serve a whole world of foods. See page 366 for healthy beef.

Next we come to the dairy group. Milk products are an excellent source of calcium, protein, and vitamins A and D. But those nutrients do not reside in the fat. Low-fat or nonfat varieties of milk, yogurt, and cheese have all the same nutrients. Often they cost less. And, if at first your taste buds don't respond favorably, give yourself a little time to get used to the idea of the light flavors of the reduced-fat dairy foods. After a while, believe it or not, one actually comes to prefer the more healthful types.

When it comes to the fruit-vegetable group, there's no limit at all to what you may eat as long as you don't start gaining weight. Orange juice for all its vitamin C, is also pretty heavy on calories. On the other hand, you've cut down on fats, you can make up for those calories with fresh fruits of all types. Go into a good food store or a fresh-fruit-and-vegetable store and treat yourself to a shopping bag full of fresh treats. "Mangos, papayas, chestnuts from the fire . . ." So goes an old Rosemary Clooney song.

Finally, the grain group. Now you can forget all the old rules about avoiding those so-called "fattening" starches. Eat rice and rolls and bread if you want to—every single day. Don't even worry about the calories. And remember, in Europe and other countries where bread is considered a staple of life and a source of national pride, no one puts butter on the bread. It takes away from the taste of the bread itself.

When it comes to pasta, go wild. Enjoy all the forms and varieties you can find. A little marinara sauce, a fresh salad, a chunk of sourdough bread, and a glass of wine all make that spaghetti dinner a memorable occasion.

Since I started to cut down on fats, I don't have to count calories. Now I can eat all the food I want, with practically no limits. Instead, I count the milligrams of cholesterol and the amount of fat in the foods I select. Following the recipes in this book will help you to get started. You'll also find that many recipes printed in today's magazines list the milligrams of cholesterol and the grams of fat in each serving. You can cut those levels even further by doing some simple alterations, such as using egg substitute for egg yolks and by using soft margarine instead of butter. And, although there's nothing wrong with enjoying beef, pork, lamb, and veal, spread your imagination beyond those types of meat. Substitute a turkey cutlet for a veal cutlet. Try ground chicken breast instead of beef in your burgers. Experiment with different types of seafood you may have avoided before. Shish kebabs made with large scallops are fantastic!

The aim is to keep your fat and cholesterol intake low, the lower the better. No matter what else one may do to reduce cholesterol levels in the blood, the place to start is with the diet.

To help you start counting those grams and milligrams, you'll find some charts of commonly eaten foods and the amounts of fats and cholesterol found in typical serving sizes in Chapter 4, "Winning by the Numbers." After just a little while, you'll begin to gravitate toward those foods with low levels of fats and cholesterol and you won't even need the guideline charts.

I love the little motto I saw on the refrigerator of a friend trying to keep her gorgeous figure. The motto read: "A moment on your lips, forever on your hips." As nice as it is to preserve that slim figure, think how much more important it is to keep those arteries clear and flowing.

Remember the conclusion of the medical authorities who state emphatically that a cholesterol reduction of 35 percent cuts the risk of heart disease in half. It's worth it!

THE PROGRAM

Lowering total cholesterol and LDL cholesterol levels sufficiently by diet alone, however, may not always be possible. The Council on Scientific Affairs of the American Medical Association states, "In carefully controlled metabolic ward situations, decreased cholesterol and saturated fat intake without altered energy intake (calories) results in a decrease of perhaps 30% in serum cholesterol concentration. In the more generally applicable circumstances of free-living subjects, the decrease in plasma cholesterol concentration is considerably less."[12] In other words, most people will not achieve sufficient lowering of serum cholesterol through diet alone.

For those with more highly elevated levels a program of diet modification, oat bran, and niacin has been shown to be dramatically effective. We'll talk more about niacin in Chapter 6.

How effective? As you'll read in Chapter 14, "The Proof of the Pudding," the program results in cholesterol levels dropping 30, 35, 40, 45, even 50 percent or more. One's risk of coronary heart disease comes tumbling down on this practical program.

Moreover, the protective HDL levels rise just as dramatically. All participants in a research study conducted to demonstrate the efficacy of this program showed an average rise of 35 percent in their HDL levels. Again, read the "Proof" chapter.

There no longer is any controversy regarding cholesterol and its deadly effect. Many people have a tendency toward elevated cholesterol levels, which are made even worse by a fatty, cholesterol-laden diet. But those cholesterol levels can be cut down to size quickly and easily, resulting in the virtual elimination of this major risk factor.

Does lowering cholesterol make a difference in longevity? Who would know that better than the actuaries at life insurance companies? They want you to stay alive so your family won't collect benefits for a long time to come. A number of insurance companies now offer discounts on life insurance for nonsmoking clients. Now one company has begun to offer 10 to 15 percent discounts for certain life insurance policies sold to clients with low cholesterol levels.

These are special policies, valued at $100,000 or more, and for those in the "pre-

ferred good health" category which also includes nonsmokers and those who have passed
a health examination. Today the only company
offering the discount is West Coast Life Insurance, based in San Francisco. I would expect
that others will follow suit in time. You can call
for additional details at (800) 366-9378. Now
is the time to find out. Don't rely on your
physician's announcement that your cholesterol levels are "normal." Learn what those
numbers mean. To help you put your own
readings into perspective, I've prepared tables
showing cholesterol levels in the population.

How to Read These Tables

In any population group or groups, there will
be an average level of fats in the blood. Data
are presented here in percentiles. Figures
given in the 5 percent category are presented
to show what low levels would be. On the
other hand, those in the 95th percentile (95
percent) in the categories of total cholesterol
and LDL cholesterol are at the greatest risk of
coronary heart disease. To help put things into
perspective, populations that have little or no
atherosclerotic cardiovascular disease often
have LDL cholesterol levels that average
below 100 mg/dl.[9] The risk of heart disease

relates clearly to increasing LDL cholesterol above the 50th percentile.[9] This would be higher than 150 mg/dl for adults.

As an example of reading these tables, look at Table 1. For adult males aged 40 to 44 years, the average total cholesterol level is 205. Only 5 percent of men have levels of 150 mg/dl. On the other end of the scale, 25 percent of men in this age group (75th percentile or 75 percent) have levels of 230 mg/dl or greater; 10 percent (90th percentile or 90 percent) have levels over 250 mg/dl; 5 percent (95th percentile or 95 percent) have cholesterol levels of 270 or more.

Bear in mind that according to these tables of data, when compared to current clinical medical opinion, half the adult male population aged forty to forty-four have cholesterol levels that should be reduced. Many physicians today still remain uninformed of the importance of lowering cholesterol levels over 200. The National Heart, Blood, and Lung Institute is now conducting an educational program to encourage doctors to rethink the cholesterol levels of their patients and to treat them appropriately. This is based on published statements that cholesterol levels over 200 mg/dl should be reduced to decrease the risk of heart disease.[12,15]

Remember also that clinical trials indicate

that each 1 percent reduction in blood choles-terol levels produces a 2 percent reduction in coronary heart disease. For example, a 5 per-cent reduction in blood cholesterol should re-duce disease rates by 10 percent. How many investments can you think of in which you can double your input?

Table 1. **Plasma Total Cholesterol (mg/dl) in Adult Males[8]**

AGE/YEARS	AVERAGE	5%	75%	90%	95%
0–19	155	115	170	185	200
20–24	165	125	185	205	220
25–29	180	135	200	225	245
30–34	190	140	215	240	255
35–39	200	145	225	250	270
40–44	205	150	230	250	270
45–69	215	160	235	260	275
70+	205	150	230	250	270

Table 2. **Plasma Low-Density Lipoprotein Cholesterol (mg/dl) in Adult Males[8]**

AGE/YEARS	AVERAGE	5%	75%	90%	95%
5–19	95	65	105	120	130
20–24	105	65	120	140	145
25–29	115	70	140	155	165
30–34	125	80	145	165	185
35–39	135	80	155	175	190

40–44	135	85	155	175	185
45–69	145	90	165	190	205
70+	145	90	165	180	185

Table 3. Plasma High-Density Lipoprotein Cholesterol (mg/dl) in Adult Males[8]

AGE/YEARS	AVERAGE	5%	10%	95%
5–14	55	35	40	75
15–19	45	30	35	65
20–24	45	30	30	65
25–29	45	30	30	65
30–34	45	30	30	65
35–39	45	30	30	60
40–44	45	25	30	65
45–69	50	30	30	70
70+	50	30	35	75

Table 4. Plasma Total Cholesterol (mg/dl) in Adult Females[8]

AGE/YEARS	AVERAGE	5%	75%	90%	95%
0–19	160	120	175	190	200
20–24	170	125	190	215	230
25–34	175	130	195	220	235
35–39	185	140	205	230	245
40–44	195	145	215	235	255
45–49	205	150	225	250	270
50–54	220	165	240	265	285
55+	230	170	250	275	295

Table 5. **Plasma Low-Density Lipoprotein Cholesterol (mg/dl) in Adult Females[8]**

AGE/YEARS	AVERAGE	5%	75%	90%	95%
5–19	100	65	110	125	140
20–24	105	55	120	140	160
25–34	110	70	125	145	160
35–39	120	75	140	160	170
40–44	125	75	145	165	175
45–49	130	80	150	175	185
50–54	140	90	160	185	200
55+	150	95	170	195	215

Table 6. **Plasma High-Density Lipoprotein Cholesterol (mg/dl) in Adult Females[8]**

AGE/YEARS	AVERAGE	5%	10%	95%
5–19	55	35	40	70
20–24	55	35	35	80
25–34	55	35	40	80
35–39	55	35	40	80
40–44	60	35	40	90
45–49	60	35	40	85
50–54	60	35	40	90
55+	60	35	40	95

Table 7. Plasma Triglycerides in Males[8]

AGE/YEARS	AVERAGE	5%	90%	95%
0–9	55	30	85	100
10–14	65	30	100	125
15–19	80	35	120	150
20–24	100	45	165	200
25–29	115	45	200	250
30–34	130	50	215	265
35–39	145	55	250	320
40–54	150	55	250	320
55–64	140	60	235	290
65+	135	55	210	260

Table 8. Plasma Triglycerides in Females[8]

AGE/YEARS	AVERAGE	5%	90%	95%
0–9	60	35	95	110
10–19	75	40	115	130
20–34	90	40	145	170
35–39	95	40	160	195
40–44	105	45	170	210
45–49	110	45	185	230
50–54	120	55	190	240
55–64	125	55	200	250
65+	130	60	205	240

Table 9. **Plasma Cholesterol and Triglycerides in Children Before Puberty**[9]

LEVELS IN MG/DL	5%	90%	95%
Total cholesterol	125	155	200
LDL cholesterol	65	95	135
HDL cholesterol	38	55	75
VLDL cholesterol	5	10	20
Triglycerides	30	55	110

2

Special Considerations for Women, Children, and the Elderly

Who has heart disease and dies of heart attacks? The typical answer would be the middle-aged male. But the truth is that no one is immune to this disease. Yes, heart disease is the number one killer of American males. But it's also the number one killer of American females. And, as we'll see very shortly, we can't ignore it in children either.

WOMEN AND HEART DISEASE

While it's true that men have three to four times more likelihood of having a heart attack during their lives, women catch up quickly after menopause. And the number of women having heart attacks and dying of heart disease is growing every year. In fact, women have a poorer chance of survival than men do after a heart attack. The bottom line is that heart disease kills seven times more women than does breast cancer. Women today conscientiously examine their breasts, see their doctors annually, and often have mammograms to detect lumps as early as possible, but they may ignore the risk factors that put them in danger of future heart attack.

Many married women, in fact, fear heart disease more as a threat to their husbands' lives than to their own; they have a false sense of security that they're safe from this killer. The same risk factors that make men susceptible to this disease apply to women.

There are some real differences between men and women in regard to heart disease. Females are more likely to develop angina pain as an early warning of the artery-clogging process; they're less likely to die suddenly of a heart attack. On the other hand, women don't appear to get the same relief from the pain of angina that surgery or medication gives men. Female patients have a shorter life span following bypass surgery in the first years after the operation, though long-term survival seems to be the same. Yet the number of bypass surgeries in women continues to grow.

The reason the medical community has largely ignored women in terms of heart disease is that women rarely have heart disease before menopause. (Exceptions are those with unusually high cholesterol owing to hereditary hypercholesterolemia, which doesn't normally respond to diet.) The explanation appears to be women's production of hormones, especially estrogen, which seems to play a protective role in guarding against heart disease.

In fact, this led to a trial in the 1950s to test if men who had had heart attacks would benefit from receiving estrogen therapy. Instead of doing better, the men did worse in terms of subsequent heart disease. Men taking estrogen also developed more prostate cancer. That was the end of that theory.

Then in the 1970s a large study was done with women after menopause. Estrogen was given to preserve youth and to relieve typical postmenopausal symptoms, such as dryness of the vagina. Of course this was all before we recognized that estrogen, given alone, had the adverse effects of increasing the incidence of cancer of the uterus. But, when the data were analyzed to see the impact of estrogen on heart disease, women were, indeed, found to be protected. Yet not all subsequent studies confirmed that finding. The facts remain, however, that estrogen therapy decreases LDL cholesterol and increases the levels of the protective HDL. Unfortunately, because of the link with cancer of the uterus, estrogens are not prescribed alone very often.

Instead, estrogens are given along with another female hormone, progestin, in order to achieve the benefits of alleviating the symptoms of menopause and of giving protection against the bone-demineralizing disease osteoporosis. But when progestin is added to the prescription, the benefits of estrogen on heart disease are not so clear. And we have no long-term data on either the safety or efficacy of such therapy. Ultimately the decision concerning hormone replacement must be a very individual one determined by a woman's personal physician after weighing all the pros and cons of this and other options.

The National Heart, Lung and Blood Institute has begun a large clinical trial called the Post-menopausal Estrogen/Progestin Intervention. This study will attempt to determine which estrogen replacement approach gives the safest and most acceptable method of preserving bone and protecting the uterus without blocking the desirable effects on heart-disease risk factors.

In the meantime, what can women do to protect themselves from future heart disease? The first and foremost step is to stop smoking immediately or, better yet, never to start. More women are smoking than ever before, and they're starting at very early ages. (Cigarette advertising can take a lot of credit for that: ads targeted directly to women show how smoking is a demonstration of freedom and liberation.) Smoking has been shown to be an independent risk factor for heart disease in a study done at the medical College of Wisconsin. In their report given at the 1988 meeting of the American Heart Association, researchers showed that cigarette smoking increased the risk of heart attack in women with minimal, moderate, and severe coronary artery disease. In other words, no matter whether you have just a little clogging of the arteries or a lot, cigarette smoking will raise the odds of your having a heart attack.

The significance of high blood pressure as a risk factor in heart disease is the same for women as for men. Even a modest increase from the ideal of 110/70 to, say, 140/90 has been shown to increase the danger of heart disease. How can one control this factor? Weight control, regular exercise, restriction of sodium in the diet, and physician-prescribed medications are all important.

Next comes the major risk factor of diabetes, the non-insulin-dependent type that occurs during adulthood. Women are particularly prone to develop diabetes if they have the hereditary predisposition to the disease. The fact is, in many if not most instances one can either completely prevent or eliminate the symptoms of this type of diabetes by a regular program of exercise and weight control. Sadly, however, few people take this advice to heart, and their continuing overweight and resultant diabetes place them at significantly increased risk of heart disease.

And finally we come to the risk factor of cholesterol. Average levels for women tend to be a bit higher than for men. But the greater amount of the artery-clogging LDL in the blood is offset in women, to one degree or another, by the protective HDL. It is, in fact, the HDL differential between men and women that many believe to be the principal reason why women are protected; higher HDL levels in women are related to estrogen production. But after menopause the estrogen production decreases and HDL levels fall while LDL levels rise.

The National Cholesterol Education Program calls for both men and women to have a cholesterol level no higher than 200. Women have as much reason to seek testing and to learn their numbers as do men. And, if those numbers are high, it's time to do something about it. But here we must make a very important distinction. Since women typically have a higher HDL level than do men, if a cholesterol screening test reveals a total level of over 200 mg/dl, further testing should be done to analyze the cholesterol for its LDL and HDL subfractions.

Unfortunately, while some women totally ignore their cholesterol levels, others have become unduly concerned about their high levels. For example, Jane Lipstone, the producer of the videotape version of this book at Video Ticket, learned that her cholesterol level was an apparently dangerous 280 mg/dl. She tried unsuccessfully to lower that number by dietary means. When, at my suggestion, she had her LDL and HDL tested as well, the results showed a protective HDL level of 106! The ratio of 2.6 protects her from heart disease, and should have put her mind at ease. Unfortunately, her physician at the time was not aware of the importance of the HDL/total cholesterol ratio and he wanted to prescribe the cholesterol-lowering drug Mevacor. After getting a second opinion from another physician and following my recommendations, she is now on a healthy diet and exercise program without drugs.

On the other hand, many women have very high total cholesterol levels without enough HDL to give full protection. In most cases, dietary means alone, especially when including soluble-fiber-rich foods such as oat bran, will be sufficient to lower the LDL levels while leaving the HDL numbers intact, thus giving a totally improved ratio.

If, after giving the diet-oat bran approach a chance, your cholesterol still remains high, you may wish to discuss the possibilities of using niacin with your physician. The benefits, along with precautions you should be aware of, are all in Chapter 6.

HEART DISEASE BEGINS IN CHILDHOOD

Heart disease is a problem for middle-aged men; we don't have to worry about cholesterol levels and other risk factors in children. Right? Dead wrong. The sad but true state of affairs is that heart disease does, indeed, begin in childhood and that today's children are developing the lifestyle and risk factors that will place them at more significant risk of heart attack and death than any previous generation of Americans. This situation is a time bomb just waiting to go off in the future.

I became acutely aware of these facts when my son, Ross, had a cholesterol check during his annual trip to the pediatrician's office prior to the new school year. His reading was higher than it should have been, placing him in the 75th percentile of children in his age group.

Although I had done a massive amount of research on cholesterol and heart disease for the first edition of this book beginning in

1984, there were many questions left unanswered about risks for children. So I plunged back into the literature.

I found that autopsies performed on American soldiers killed during the Korean and Vietnam wars showed the presence of significant clogging of the arteries. The majority of these soldiers were in their late teens to early twenties. Not surprisingly, autopsies on enemy soldiers, who consumed a much different diet, revealed no such blockage.

A number of studies have subsequently been done with our American children, and with children around the world. The findings are very similar. Children in Western cultures have elevated cholesterol levels, placing them at future risk of heart disease.

Probably the most revealing research of all was the Bogalusa Heart Study conducted with children in Bogalusa, Louisiana. Each year children were given cholesterol tests along with other examinations, and careful records were kept. Significant numbers of youngsters, both black and white and of both sexes, were shown to have elevated cholesterol levels. During the course of that sixteen-year study, a number of children died of accidents, suicides, and homicides. Autopsies revealed the beginnings of artery blockage in children as young as ten years of age. And the blockage was directly related to the levels of cholesterol in the children's records. The founder of that study, Dr. Gerald Berenson of Louisiana State University, stated unequivocally that heart disease begins in childhood.

During its annual meeting in 1988, the American Academy of Pediatrics issued a statement recommending that pediatricians test the cholesterol levels of all their patients with histories of heart disease in the family or knowledge of elevated cholesterol levels in parents. The World Health Organization went even further during its 1988 session held in Geneva, Switzerland, urging the testing of all children. And in his research Dr. Dennis Davidson of the University of California at Irvine has shown that elevated cholesterol levels in half of all children who have them would be missed if testing were limited to only those with established medical histories. The handwriting is on the wall: test the children for this major risk factor. The best time to do so is when your children reach school age.

Cholesterol levels for children will be lower than for adults. We can extrapolate from those numbers that, say, a child in the 90th percentile for his or her age will likely grow up to be an adult in the same risk stratum. Ideally we'd like to see all the children with cholesterol levels in the 140 to 150 mg/dl range. Those numbers correspond to adult values under 200mg/dl.

If your children or grandchildren are found to be in the safety zone, that's wonderful. Keep them on a healthful lifestyle regimen, including a good diet, plenty of exercise, and, of course, lots of hugs and kisses.

If your kids test high for cholesterol, this is the time to start doing something about it. There is no need to panic or to make children feel they have some disease. They don't. Their arteries are currently clear and you simply want to keep them that way.

Diet does seem to make a difference. A study of rural Guatemalan children showed that an increase in cholesterol in the diet for just one month resulted in a significant increase in cholesterol levels in their blood.[1] In an American study, when the average daily cholesterol level in the diet was decreased from 720 to 380 milligrams with total calories from fat decreased from 38 percent to 33 percent, there was an average decrease in cholesterol levels of 15.6 percent.[1] The higher the original level, the greater the decrease. Thus some children have the tendency early in life to develop elevated levels, and those are the children who respond most to dietary changes.

You talk to your children about not getting into cars with strangers and about looking both ways before crossing the street. Of course you don't try to frighten them when having such discussions. And the same applies to talks about diet. Stress the positive aspects of eating a good, low-fat variety of foods—in terms of health, athletic performance, and weight control.

Then start getting the kids involved with food. At the supermarket, plan an extra twenty minutes or so when you bring the children along. Allow them to pick out fruits and vegetables. Teach them to read the food labels found on most foods, and to avoid high-fat items as well as those made with offenders such as coconut and palm oils. You'll be amazed at how quickly they'll pick up on all this. My daughter Jenny can now read food labels better than most adults, and she's only seven!

Involve them in the kitchen as well. They'll enjoy the independence of being able to whip up their own Egg Beaters omelets, spaghetti, and other meals. Most brands of egg substitutes today have removed not only the cholesterol, but also the fat. See which you like best. Together you can learn to cook and bake with oat bran, which, as you'll see in Chapter 5, has marvelous cholesterol-lowering properties.

Probably the most important aspect of changing eating habits during childhood is that you're establishing a lifestyle for the future. And, in any effort that will have long-lasting effects, you'll want to take things one step at a time.

Most pediatricians and nutritionists feel, and I agree, that there's no reason to change dietary habits in those younger than two years of age. In fact, since there's such a growth spurt during the first two years of life, it's probably best to stay with whole milk, cheeses, and meats until the child's second birthday.

On the other hand, there's no reason to introduce such unnecessary foods as Twinkies or potato chips to children of any age. There's no Minimum Daily Requirement for such snack foods. Infants and toddlers don't ask for these until their parents start bringing them into the house. Don't start bad habits in those you love.

But cholesterol control is only part of giving children a future free of heart disease. Centuries ago, the Greeks educated both the mind and the body; physical fitness was a natural part of life. We can learn much from that ancient wisdom. Encourage your children to get plenty of exercise. Praise their physical accomplishments. Do everything in your power to keep your children from smoking, beginning, of course, with your own good example. Encourage your children never to start—or to stop now if they've already begun.

If you have children or grandchildren, you may wish to learn more about controlling their cholesterol and other heart-disease risk factors. I've written about my own experiences with my children, along with tips on how to deal with parties and holidays and how to prepare low-fat foods that children love, in a book called *Cholesterol & Children: A Parent's Guide to Giving Children a Future Free of Heart Disease.*

HEART DISEASE AND THE ELDERLY

Just as it's never too early to start a lifestyle of heart disease prevention, it's also never too late. Not too long ago, medical students were taught that normal cholesterol levels were "200 plus the patient's age." As we've learned, the advice today from the National Cholesterol Education Program is that the ideal of 200mg/dl or less applies to men and women *of all ages*. And a panel of experts convened at the 1988 meeting of the American Heart Association agreed that more attention should be paid to cutting risk factors for the older individual, noting that risk reduction in the elderly can increase the quality as well as the quantity of life.

According to Dr. Russell Luepker of the University of Minnesota, there's no question that elevated cholesterol levels "confer added risk" to all patients, including men and women over fifty years of age. "You cut the cholesterol levels and you cut the coronary heart disease rates," he said.

Dr. Nanette Wenger of Emory University noted that the number of elderly heart-disease patients is rising, and that actually the greatest occurrence of coronary heart disease, heart attacks, and coronary bypass surgery is in those over sixty-five. Dr. Wenger advocates cholesterol-lowering diets as well as regular exercise. As to the type of exercise, she feels it should be fun, not a chore. Walking at a 3- to 3.5-mile-per-hour rate, especially when in a group in which individuals can talk as they walk, is a good approach.

And Dr. John LaRosa of George Washington University Medical Center said blood pressure and smoking should also be targeted in the elderly. Unlike younger patients, elderly individuals are at greater risk when the systolic blood pressure rather than the diastolic pressure rises. The systolic pressure is the number on top, as in 130 over 90. Regarding smoking,

Dr. LaRosa noted that, while older men and women may be more addicted, they are also more receptive to suggestions to make changes that can improve health.

On a very upbeat note, pathologists today are seeing less plaque in the arteries of the elderly population. We can expect this trend to get better and better as the years go on, resulting in a healthier population of older men and women.

As I've traveled through the country giving presentations regarding the 8-week cholesterol cure, I've found that my audiences are largely elderly, often well into their seventies and eighties. They know something that many younger people don't realize: life is precious, short, and worth improving.

High cholesterol levels are a risk factor for older folks as much as for their sons and daughters. And those numbers can come down safely and effectively through this program, with the additional benefits of weight control and blood control. If you're into your sixties or beyond, you've worked hard all your life to come to an enjoyable retirement. Enjoy it in the best possible health.

The bottom line is that, despite special considerations, the advice to control cholesterol, exercise regularly, maintain ideal weight, control stressful situations, and enjoy life in order to prevent future heart disease applies equally to all men, women, boys, and girls of all walks of life, of all races, and of all ages. It's never too early and never too late to start a heart-healthy lifestyle.

3

Testing Your Cholesterol Level

The National Cholesterol Education Program has recommended that everyone over twenty should have his or her level tested and that everyone should aim for a measurement of 200 mg/dl or less.

When I first became interested in cholesterol there was only one way to learn one's cholesterol level, and that was to make an appointment through one's physician to have a test done at a hospital or laboratory. Today, however, testing has become far more widespread. In addition to those traditional settings, where samples of blood are drawn by needle through a vein in the arm, supermarkets, shopping malls, and health fairs host fingerprick testing sessions, during which one can learn his or her cholesterol level in minutes.

Unfortunately, such convenience brings with it a few problems. The fingerprick test may or may not be accurate and it doesn't give the important HDL/total cholesterol ratio. Some people are erroneously frightened into cholesterol-reducing programs or treatments, while others are wrongly reassured that their cholesterol levels are just fine, and so they continue with current lifestyles. And even the standard tests are not always accurate.

Picture a few scenarios. A woman learns that her cholesterol level tops out at 240 mg/dl and, fearing impending heart attack, she drastically changes her diet, giving up the foods she loves, which are rich in nutrients. What she doesn't know, since the fingerprick test she took reveals only the total cholesterol, is that her protective level of HDL cholesterol soars to 80 mg/dl, thus giving her a ratio of 3.0 and shielding her from atherosclerosis.

Across town in a physician's office, a man learns his cholesterol, coming in at 270 mg/dl, puts him at risk. The doctor immediately pulls out a prescription pad and puts the man on Mevacor without retesting to be certain the first test was accurate, and perhaps without testing to determine HDL levels.

At a shopping mall a man pays his $6 fee for a fingerprick test, which measures his cholesterol at 250. He immediately goes to a health-food store to buy a supply of oat bran and niacin. Two months later he returns to the mall to find to his delight that his cholesterol level has fallen to a safe 175. And during this entire process the man never bothers to consult with his physician. Unfortunately, then, he never learns that niacin is contraindicated for those with gout. He suffers an acute gout attack, winds up in his doctor's office, and pays for a series of tests as the physician tries to learn why the man's uric acid levels have risen to bring on the gout.

These three examples point out the need for a little common sense when it comes to cholesterol testing and the decisions that follow. Cholesterol levels are a measurement of complex and often confusing factors involved with a major cause of death in this nation. Cholesterol is far too important to be taken lightly or to be self-treated. Efforts at cholesterol reduction should be made under medical supervision in order to be safe and effective.

But, you might ask, isn't this a self-help book? Can't one simply read about cholesterol and methods of reduction without involving one's doctor? The answer is that the book works best when it acts as a bridge between doctor and patient. Working together, with the knowledge gained about cholesterol, fats, the diet, oat bran, and so on, the doctor-patient team can completely eliminate the cholesterol risk factor. To paraphrase the famous saying about individuals acting as their own lawyers, the patient who treats himself has a fool for a physician.

With that said, let's take a look at what the National Cholesterol Education Program guidelines specify for interpreting cholesterol tests, regardless of where or when those tests are done. We know that the NCEP recommends that every man and woman, regardless of age, should have a cholesterol level that does not exceed 200 mg/dl. Ideally, the total count should be lower than 200, with authorities agreeing that while a significant rise in heart-disease deaths occurs as levels exceed that number, there is a notable rise in heart attacks and heart-disease deaths in individuals whose levels go over 180. These recommendations, the NCEP believes, are realistic and attainable for the entire population. But for those with the motivation and commitment to make them, greater cuts into cholesterol levels can be expected to provide even better protection.

The NCEP suggests that those who test out at lower than 200 mg/dl should have a repeat cholesterol measurement within five years or at the next physical examination performed by a physician. Those with such desirable levels are encouraged to keep up the good work in terms of diet and lifestyle in order to maintain lower cholesterol counts.

The NCEP considers a level between 200 and 239 as a borderline-high cholesterol reading. They do not ignore the fact that many if not most patients suffering heart attacks have cholesterol levels between 210 and 215. So why are the assigned numbers in this borderline-high category so high? Those falling into this bracket are divided into two groups and given appropriate advice.

In the first group are those who have no other risk factors for heart disease whatsoever. They are to be given information regarding ways to improve the diet to further reduce cholesterol levels to the desirable zone, and are advised to have other cholesterol tests performed annually. They may even be advised to have a repeat test to make sure the first one was accurate. We'll look more at expectations for accuracy a bit later in this chapter.

In the second subgroup of those with a borderline-high cholesterol of between 200 and 239 are individuals with either known coronary heart disease or two additional risk factors for the disease. Such factors include male sex, family history of heart disease, smoking, high blood pressure, diabetes, and obesity in excess of 30 percent over ideal weight. Those in this group should have what is known as a lipoprotein analysis, which breaks down the total cholesterol into its component parts (LDL and HDL) and also measures triglycerides.

Those with a high blood cholesterol level of more than 240 mg/dl are also advised to have more extensive testing performed to further determine risk. This, in turn, brings us to the NCEP recommendations regarding LDL cholesterol levels. Remember that it is the LDLs, the low-density-lipoprotein molecules carrying cholesterol through the blood, that are responsible for the buildup of atherosclerotic plaque in the arteries.

To have the lipoprotein analysis done, patients should fast for twelve to fourteen hours prior to having their blood drawn in the laboratory. While the food eaten just prior to testing will have little if any influence on cholesterol levels as such, food will elevate triglycerides, which are the storage form of fats in the blood. Those triglycerides, in turn, are used in the laboratory to calculate the amount of LDL cholesterol. The formula used for this calculation is:

$$\text{LDL cholesterol} = \text{total cholesterol} - \text{HDL cholesterol} - \frac{\text{triglycerides}}{5}$$

For example, let's look at a person whose blood sample shows a total cholesterol of 235, HDL cholesterol of 40, and triglycerides of 190. Plugging those numbers into the equation we get:

$$\text{LDL cholesterol} = 235 - 40 - \frac{190}{5} = 157$$

With an LDL level of 157, the individual finds himself in the borderline-high category for risk of coronary heart disease, as seen in Table 10 on page 108.

If lipoprotein analysis reveals the LDL to be less than 130, the person should be told to get a repeat cholesterol measurement within five years, and to follow a low-fat, low-cholesterol diet to improve the cholesterol profile even more.

Those in the borderline-high range of 130–159 LDL cholesterol also fall into two categories. Anyone with two additional heart-disease risk factors is advised to begin the National Cholesterol Education Program's Step I diet. This calls for total fat intake equaling no more than 30 percent of total calories and dietary cholesterol less than 300 mg. These patients are to be reevaluated annually.

Those borderline-high LDL patients with two risk factors *plus* the presence of heart disease are designated for clinical evaluation, during which a medical history is taken, a physical examination is performed, and laboratory tests are done. The physician should evaluate the patient for secondary causes of high cholesterol levels, such as hypothyroidism, should check for hereditary lipid disorders, and should consider the influences of age, sex, and other risk factors. Patients are then advised to begin making dietary changes to reduce those elevated cholesterol levels.

Those individuals who are tested at greater than 160 mg/dl LDL cholesterol are treated the same as those borderline-high patients with two additional risk factors plus known heart disease. Known heart disease is determined by a history of heart attack, angina pectoris, or a positive treadmill stress test showing cardiac insufficiency (that is to say, the heart is not receiving enough oxygen through the occluded coronary arteries).

Dr. Basil Rifkind of the National Heart, Lung, and Blood Institute has stated unequivocally that "no individual should be placed on a lifelong program of cholesterol reduction without determining whether in fact the LDL level is elevated." He explains that there can be instances in which the potential risk of the total elevation of cholesterol can be mitigated by the presence of elevated HDLs. This is particularly true in women, in whom HDL levels tend to be higher. Dr. Scott Grundy of the University of Texas Health Science Center has reported that the greatest number of patients taking the prescription cholesterol-lowering drug Mevacor are elderly women. Many such patients, if properly tested and diagnosed, are not candidates for drug therapy at all. Some may not even be at risk of heart disease, owing to the protection of high HDL levels. And most should first be advised to use dietary measures to reduce total cholesterol.

Ultimately, anyone who has been found to have a total cholesterol level much over 200 should have a more revealing lipo-protein analysis performed to determine the HDL and LDL levels.

We've seen the importance in diagnosis of the LDL levels and the vital role played by HDL cholesterol. Simply stated, even those with relatively low total cholesterol levels may well be at significant risk for heart disease owing to low levels of HDL. Certainly anyone with a family history of heart disease should be tested to determine HDL levels, as should those with other risk factors for heart disease. As discussed in Chapter 1, many authorities have questioned the current NCEP recommendations in light of what we've since learned about HDLs, and have suggested that the recommendations be revised to include advice regarding those HDLs in order to take this independent risk factor into consideration.

In order to avoid errors, authorities now strongly recommend that individuals who find themselves at supposed risk as the result of a cholesterol test ought to have the test repeated. There are many reasons for this, from individual variations in cholesterol levels to the all-too-real potential for testing error. Let's look at some of the personal influences that cause cholesterol levels to fluctuate.

INDIVIDUAL VARIATIONS IN CHOLESTEROL LEVELS

First of all, cholesterol levels vary in each of us by an average of 6 percent from day to day. For some people, that number may be as low as 4 percent, while for others it may be as high as 11 percent. Next, cholesterol levels vary with the seasons, with winter bringing the highest numbers. But we don't really know whether those seasonal differences are the result of dietary modifications, that is, our tendency to eat lighter foods in the summer, while winter meals often contain more fat.

Current stress levels also take their toll. The more stress one experiences, the higher the cholesterol level tends to be. Medical students have demonstrated higher counts during examination periods, and in one study accountants' measurements were significantly higher before the April 15 tax deadline than a few weeks after. The actual effect of stress on cholesterol levels is difficult to predict accurately, however, since each individual responds differently.

Menstrual cycles have a definite impact on women's cholesterol levels. Tests done at Brown University show that lipid levels tend to increase within five to ten days after menstruation, with statistically significant changes for total and LDL cholesterol. The researchers feel the variation in plasma volume is responsible for at least half of the cholesterol variation. That is to say, after menstruation there is a lower volume of blood, and thus the cholesterol is more concentrated at that time. Most likely hormonal influences are responsible for the other half of the change.

Women's cholesterol levels are also increased during pregnancy, so tests are unlikely to be accurate until several weeks after pregnancy. Breast feeding may also have an influence.

The state of your general health will also have an impact. Researchers at Stanford University studied the total and HDL cholesterol levels of 6780 men and women. Of those, 7 percent reported having a minor illness such as a cold. Scrutiny of the data revealed that those reporting a cold tended to have a lower total and HDL level. The average total cholesterol for those with colds was 195, compared to 201 for those in good health. HDLs for persons with colds averaged 51, while those without colds scored 52.

Recent myocardial infarctions, or heart attacks, lower cholesterol levels. Dr. Basil Rifkind points out that this variation played a role in the resistance of doctors at first to recognizing the importance of cholesterol levels in heart disease. Cholesterol levels return to normal five to six weeks following heart attacks.

One should also take prescription medications into consideration. Drugs used to lower blood pressure tend to elevate cholesterol levels. The same holds true for hormone therapy and for anabolic steroids. And it's quite possible that in the future other medications will be shown to have an influence on cholesterol levels.

Even the position of the body plays a role. Cholesterol levels tend to fall when one is lying on one's back, because the volume of blood shifts in the body. Authorities recommend that blood samples should be taken in the sitting position after at least a five-minute resting period. Some feel that a rest as long as ten to fifteen minutes would be better.

Of course, diet has a major impact on your cholesterol levels. But don't expect last night's steak dinner to show up on today's test; it takes about two and a half days for the effect of food intake to register on measurements of cholesterol. Triglycerides, on the other hand, rise very rapidly in response to foods. That's why it's essential to fast for twelve to fourteen hours before cholesterol testing that will measure triglycerides. And, since triglycerides are used as part of the equation to calculate LDL cholesterol, foods eaten prior to lipoprotein analysis will influence those measurements. While fats and dietary cholesterol are the culprits in raising cholesterol levels in the blood, sugars, starches, and alcohol are more influential on triglyceride levels.

Adding up all these individual variations, one can expect quite a shift in total cholesterol readings from day to day. That's why it's important not to take just one reading as being a definitive measurement. Only after a few tests can one determine a predictable level.

Testing Methods and Their Accuracy

Apart from individual variation in cholesterol levels, we must also consider the problem of accuracy in the testing itself. The two most common kinds of testing methods as of this writing make use of standard laboratory equipment, as in hospitals, medical labs, and in some physicians' offices, and the newer portable fingerprick devices, used in some doctors' offices, by cholesterol-testing firms, and at health fairs, health clubs, and shopping malls.

Federal Standards

National government standards call for accuracy of 5 percent for hospital and laboratory testing equipment and for all the portable fingerprick testing devices; a 3 percent margin went into effect in 1990. Most of the better labs do better than 5 percent already. Unfortunately, laboratory equipment in physicians' offices are not subject to the federal standards.

While a 5 percent margin for error may not seem like much at first, it can make a significant difference when added to the already present individual variation of between 4 and 11 percent. Let's take an individual who has a true cholesterol level of 200 mg/dl. He or she will have an individual daily variation of plus or minus 5 percent on average. Now add the additional potential of 5 percent plus or minus error from the test itself. That's a total of 10 percent error. So that person's cholesterol level could be measured at 180 on one day and 220 on another. Take into account the other variations mentioned earlier and you begin to see the problem.

Before you throw up your hands in despair, however, be somewhat reassured that if you have two or three tests done you'll start to see a clear trend. If the results of three tests are, let's say, 210, 215, and 175, you can be fairly confident that your true level is above 200. And, if that's the case, you'd be well advised to have a more complete lipoprotein analysis performed to determine your LDL and HDL as well as your total cholesterol.

Is there any way to have confidence in any given test? Fortunately the answer is yes. The Laboratory Standardization Panel of the National Heart, Lung and Blood Institute has established a proven reference standard that can be used by laboratories. This reference standard consists of a sample containing a proven amount of cholesterol. It was developed by the Centers for Disease Control using the Abel-Kendall method of analysis, which is accepted by authorities as being the gold standard. Laboratories can (but are not required to) use this reference standard to determine whether their equipment measures the sample accurately and precisely and, if not, to make appropriate calibration adjustments. Accuracy, simply enough, means whether the testing equipment comes up with the right number. Precision, on the other hand, means that the equipment will register that number time after time. Other reference standards are also available to laboratories and to manufacturers of portable cholesterol-testing machines.

Standard Laboratory Equipment: at Hospitals, Medical Laboratories, and Physicians' Offices

Because of the federal standards that apply to hospital and medical labs, and because tests taken with this equipment can give figures for HDL, LDL, and triglycerides, this is a good way to go when having your cholesterol tested. By finding out if a given laboratory uses the standard reference, you can assure yourself of even greater accuracy.

More and more doctors are doing their own testing, since this offers both patient convenience and additional profit. Some use the portable machines, and others have more sophisticated laboratory equipment. Testing in physicians' offices is excluded from federal standards. Furthermore, published research points to greater reliability from lab-trained medical technologists, although nurses can also perform well if given proper instruction. In many physicians' office labs, doctors, nurses, or nonmedical personnel with no specific laboratory training perform the tests.

You have a right to the best possible testing, but you'll have to speak up for that right. Don't blindly accept your doctor's recommendations of a laboratory. Ask your doctor or the personnel at the laboratory itself whether the reference standard is being used. If not, find another lab that does use it.

Portable Fingerprick Tests

We can expect that cholesterol testing will develop into quite an industry as public interest and education in this area increases. To meet that increased demand, companies that provide public cholesterol screenings have been formed and continue to proliferate, giving tests at health fairs, shopping malls, and health clubs. Some doctors' offices use the same type of equipment.

Typically cholesterol-testing firms use one of three portable machines, the Reflotron made by Boehringer Mannheim, the Kodak Ektachem, and the Abbott Vision. You'll see the Reflotron most often since it is the most portable and the least expensive. All use a fingerprick to get a small blood sample. Most portable testing machines provide only total cholesterol readings.

How accurate are these machines? That depends on whom you ask. A number of studies have been done comparing the results from the portable analyzers with those from more sophisticated laboratory machines.

In a study done at Baylor College of Medicine in Houston, researchers reported that the Reflotron device provided results that were not only precise and accurate, but similar to those obtained by the Centers for Disease Control standardized reference methods. Similarly, Dr. Paul Bachorik of Johns Hopkins University School of Medicine reported that the Reflotron and laboratory methods yielded highly correlated results. The Reflotron readings, he found, might be 1 percent to 4 percent lower than laboratory findings. Using the Kodak portable model, Dr. G. Russell Warnick of the University of Washington's Northwest Research Center in Seattle found the device to provide data comparable to those obtained from CDC standardized labs.

There were a number of studies reported at the First National Cholesterol Conference held in the fall of 1988 that compared and evaluated portable cholesterol-testing machines. Dr. Robert Wones of the University of Cincinnati, looking at the precision and accuracy of total cholesterol measurements by the Abbott Vision, concluded that "fingerstick sampling and testing in field settings lessens the precision and accuracy of cholesterol measurements; even so, when appropriately calibrated, the Vision provides total cholesterol measurements in all settings that are within NCEP standards."

The Abbott Vision has received good reviews elsewhere as well. Dr. Herbert Naito, chairman of the NCEP panel on cholesterol screening, has said that this device provides a "valuable and highly accurate tool to the primary care physician."

One reason for praises of the Abbott device is that it is the only portable cholesterol-testing machine that is entirely nondependent on the testing personnel's expertise. That makes it particularly useful in a doctor's office, where the personnel doing the tests may be more or less trained in laboratory procedures.

Another advantage of the Vision is that it provides a printout of cardiac risk assessment based on the patient's medical history and lifestyle. The printout provides the estimated risk of having a heart attack during the next six years. And this printout becomes a permanent record of the patient's cholesterol level. The Kodak apparatus also provides a printout of the total cholesterol reading. The Reflotron, on the other hand, gives the reading only on the digital screen. During crowded testing situations, it has been suggested, personnel might make a mistake in writing the number on the patient's report. That may or may not be a real problem. But, in any case, if you are tested using the Reflotron, take a look at the screen for your numbers to appear rather than relying entirely on any written report given to you.

Despite the generally favorable reports on portable cholesterol-testing devices, there has been some criticism. In standardized laboratory methods, blood is simultaneously drawn by fingerprick and by needle through a vein in the arm, and the blood samples are compared. And all testing is performed by trained laboratory personnel. In other words, the best of conditions are employed.

That may not always be the reality when the portable devices are used in the field, whether at a local health fair or at a shopping mall. In such situations, except when the Abbott device is being used, accuracy will largely depend on the experience and expertise of the personnel.

Fortunately, we can expect that cholesterol testing will become more sophisticated as a number of companies already involved in this emerging industry hone their abilities.

It's perfectly acceptable to ask about testing techniques before you have your fingerprick, to see how reliable the company or organization is. Personnel should be laboratory trained. Requirements for testing personnel vary from state to state. Find out how much testing experience the staff has; the more the better. Next, ask how often the equipment is checked for accuracy and precision.

When it's time to have your test done, rest for about five to ten minutes. Then make sure your hands are nice and warm. If the fingers are cold, blood won't flow very well and the technician may try to "milk" blood from the fingertip. This compromises accuracy by giving readings significantly lower owing to the dilution of the sample.

Virtually every authority agrees that one should trust a trend in cholesterol values rather than a single reading. Fingerprick testing can certainly provide that kind of trend, and is valuable in terms of screening the public and for monitoring one's progress.

To find out where you can get a fingerprick test in your area you can call the local office of your chapter of the American Heart Association.

The next step in cholesterol testing will require no equipment whatsoever. A number of companies have developed or are developing instant test kits, which can be used in physicians' offices or at cholesterol-screening sites.

One such company, Home Diagnostics, Inc., has introduced a test called LipoScan TC.

The LipoScan instructions call for a finger-prick drop of whole blood placed on a small disposable, color-changing strip. After one minute, the strip changes color in response to the total cholesterol content of the blood. The user then visually compares the color of the strip with a numerically coded color chart. The chart breaks down 13 different total cholesterol values from 100 through 550 mg/dl in 25 mg/dl increments. Currently, one must rely on the visual interpretation to determine a cholesterol reading. The company is expected to introduce an electronic, digital reflectance meter capable of reading the test strips in 1 mg/dl increments. However, none of the companies involved in this area plan to make the cholesterol testing kits available for home use anytime in the near future.

With a 25 mg/dl increment between cholesterol readings, the value of this type of kit is relatively limited to broad screenings to identify those individuals at significant risk of heart disease. One can expect, however, that with electronic reading techniques and improvements in both accuracy and precision of the approach, this will become a part of cholesterol technology for tomorrow.

Another approach for the future, called

apolipoprotein analysis, provides more accurate measurements of heart-disease risk through analysis of the lipoproteins that carry the cholesterol molecule through the bloodstream. Dr. Herbert Naito of the Cleveland Clinic has stated that measuring the apolipoproteins provides prediction of heart disease four times more reliable than standard cholesterol testing. Such testing is not widely available today; it is limited to the certified standardization laboratories established by the National Cholesterol Education Program. For this test patients can be referred to the laboratories by their physicians.

Laboratories for apolipoprotein analysis have been set up at the following eight locations: Baylor College of Medicine in Houston; Cleveland Clinic in Cleveland; Minnesota Lipid Research Clinic in Minneapolis; New York State Department of Health in Albany; Northwest Lipid Research Clinic in Seattle; Pennsylvania State Department of Health in Philadelphia; Wisconsin State Department of Health in Madison; and the Yellow Springs Instrument Company in Yellow Springs, Ohio.

Short of being referred to one of those laboratories, you can be fairly confident of cholesterol readings provided by major hospital laboratories close to home. Even then, be sure to ask whether the laboratory uses the nationally established reference standard based on the Abel-Kendall method of cholesterol determination. And remember to be aware of individual variations as discussed earlier.

Whether your cholesterol measurement comes from a big hospital laboratory or a simple fingerprick test, it will give one number for you to consider as part of a trend. Once you know the typical range of your own cholesterol level, you can use either test with a fair degree of confidence to monitor your progress.

Remember that while cholesterol testing is not 100 percent foolproof it remains the only way we have to gauge our risk of heart disease from cholesterol levels.

How often should one have a cholesterol test? If you've begun to follow the program in this book, you can expect results at the end of just eight weeks. And if you stay on the program, you can expect your cholesterol levels to remain reduced, so an annual test is all you'll need. The best place to go for that annual check is a major laboratory your physician will suggest for you. That way you'll also learn about the status of HDLs, LDLs, and triglycerides. And, if you're taking niacin, you'll also want to have a liver enzyme test to make sure your liver is tolerating the added burden of the niacin without difficulty.

From time to time you might begin to experiment with your diet. I know that I do. You might cut back on certain kinds of fats, or increase your consumption of various kinds of foods. For example, what would happen if you had an additional dollop of olive oil daily? Or how would your cholesterol level respond to an extra oat-bran muffin eaten as an evening snack? The only way you'll know is by way of the cholesterol test.

If your cholesterol has gone up a bit, you'll want to know so you can make appropriate modifications in your diet. If those levels have dropped a little, you'll be pleased to find out so you can keep up whatever you've been doing. There's no greater satisfaction than getting back a wonderful report from your doctor saying that you've beaten the cholesterol culprit.

Table 10. **Recommendations of the Adult Treatment Panel of the National Cholesterol Education Program for Classification of Patients**

CLASSIFICATION BASED ON TOTAL CHOLESTEROL	CLASSIFICATION BASED ON LDL-CHOLESTEROL
less than 200 mg/dl desirable blood cholesterol	less than 130 mg/dl desirable LDL-cholesterol
200–239 mg/dl border-line-high cholesterol	130–159 mg/dl border-line-high-risk LDL
more than 240 mg/dl high blood cholesterol	more than 160 mg/dl high-risk LDL-cholesterol

4

Winning by the Numbers

More than twelve separate clinical trials have established that lowering levels of blood cholesterol can reduce the incidence of cardiovascular disease. Adults should shoot for a total cholesterol level of less than 200 mg/dl. The National Institutes of Health in January 1985 stated that "one-half of the U.S. population is at risk of coronary heart disease, with blood cholesterol levels above 200 mg/dl."

The program in this book is designed—and proven—to lower cholesterol levels by 20, 30, even 40 percent or more. That's because this is the only program to consider all three reasons for elevated cholesterol. You've been eating too much fat and cholesterol, so I'll show you some delicious ways to cut back on those culprits. Your body doesn't excrete sufficient cholesterol in the form of bile salts and bile acids through your intestine, so eating oat bran will increase the amount of cholesterol excreted. And your liver has been producing too much cholesterol, so by taking some niacin you'll short-circuit that production. By considering all three aspects, the program is effective although it calls for only moderate dietary modification, a small amount of oat bran, and reasonable doses of niacin.

It's fairly straightforward to suggest eating three oat-bran muffins a day. And you can count the niacin tablets you swallow daily. But for most people, when it comes to percentages and figures and numbers about nutrition, the eyes just glaze over. Who can understand or remember all those numbers?

For example, the American Heart Association says that everyone in the United States should limit their cholesterol intake to no more than 300 milligrams a day. And the fat intake should be no more than 30 percent of total calories, with 10 percent each coming from saturated fat, polyunsaturated fat, and monounsaturated fat. Confusing? You bet. What does all that mean in the real world of shopping for and eating food?

Most people find it tough just to remember how many calories different foods have; it's difficult to memorize calorie charts. The majority of us just learn that some foods are more "fattening" than others.

Even then, there are ions of misconceptions. For example, that butter has more calories than margarine; actually they are identical. Or that pasta and baked potatoes are fattening. Actually, it's only the fats we may put on those foods that add up the calories.

But, even if we don't know *anything* about calories, we can see the results in the mirror and on the bathroom scale. It's not quite so simple with cholesterol. Too many people don't know their levels are dangerously high until the doctor says it's time for bypass surgery.

Before we get into the actual details of how to win by the numbers, I want you to think about something obvious. We all learn things a little bit at a time. Today we can all tell the difference between an inch and a mile, and between an ounce and a gallon. We know that something weighs "about a pound," and that another thing is "about six inches long." We've learned those things by experience over the years.

It'll take a little time, but you can also learn the numbers that can help you live a long life. It's worth the effort. So let's start with something very basic: how to figure out how much food to eat to stay healthy and at ideal body weight.

As adults, we're no longer growing in the same way children grow. Our bones, skin, and muscles are pretty much developed. Therefore, we need far less food, in proportion, than we did when we were younger. But how much?

Only two variables come into play: first, whether you're a man or woman; second, whether you're sedentary, moderately active, or very active. Then decide your ideal weight. The weight table (pages 283–84) was adapted from the Metropolitan Life Insurance Company of New York, and specifies weights most health authorities have accepted as beneficial for optimum health.

The next step is to decide to feed *only* your ideal weight, *not* the weight you have today—unless, of course, you are already at ideal weight. If you weigh, let's say, 175 pounds and should weigh 150 pounds, then feed only your 150-pound self—let the other 25 pounds slowly drift away.

An adult man with a moderately active lifestyle will require 15 calories for every pound of his weight. If he starts to become involved with a really strenuous exercise program, he may need an extra calorie per pound. If he becomes sedentary, like so many men in the United States, he'll be able to burn even fewer than 15 calories per pound.

Despite all requests for equal rights, women unfortunately have different metabolisms, and, for the most part, they burn fewer calories per pound. A moderately active woman needs only 12 calories per pound of ideal body weight.

The calculations, then, are rather simple:

Moderately active man
  150 pounds × 15 calories/pound = 2250 calories/day
Relatively inactive man
  150 pounds × 13 calories/pound = 1950 calories/day
Moderately active woman
  120 pounds × 12 calories/pound = 1440 calories/day
Relatively inactive woman
  120 pounds × 10 calories/pound = 1200 calories/day

Obviously, if you are greatly overweight, or if you get turned on to heavy-duty exercise, your caloric needs will be different. Read Chapters 8 and 9, on weight loss and exercise, for more specifics. But, for the most part, these are the caloric needs for the male and female examples I've chosen. Now do the calculations for yourself.

Counting calories is fairly simple. Most foods today have very complete nutrition labels. Many magazines today provide complete nutrition breakdowns along with their recipes, listing the amount of fat, cholesterol, sodium, and calories provided per serving. *Family Circle* and *Woman's Day* are two good examples. The chart at the end of this chapter lists fat, cholesterol, sodium, and calories found in many commonly consumed foods. And you may wish to purchase a complete calorie counter in booklet form. These are available at most supermarket checkout stands. You'll quickly see that foods with the most calories also have the most fat.

Carbohydrates and proteins contain just 4 calories per gram. There are about 28 grams to an ounce, for those who don't "think metric." But fat contains 9 calories per gram! If you just cut down on the amount of fat you eat, you'll automatically and dramatically reduce calories.

Which brings us to the very important consideration of how to determine how much fat to include in our daily food intake.

First, the average American diet is between 40 and 50 percent fat. And every medical authority agrees that's too much. The American Heart Association recommends 30 percent for the general population. Many feel that those with an elevated cholesterol level should cut down to less than 30 percent. And those at real risk should cut down to just 10 percent. With this complete program I was able to bring my own cholesterol level down by taking the middle-ground level of 20 percent fat intake. Thousands of others have proved that anyone can do the same. So shoot for that 20 percent number, or 30 percent if your cholesterol is not too high, and here's how to do your calculation for your own body.

Let's take the example of the 150-pound man who's moderately active. He needs 2250 calories daily in order to neither gain nor lose weight. And because he's on this program to dramatically reduce his cholesterol level he's decided to consume only 20 percent of calories as fat.

So we multiply 2250 calories by 20 percent to get a total of 450 calories as fat. What does that mean? How can we tell how much food provides 450 calories as fat?

Fat, as you'll recall, provides 9 calories per gram. The man in our example wants to eat no more than 450 calories as fat. Therefore we divide 450 calories by 9, the number of calories per gram, to give us 50 grams. So our man can now limit himself to 50 grams of fat daily. That's a good target, even if he misses by a bit.

Personally, I have found the 20 percent level, providing 50 grams of fat daily, to be right for me. It's right because my regular blood cholesterol tests indicate that my serum cholesterol remains in the safe zone. But will this be right for you? Each of us has a slightly different body, with its own metabolism. You may find that you can increase the percentage to, say, 25 percent of calories as fat. Start with that 20 percent level and go from there.

Again, it's the combination of the aspects of this program that allows us to modify the diet only moderately. Other authorities, including the late Nathan Pritikin, say it is an all-or-nothing situation. Until this program came along, they were right. And that deserves some explanation.

Researchers have found that the body has what they call a saturation level for fat and cholesterol intake. Some people have a relatively low blood cholesterol level even though they consume a lot of dietary fat and cholesterol. Others, including myself, don't metabolize fat and cholesterol as well. But dietary intake does have impact on everyone to one degree or another.

If one were to find a group of normal, healthy men and women whose cholesterol levels were, say, an average of 170 and feed them an extra egg daily, their cholesterol levels would go up. The same would apply if one added several extra grams of fat daily. But if another group had an already elevated level of, for example, 250, the extra fat or cholesterol would not have as much effect, if any. Those persons would be at their saturation levels and it would take a considerable amount of additional fat and cholesterol to drive their levels in the blood higher.

The converse also applies. If one has an elevated cholesterol level and cuts back only a bit, there will be little or no effect. That's why so many people over the years have claimed that dietary cholesterol has little to do with serum cholesterol. Eliminate egg yolks, eat very little meat, and do all the other modifications, and there still will be an elevated level. It's only when one almost completely eliminates fat and cholesterol from the diet that an elevated cholesterol level can be brought back down to truly safe levels of between 150 and 180.

That's why the Pritikin diet and others require such strict adherence. For persons with elevated cholesterol levels that put them at risk, the saturation points are very low. The diet, therefore, must be all-or-nothing.

The 8-Week Cholesterol Cure, however, considers all three aspects of elevated cholesterol. Diet is only one of those three aspects. While it is still very important to modify the diet, eating oat bran and supplementing the diet with niacin will complete the cholesterol-lowering effect we all want.

The next part is really quite simple, although like any other learning situation, it may not seem so at first. What our man should do is to start looking at those food labels in the supermarket.

Several years ago a law was passed requiring a prominently featured label of nutrient content on a number of foods. You'll find the label on canned or frozen vegetables, crackers, dairy foods, and practically everything else that is processed or that makes some sort of nutrition claim such as being low-calorie or high-protein or whatever. Unprocessed foods, such as meats and fruits and vegetables, do not have to be labeled, but many stores now feature little placards alongside the produce spelling out the nutrient components.

On those labels you'll find the number of calories per serving size and the amount of protein and fat listed in grams. Or you can look the food up in the charts in this book. Since the man in our example knows he needs no more than 50 grams of fat each day, he can simply look at the nutrient label of foods to see how many grams that particular food supplies.

Does he have to think about every single food he eats? Not at all. Other than avocados and nuts, most plant foods do not contain a substantial amount of fat. Fat in the diet comes from (1) animal foods, (2) baked goods, (3) processed foods, and (4) added fats in the form of oil, margarine, butter, mayonnaise, and so forth.

The table at the end of this chapter clearly

states the amount of both fat and cholesterol found in commonly used foods. Some shellfish have considerable amounts of cholesterol, though still much lower than previously believed. These foods, however, have very low levels of fat. So they can be enjoyed in moderation as long as they are not fried.

Do some other comparisons in the chart. Note that while turkey breast and beef cuts contain just about the same amount of cholesterol in a 3 ½-ounce serving, the difference in the amount of fat is enormous. One serving of turkey provides less than 2 grams, while the same weight of porterhouse steak gives you nearly 15 grams!

But does that mean you can't ever have a piece of beef? Certainly not. Just remember that you want to keep your total fat consumption and cholesterol intake down on a daily basis. If you want a piece of steak for the evening meal, cut down on fat in the rest of your foods that day. And choose the cuts of beef lower in fat content.

I grew up in Chicago, a city famous for its steaks. There the fine steak houses took pride in their 24-ounce sirloins, or the porterhouses they delivered on an oversized platter. That's just totally unacceptable for *anyone* today. There's no reason in the world to eat that much meat at one sitting—even the National

Live Stock and Meat Board in Chicago agrees!

On the other hand, a 3 ½-ounce piece of meat may not be enough to satisfy that urge for an occasional rare steak. So double the amount. Sure, it's o.k. to do it now and then. You'll be consuming 140 milligrams of cholesterol, and, for a T-bone steak, 28.4 grams of fat. Just know what you're doing. Then, to make up for that intake, avoid sour cream on the potato, pass up butter with your bread, and have just a touch of oil and vinegar dressing on your salad.

Take a few moments right now to calculate your own calorie and fat intake for the day. Use paper and pencil to figure out the numbers for yourself. This is important, so don't skip it. Here's how to determine your daily fat intake in grams.

Write down the weight you would like to maintain.

ideal weight

Now, depending on the amount you exercise, multiply that weight by the appropriate number of calories. Multiply by 10 calories if you are a sedentary adult woman; by 11 calories if you are a sedentary adult man; by 12 calories if you're a moderately active woman;

or by 15 calories if you are a moderately active man. By multiplying your ideal weight by the appropriate number of calories per pound, you'll have the number of calories you need to maintain your ideal weight. If you weigh more than the ideal weight and still eat only enough calories to maintain the ideal weight, the extra weight will gradually disappear.

(ideal weight) x (calories per pound) = daily calorie intake

Now let's determine how many of those calories will come from fat. Ideally, we want to consume 20 percent of our calories as fat. So we multiply our daily calorie intake by 20 percent.

(daily calorie intake) × .20 = daily calories as fat

Each gram of fat provides nine calories. So to determine your daily allowance of fat as measured in grams, divide the calories eaten as fat by nine.

(daily calories as fat) ÷ 9 = daily allowance of fat in grams

Now that you know how many grams of total fat you should limit yourself to, remember that there are three kinds of fat to choose from. Medical authorities recommend that you divide your fat intake evenly among saturated fats, polyunsaturated fats, and monounsaturated fats. See page 129 for a list of where those fats are found. You'll notice that not many foods provide monounsaturated fats. So for all practical purposes, and this is a practical book, you can really divide your fat grams between animal and plant sources. Emphasize vegetable fats. With one little exception: watch for the labels that tell you the fat is from coconut, palm, or palm kernel oil. Those fats are saturated and belong in the same category as fats from animal sources.

There are so many terrific alternative recipes around that you'll wonder why anyone would ever complain about modifying the diet. This is modification, far, far, far from deprivation!

Even if recipes don't specifically list the fat and cholesterol, it's fairly easy to see if the foods in question are o.k. Just use Table 11 at the end of this chapter.

What if you see recipes that are particularly appealing but are laden with no-nos? Or what about those cherished family recipes that you really love? Do you have to give them up? Never! Just substitute ingredients.

There are very few foods that don't have

very acceptable low-fat, low-cholesterol substitutes. And you'll find that, if a recipe calls for ½ cup of oil, ¼ cup will do just as well. Maybe you'll even be able to get by with just ⅛ cup. As your tastes start to change, and believe me and everyone else who's done it, they will, you'll actually *prefer* the lighter, lower-fat versions.

Here are some helpful tips for substitutions in your recipes:

One whole egg = two egg whites
One egg yolk = one ounce egg substitute
Cream = evaporated skim milk
Whole milk = nonfat milk
Butter = soft margarine or corn oil
Oil to fry = Pam cooking spray
Shortening in baking = substitute ripe
    banana for half the shortening

You'll find many more hints about how to fill your pantry shelves with terrific foods and food substitutes in Chapter 13, "Let's Go Shopping." There are a number of fine foods available if you know what to look for in the supermarket. But by all means, when you go shopping, be sure you have the time to read those labels. Don't just rush out. Especially at the beginning when you're learning to recognize the hidden fats, schedule plenty of shopping time into the week.

Here's how the typical nutrition information panel looks on hundreds of foods in your supermarket:

NUTRITIONAL INFORMATION PER SERVING

Serving size . . . . One cup
Servings per container 8
Calories 150
Protein . . . . 8 grams
Carbohydrate . . . . 11 grams
Fat . . . . 8 grams

PERCENTAGE OF U.S. RECOMMENDED DAILY ALLOWANCES (U.S. RDA)

Protein 20
Vitamin A 4
Vitamin C 4
Thiamin 6
Riboflavin 25
Niacin . . . . *
Calcium 30
Iron . . . . *

Note that if a food contains less than 2 percent of the U.S. RDA of a given nutrient it is marked with an asterisk.

Don't stop reading when you've finished the nutrient label. Find the ingredient listing on the side of the package. Ingredients are listed *in order by weight*. Don't forget that. If water is listed first, that means there's more water than anything else. If sugar tops the list, then you know you're getting a lot of sugar.

Recently a number of my friends were getting "into" a trendy new confection called To-futti, which was advertised and promoted as ice cream without guilt. What could be healthier than eating tofu? But read the label: tofu is listed *fourth*! There is more sugar and fat than tofu. Low-fat frozen yogurt is a far better choice.

For your first comparison-shopping trip, pick up a number of foods to choose from. Look at the labels for both whole milk and nonfat milk. Not only do you have the problem of fat and cholesterol, a serving of whole milk provides 150 calories while nonfat milk has only 89. While you're at the dairy case, you'll also notice that buttermilk is low in fat and calories. It gets its thickness through the process of acidification. Now turn to the yogurt. Not all are the same, by a long shot. Opt for the low-fat or nonfat varieties. Look at the number of grams of fat contained in each.

When I began my own heart-health quest in 1984, cheese posed a real problem. Most cheese is extremely high in fat, especially the deadly saturated kind. Vegetarian cheeses, made with soy, didn't taste very good. And the fat-free varieties that came later bore little resemblance to real cheese, either in taste or in ability to melt.

Happily, today there is a compromise. Several brands and varieties of low-fat cheeses line the dairy aisle. My favorite cheese slices come from Borden, with just a single gram of fat. And Sargento makes wonderful cheese shreds in mozzarella flavor for pizzas and cheddar for Mexican dishes.

Since few foods, however, list cholesterol content, take some time to learn where that cholesterol lurks. You are shooting for less than 250 milligrams daily. For some foods, that's a real problem while for others it's not at all. An egg yolk contains up to 250 milligrams of cholesterol all by itself. You have two choices: either find an egg substitute, or eat just one egg yolk as your source of total cholesterol for the day. I personally don't feel that eating one egg yolk is worth giving up everything else for the day, so I've simply cut egg yolks out entirely. But my shopping cart is always loaded with eggs. I use just the whites. When it comes to cost, you'll find that using only the whites and tossing out the yolks is just about as much as buying the egg substitutes.

You'll be surprised how quickly you'll learn the cholesterol levels of foods so that you won't have to consult the chart every time you bite into something. At the beginning, though, you'll also be surprised to see cholesterol in foods you never even thought of as culprits. Today you can block cholesterol. See pages 371 and 442.

How much cholesterol could there be in cornbread made from a mix? After all, there's no cholesterol in corn. But, thanks to other things added, like lard and dried egg yolks, cornbread and other bakery mixes are significant sources of fat and cholesterol. Pancakes have about 33 milligrams each. That's *each* pancake; how many do you have in a stack? But all is not lost. Just start making your pancakes with egg whites instead. No problem; they're delicious. And French toast made with egg substitute can't be told from those slices made with whole eggs. The recipe chapters contain all the suggestions you'll need for months of delicious, low-fat, low-cholesterol eating.

You'll have to know how *much* you're eating to successfully modify your diet. How big is a serving? For many people a steak, no matter how large, is a serving. In realistic terms, a serving of meat should be about four ounces. Don't forget: that's a whole quarter of a pound! Some hamburgers brag about being that large. If you don't know how much four ounces is, make a small investment in a food scale for the kitchen. After a while your eye will become trained to make accurate estimates.

Many individuals must also restrict the amount of sodium in the diet owing to high blood pressure, hypertension. The role of sodium is discussed fully in Chapter 7.

And nutrition isn't just a mater of learning what *not* to eat. This also means increasing the amounts of certain foods. Most women, for example, need far more calcium and iron than their present diets offer. That's spelled out in Chapter 12.

You'll be amazed, as time goes by, how easy it will be to choose one food over another because of the numbers you'll learn. Whether eating at home, in a restaurant, or at friends' homes, you'll come out a winner. There's nothing like the feeling of satisfaction you'll get when the doctor announces how dramatically your cholesterol level has dropped. *That's* winning by the numbers!!

Type of Fat Found in Foods

Saturated Fat
Most fat from animal sources: beef,
    pork, lamb, veal, and poultry
Coconut oil
Palm oil
Palm kernel oil
Hydrogenated or partially
    hydrogenated vegetable oil

Monounsaturated Fat
Olives and olive oil
Peanuts and peanut oil
Canola (rapeseed) oil (Puritan and
    other brands)
Avocados

Polyunsaturated Fat
Vegetable oils other than those
    listed above

Note: Cholesterol is found only in animal sources.

These charts give a representative look at foods you probably eat regularly. Don't try to memorize them, but do become familiar with trends in composition for types of foods. Certainly it is not possible to list all the thousands of foods found in the supermarket. If you'd like to have a more complete listing, I'd recommend the book *Food Values of Portions Commonly Used* by Jean A. T. Pennington and Helen Nichols Church. The book, published by Perennial Library, is considered a bible by anyone involved in food and nutrition.

Table 11. Calorie, Fat, Cholesterol, and Sodium Content of Foods

FOOD	SERV. SIZE	CAL.	FAT (GRAMS)	CHOL. (MGS.)	SODIUM (MGS.)
CANDY					
Carnation Breakfast Bar	1 bar	210	11.0	1	140–220
Milk chocolate bar or 6–7 kisses	1 oz.	150	9.2	5	7
Milk chocolate with almonds	1 oz.	155	9.3	4	22
CHEESE					
American	1 oz.	105	8.4	27	318
Blue	1 oz.	103	8.5	21	390
Brick	1 oz.	103	8.5	25	157
Brie	1 oz.	94	7.8	28	176
Camembert	1 oz.	84	6.9	20	236
Cheddar	1 oz.	112	9.1	30	197
Colby	1 oz.	110	9.0	27	169
Cottage (1% fat)	½ cup	82	1.6	5	460
Cottage (2% fat)	½ cup	100	2.2	9	460

FOOD	SERV. SIZE	CAL.	FAT (GRAMS)	CHOL. (MGS.)	SODIUM (MGS.)
Cottage (4% fat)	½ cup	120	4.7	12	460
Cream cheese	2 tbsp.	99	9.9	34	84
Edam	1 oz.	87	5.7	25	270
Feta	1 oz.	74	6.0	25	312
Gouda	1 oz.	100	7.7	32	229
Gruyère	1 oz.	115	8.9	31	94
Monterey Jack	1 oz.	105	8.5	30	150
Mozzarella	1 oz.	79	6.1	22	104
Mozzarella (part skim)	1 oz.	78	4.8	15	148
Muenster	1 oz.	104	8.5	27	178
Neufchâtel	1 oz.	73	6.6	21	112
Parmesan (grated)	1 tbsp.	23	1.5	4	93
Parmesan (hard)	1 oz.	111	7.3	19	454
Provolone	1 oz.	98	7.3	19	245
Ricotta (13% fat)	½ cup	216	16.1	63	104
Ricotta (8% fat)	½ cup	171	9.8	40	155
Romano	1 oz.	110	7.6	29	340
Roquefort	1 oz.	105	8.7	26	513
Swiss (pasteurized processed)	1 oz.	95	7.1	26	388
Cheezola	1 oz.	89	6.4	1	448
Countdown	1 oz.	39	0.3	1	434
Lite Line	1 oz.	50	2.0	10	410
Light n' Lively	1 oz.	70	4.0	15	350+
Cheeze Whiz spread	1 oz.	80	6.0	15	490

Table 11 (continued)

FOOD	SERV. SIZE	CAL.	FAT (GRAMS)	CHOL. (MGS.)	SODIUM (MGS.)
Lo-Chol	1 oz.	105	9.0	4	130
Formagg	1 oz.	70	5.0	0	140

COMBINATION FOODS

Beefaroni	7 oz.	229	7.9	50	1044
Beef pot pie	1 pie	443	25.4	41	1008
Beef stew	1 cup	186	7.3	33	966
Chicken & noodles	6 oz.	15	14.9	20	816
Dennison's Chili con Carne	16-oz. can	320	17.0	30	10
Egg roll	3½ oz.	210+	6.7+	12+	530+
Morton Salisbury Steak Dinner	1 oz.	373	15.6	47	1213
Franco-American Macaroni and Cheese	1 cup	180	8.0	26	900
ARMOUR CLASSIC LITE DINNERS:					
Beef Pepper Steak	1	270	9.0	55	900
Chicken Burgundy	1	230	4.0	75	920
Chicken Oriental	1	240	4.0	75	730
Fillet of Cod Divan	1	280	7.0	80	990
Chicken Breast Marsala	1	270	7.0	NA	NA
Seafood, Natural Herbs	1	240	5.0	25	1440
Sliced Beef with Broccoli	1	280	7.0	70	2140

FOOD	SERV. SIZE	CAL.	FAT (GRAMS)	CHOL. (MGS.)	SODIUM (MGS.)
Turf n Surf	1	260	8.0	105	690
Turkey Parmesan	1	260	7.0	75	960
Veal Pepper					
Steak	1	280	8.0	90	480
LEAN CUISINE:					
(Stouffer's)					
Cheese Cannelloni	1	270	10.0	45	950
Chicken					
& Vegetables					
with Vermicelli	1	260	7.0	40	1250
Chicken					
Cacciatore					
with Vermicelli	1	280	10.0	40	1040
Chicken Chow					
Mein	1	250	5.0	25	1160
Fillet of Fish					
Florentine	1	240	9.0	100	800
Glazed Chicken	1	270	8.0	55	840
Linguini/Clam	1	260	7.0	40	860
Meatball Stew	1	250	9.0	65	1165
Oriental Beef	1	260	8.0	35	1270
Oriental Scallops	1	220	3.0	20	1200
Spaghetti	1	280	7.0	20	1400
Stuffed Cabbage	1	210	9.0	40	830
Zucchini Lasagna	1	260	7.0	20	1050
KRAFT					
Macaroni					
& Cheese	3/4 cup	290	13.0	5	530
Spiral Mac.					
& Cheese	3/4 cup	330	17.0	10	560

Table 11 (continued)

FOOD	SERV. SIZE	CAL.	FAT (GRAMS)	CHOL. (MGS.)	SODIUM (MGS.)
Egg Noodles & Cheese	³/₄ cup	340	17.0	50	630
Egg Noodles & Chicken	³/₄ cup	240	9.0	35	880
Spaghetti Dinner	I cup	310	8.0	5	730
Spaghetti Dinner Meat Sauce	I cup	370	14.0	15	720
Velveeta Shells & Cheese	³/₄ cup	260	10.0	25	720

CONDIMENTS

FOOD	SERV. SIZE	CAL.	FAT	CHOL.	SODIUM
Mayonnaise	I tbsp.	100	11.0	5	80
Tartar sauce	I tbsp.	95	10.0	10	141
White sauce	2 tbsp.	54	4.1	4	125
Diet mayo.	I tbsp.	45	5.0	5	90
Imitation mayo.	I tbsp.	60	4.0	10	100
Miracle Whip	I tbsp.	70	7.0	5	85
Kraft sandwich spread	I tbsp.	50	5.0	5	75

DAIRY FOODS

FOOD	SERV. SIZE	CAL.	FAT	CHOL.	SODIUM
Whole milk	I cup	150	8.1	34	120
Low-fat milk	I cup	122	4.7	20	122
Skim milk	I cup	89	0.4	5	128
Nonfat dry	I cup	81	0.2	4	124
Canned evaporated skim	I oz.	23	trace	I	35
Buttermilk (skim)	I cup	88	0.2	10	318
Goat milk	I cup	163	9.8	27	83

FOOD	SERV. SIZE	CAL.	FAT (GRAMS)	CHOL. (MGS.)	SODIUM (MGS.)
Yogurt (nonfat)	1 cup	127	0.4	4	174
Yogurt (low-fat)	1 cup	143	3.4	14	159
Yogurt (whole-milk)	1 cup	141	7.7	30	107
Half & half	1 tbsp.	20	1.7	6	6
Light cream	1 tbsp.	29	2.9	10	6
Medium cream	1 tbsp.	37	3.8	13	6
Light whipped cream	1 tbsp.	44	4.6	17	5
Heavy whipped cream	1 tbsp.	52	5.6	20	6
Sour cream	1 tbsp.	26	2.5	5	6
Aerosol whipped-cream topping	1/4 cup	25	2.0	10	10

DESSERTS

FOOD	SERV. SIZE	CAL.	FAT (GRAMS)	CHOL. (MGS.)	SODIUM (MGS.)
Cinnamon roll	1 ave.	174	5.0	39	214
Brownie	1 ave.	146	9.4	25	75
Angel-food cake	2 oz.	161	0.1	0	170
Carrot cake	3 1/2 oz.	356	20.4	30	246
Devil's-food cake	3 oz.	323	15.0	37	357
Gingerbread	2 oz.	175	4.3	0.6	190
Marble cake	3 oz.	288	7.6	40	225
Choco-chip cookies	1 ave.	52	2.3	6	44
Ladyfingers	1 large	50	1.1	50	10
McDonald's cookies	1 box	292	10.5	9	328
Oatmeal cookies	1 ave.	63	2.2	7	23

Table 11 (continued)

FOOD	SERV. SIZE	CAL.	FAT (GRAMS)	CHOL. (MGS.)	SODIUM (MGS.)
Peanut-butter cookies	I ave.	57	2.3	7	21
Hostess Devil's Food Cupcakes	I	185	6.0	5	282
Hostess Ding Dongs	I	187	10.5	10	121
Hostess Ho Hos	I	118	6.0	14	63
Hostess Suzy Qs	I	256	10.9	10	301
Hostess Twinkies	I	152	6.2	20	203
Custard mixes	½ cup	143	4.6	19–24	125+
Doughnuts	I ave.	125+	6–12	8–100+	75+
Ice Cream:					
16% fat	I cup	349	23.8	84	108
10% fat	I cup	257	14.1	53	116
sandwich	I	238	8.5	34	100+
Eskimo Pie	I	270	19.1	35	100+
Ice milk	I cup	222	4.6	13	163
Frozen yogurt	I cup	244	3.0	10	121
Tofu dessert	I cup	130	10.8	0	95
Sherbet	I cup	268	4.0	7	92
Pies:					
Hostess Apple	3½ oz.	331	18.1	35	320
Hostess Cherry	3½ oz.	352	17.1	10	180
Sara Lee Bavarian Cream	3½ oz.	352	25.1	23	80
Morton Coconut Custard	3¼ oz.	290	15.0	60	150
Lemon meringue	3½ oz.	227	7.5	93	282
Morton Peach	3½ oz.	260	12.0	10	230
Morton Pumpkin	3½ oz.	210	8.0	40	270

FOOD	SERV. SIZE	CAL.	FAT (GRAMS)	CHOL. (MGS.)	SODIUM (MGS.)
Puddings:					
Canned tapioca	3½ oz.	129	3.1	53	185
Vanilla					
(whole-milk)	½ cup	175	4.1	16	251
Vanilla (skim-milk)	½ cup	147	0.3	3	258

DIPS:

FOOD	SERV. SIZE	CAL.	FAT	CHOL.	SODIUM
Kraft Premium					
(various types)	1 oz.	50	4.0	10–20	150+
Guacamole	2 tbsp.	50	4.0	0	210
Buttermilk	2 tbsp.	70	6.0	0	240
French onion	2 tbsp.	60	4.0	0	260
Green onion	2 tbsp.	60	4.0	0	170
Bacon-horseradish	2 tbsp.	60	5.0	0	200
Clam	2 tbsp.	60	5.0	0	250
Garlic	2 tbsp.	60	4.0	0	160

EGGS & SUBSTITUTES

FOOD	SERV. SIZE	CAL.	FAT	CHOL.	SODIUM
Whole egg	1 med.	78	5.5	250	59
Egg yolk	1 med.	59	5.2	250	12
Egg white	1 med.	16	trace	0	47
Eggnog	1 cup	352	19.0	149	138
Egg Beaters	¼ cup	25	0	0	80
Eggstra	¼ cup	30	0.8	23	56
Eggtime	¼ cup	40	1.0	0	120
Lucem	¼ cup	50	2.0	trace	NA
Second Nature	¼ cup	35	1.6	0	79
Scramblers	¼ cup	60	3.0	0	150

Table 11 (continued)

FOOD	SERV. SIZE	CAL.	FAT (GRAMS)	CHOL. (MGS.)	SODIUM (MGS.)
FAST FOODS					
McDonald's:					
Big Mac	1	541	31.4	75	963
Egg McMuffin	1	352	20.0	191	911
Fish fillet	1	402	22.7	43	707
French fries	1 serv.	211	10.6	14	112
Hamburger	1	257	9.4	26	525
Hamburger with cheese	1	306	13.3	41	724
Apple pie	1	295	18.3	14	408
Quarter Pounder	1	418	20.5	69	278
Quarter Pounder with cheese	1	518	28.6	95	1206
Vanilla shake	1	324	7.8	29	250
Kentucky Fried Chicken:					
Original recipe chicken	3½ oz.	290	17.8	133	535
Extra-crispy chicken	3½ oz.	323	20.8	116	446
Cole slaw	1 serv.	110	5.9	4	237
Mashed potatoes w/gravy	1 serv.	74	2.0	3	353
Dinner roll	1	52	1.1	trace	83
FATS & OILS					
Bacon fat	1 tbsp.	126	14.0	11	150+
Beef suet	1 tbsp.	216	23.3	21	18
Chicken fat	1 tbsp.	126	14.0	9	0
Lard	1 tbsp.	126	14.0	13	0

FOOD	SERV. SIZE	CAL.	FAT (GRAMS)	CHOL. (MGS.)	SODIUM (MGS.)
Vegetable oil	I tbsp.	120	13.5	0	0
Butter	I tbsp.	108	12.2	36	124
Margarine	I tbsp.	108	12.0	0	Var.
Butter Buds	I oz.	12	0	0	NA

FISH & SHELLFISH

FOOD	SERV. SIZE	CAL.	FAT	CHOL.	SODIUM
Caviar (sturgeon)	I tsp.	26	1.5	25	220
Clams (canned)	½ cup	52	0.7	80	36
Clams (raw)	3½ oz.	82	1.9	50	36
Cod (raw)	3½ oz.	78	0.3	50	70
Crab (king)	3½ oz.	93	1.9	60	Var.
Fish sticks (frozen)	3½ oz.	176	8.9	70	180
Flatfish	3½ oz.	79	0.8	61	78
Haddock	3½ oz.	141	6.6	60	71
Halibut	3½ oz.	214	8.8	60	168
Herring	3½ oz.	176	11.3	85	74
Lobster	3½ oz.	91	1.9	100	210
Mackerel	3½ oz.	191	12.2	95	148
Oysters	3½ oz.	66	1.8	50	73
Salmon	3½ oz.	182	7.4	47	50
Salmon (canned chinook)	3½ oz.	210	14.0	60	300+
Sardines (canned in oil)	3½ oz.	311	24.4	120	510
Scallops	3½ oz.	81	0.2	35	255
Shrimp	3½ oz.	91	0.8	100	140
Trout (brook)	3½ oz.	101	2.1	55	50
Trout (rainbow)	3½ oz.	195	11.4	55	50
Tuna (raw)	3½ oz.	133	3.0	60	37

Table 11 (continued)

FOOD	SERV. SIZE	CAL.	FAT (GRAMS)	CHOL. (MGS.)	SODIUM (MGS.)
Tuna (canned in oil)	3½ oz.	197	8.2	63	800+
Tuna (canned in water)	3½ oz.	127	0.8	63	41

GRAIN PRODUCTS
Breads:

FOOD	SERV. SIZE	CAL.	FAT (GRAMS)	CHOL. (MGS.)	SODIUM (MGS.)
Cracked-wheat	1 slice	66	0.6	0	132
English muffin	1 slice	133	1.0	0	203
French	1 slice	75	0.5	0	140
Pita (pocket)	1 slice	145	1.0	0	86
Pumpernickel	1 slice	79	0.4	0	182
Raisin	1 slice	66	0.7	0	91
Rye	1 slice	61	0.3	0	139
White	1 slice	68	0.8	0	127
Whole-wheat	1 slice	61	0.8	0	132
Crackers:					
Matzo 1	118	0.3	0	10	
Melba toast	3	60	2.0	0.6	2
Saltines	4	48	1.3	1.0	123
Egg noodles	1 cup	200	2.4	50	3
Pancake mix	1 ave.	367	5.0	33	1192
Stuffing mix	½ cup	198	8.0	45	515

MEATS
Beef: Cooked, well-trimmed

FOOD	SERV. SIZE	CAL.	FAT (GRAMS)	CHOL. (MGS.)	SODIUM (MGS.)
Composite	3 oz.	192	9.4	73	57
Eye round steak	3 oz.	158	6.0	59	52
Top round steak	3 oz.	166	5.9	72	52

FOOD	SERV. SIZE	CAL.	FAT (GRAMS)	CHOL. (MGS.)	SODIUM (MGS.)
Tip roast	3 oz.	167	7.0	69	55
Bottom round	3 oz.	201	9.3	81	44
Sirloin steak	3 oz.	185	8.3	75	56
Top sirloin	3 oz.	182	8.7	65	57
Rib steak	3 oz.	200	10.9	68	58
Rib roast	3 oz.	217	12.9	68	62
Blade pot roast	3 oz.	241	14.3	90	60
Arm pot roast	3 oz.	205	9.3	85	56
Brisket	3 oz.	230	14.3	77	66
Tenderloin	3 oz.	183	8.9	72	54
Ground beef (27% fat)	3 oz.	251	16.9	86	71
Ground beef (18% fat)	3 oz.	233	14.4	86	69
Lamb Composite cooked, trimmed	3 oz.	176	8.1	78	71
Lamb shank	3 oz.	156	6.0	81	54
Lamb loin chop	3 oz.	188	8.9	82	71
Lamb blade chop	3 oz.	195	10.9	82	80
Lamb rib roast	3 oz.	211	12.9	78	67
Pork Composite, cooked, trimmed	3 oz.	198	11.1	79	50
Leg roast	3 oz.	187	9.4	80	55
Top loin chop	3 oz.	219	12.7	80	57
Top loin roast	3 oz.	208	11.7	67	39
Shoulder blade	3 oz.	250	15.0	99	64
Spareribs	3 oz.	338	25.8	103	79
Center loin chop	3 oz.	196	8.9	83	66
Tenderloin	3 oz.	141	4.1	79	57
Sirloin roast	3 oz.	221	11.1	94	50

Table 11 (continued)

FOOD	SERV. SIZE	CAL.	FAT (GRAMS)	CHOL. (MGS.)	SODIUM (MGS.)
Center rib chop	3 oz.	219	12.7	80	57
Center rib roast	3 oz.	208	11.7	67	39
Bacon	1 slice	40	3.0	5	120
Ham (3% fat)	3 oz.	120	6.0	45	240
Chicken:					
Light, no skin	3 oz.	153	4.2	66	54
Dark, no skin	3 oz.	156	5.4	78	72
Dark & white,					
with skin	3 oz.	210	12.6	75	66
Chicken gizzard	1 cup	215	4.8	283	83
Chicken liver	1 cup	200	5.0	800	68
Turkey:					
Light, no skin	3 oz.	153	4.2	66	54
Dark, no skin	3 oz.	156	5.4	78	72
Light & dark,					
with skin	3 oz.	210	12.6	75	66
Bologna, franks	1 oz.	71	5.4	37	336
Ham	1 oz.	40	1.5	28	280
Pastrami	1 oz.	34	1.6	29	525
Salami	1 oz.	50	3.5	26	454
Veal:					
Lean only					
(leg, loin, cutlet)	3 oz.	120	2.7	84	48
Lean & fat					
(most cuts)	3 oz.	183	9.0	84	39
Lean & fat					
(rib, breast)	3 oz.	267	23.1	87	42
Duck:					
Flesh only	3 oz.	141	6.9	62	63
Flesh & skin	3 oz.	276	24.3	60	63

FOOD	SERV. SIZE	CAL.	FAT (GRAMS)	CHOL. (MGS.)	SODIUM (MGS.)
Goose:					
Flesh only	3 oz.	135	6.0	63	72
Organ meats:					
Beef kidney	3½ oz.	252	12.0	375	253
Beef liver	3½ oz.	140	4.7	300	73
Chicken liver	3½ oz.	165	4.4	746	61
Beef tongue	3½ oz.	244	16.7	140	61
Beef heart	3½ oz.	179	5.7	274	104
Brains	3½ oz.	106	7.3	2100	106
Sweetbreads	3½ oz.	90	6.6	132	99
Luncheon meats:					
(Oscar Mayer)					
Bologna	1 oz.	88	8.1	15+	292
Canadian bacon	1 oz.	45	2.0	13	384
Chopped ham	1 oz.	64	4.8	14	387
Ham & cheese					
loaf	1 oz.	70	5.6		372
Headcheese	1 oz.	55	4.1	28	
Honey loaf	1 oz.	39	1.7	8	377
Liverwurst	1 oz.	139	9.1	35	81
Olive loaf	1 oz.	64	4.5	10	416
Salami (dry)	1 oz.	112	9.8	22	540
Spam (Hormel)	1 oz.	87	7.4	15	336
Hot dog	1.6 oz.	142	13.5	23	464
Ham	3½ oz.	120	5.0	50	1527

Table 11 (continued)

FOOD	SERV. SIZE	CAL.	FAT (GRAMS)	CHOL. (MGS.)	SODIUM (MGS.)
SALAD DRESSINGS					
Blue cheese	1 tbsp.	71	7.3	4–10	153
Green goddess	1 tbsp.	68	7.0	1	150
Russian	1 tbsp.	74	7.6	7–10	130
Thousand Island	1 tbsp.	70	7.0	9	98
French	1 tbsp.	66	6.2	0	219
Italian	1 tbsp.	83	9.0	0	314

5

Getting the Scoop on Oat Bran

Other than a few hermits living in caves up in the hills, I don't imagine there's a single American man, woman, or child who hasn't heard about the benefits of fiber in the diet. Everywhere you turn, someone's telling you to increase your fiber intake.

In case you haven't paid really close attention, the whole thing began in 1972 when Dr. Dennis Burkitt, who had been studying primitive tribes in Africa, wrote a landmark paper published in the British journal *The Lancet*.[1] He observed that when the diet contains a lot of roughage, stools are softer and larger, and bowel movements are far more frequent. His conclusion, comparing the health of Africans with that of Westerners, was that dietary fiber has a role in the prevention of certain large-intestine diseases, including cancer of the colon and diverticulitis. He also noted that "the serum-cholesterol rises when fibre is removed from the diet. Eating a fibre-rich diet or adding cellulose to the diet lowers the serum-cholesterol."

That began a series of scientific discussions and research studies that have continued to this day. Dr. David Kritchevsky, working at the Wistar Institute in Philadelphia, found that alfalfa did a good job of keeping cholesterol levels down in rabbits. Of course, humans couldn't eat alfalfa, but the work went on.

The story of fiber became a favorite with the media. There were high-fiber recipes in magazines and newspapers and pep talks on TV. Books were published on how to get more fiber into practically everything we eat. Quickly responding to the strong public demand, the food industry began actively marketing fiber in a wide variety of foods. Advertising pointed out the fiber benefits of breads and cereals, especially breakfast cereals.

But, while a rose is a rose is a rose, not all fiber is the same. It's not that any harm can be done by consuming one fiber rather than another. Rather, different fibers accomplish different health benefits. For example, wheat fiber is excellent for speeding up the "transit time" it takes for food to move through the digestive tract.[2] Such fiber is the ultimate natural laxative. In fact, a number of different kinds of fiber from a wide variety of food sources will achieve that same goal.

Unfortunately, however, the same does not hold true for the ability of all fiber to lower cholesterol levels. Research findings have been building over the past few years until now we have conclusive evidence that oat bran is the fiber of choice for those who want to keep their cholesterol levels out of the risk zone. It's a fascinating story that's worth telling.

Most of us are familiar with oatmeal, or rolled oats, from that familiar cylindrical container with the smiling Quaker face that today seems so wholesome. That oatmeal is made by treating the whole grain with steam and then passing the grains between rolls to produce flakes. Grinding the oat flakes and sifting results in two milling fractions. There's a fine fraction, flour, and a coarse fraction known as oat bran. For a long time oat bran was available only in health-food stores, but because of greater demand you can now find it in most supermarkets as well.

The difference between oat bran and wheat bran is that oat bran contains a large portion of soluble fiber whereas wheat has mainly insoluble fiber. It's the soluble fiber that is capable of lowering cholesterol levels.[3]

Table 13 on pages 176–77 lists the fiber content of various foods. Not that wheat bran has the most total plant fiber, but most of it is insoluble. Oat bran, on the other hand, has more soluble fiber than any other food.

But fiber is only part of oat bran's appeal nutritionally. A look at the nutrition information on the side of the oat-bran box shows that a one-ounce serving has a substantial amount of protein, energy-providing carbohydrate, and the B-vitamin thiamin. Some manufacturers, competing in a kind of "nutrient war," have fortified their cereals with vitamins and minerals, claiming the result is a better product than naturally nutritious cereals. That's nonsense. Rely on a balanced diet for all the nutrients you'll need.

Before describing in detail what oat bran does and the research studies that back up its claims, here's an overview of just what can be expected by making oat bran a part of the daily diet. Oat bran significantly lowers both total cholesterol and LDL cholesterol while not at all lowering the protective HDL levels. As a side benefit, oat bran helps maintain a normal glucose level in the blood of diabetic patients.

Investigations regarding oat bran have been conducted all over the world. Both animal and human studies have consistently demonstrated the significant effect oat bran has on cholesterol levels in the blood. As is true with almost all breakthroughs in human nutrition and medicine, the first discoveries about the benefits of oat bran took place in laboratories where researchers studied animals. The first observation, made in the Netherlands in 1963, showed that rolled oats significantly lowered the cholesterol levels of rat.[4] Seeing these results in his rat study, Dr. A. P. DeGroot and his associates in Utrecht then worked with human volunteers, who ate an oatmeal bread instead of their regular bread for three weeks. Cholesterol levels fell from an average of 251 to 239 in just three days, and then down to 223 at the end of the three weeks. When regular bread replaced the oatmeal bread, cholesterol levels rose back to original levels.

Then in 1967 scientists at Rutgers University in New Jersey determined that it was the fiber in oatmeal that was the effective portion.[5] The Quaker Oats Company, understandably interested in these findings, began doing its own studies and found that the specific element that lowered cholesterol was the gum fraction of oat bran. Over the years, numerous investigations on a wide variety of animals confirmed the initial discovery: that oat bran has a strong hypocholesterolemic effect—it lowers cholesterol. One of the most active researchers during the early animal studies was Dr. James Anderson at the Department of Medicine at the University of Kentucky in Lexington. His work and that of his colleagues really laid the foundation for human investigations to follow.

Interestingly, Dr. Anderson first looked at

oat bran as a food for controlling glucose levels in diabetic patients. He found that those patients also benefited in terms of reduced cholesterol levels.

To look more closely at just how oat bran works, Dr. Anderson has done a number of metabolic studies with men who have high cholesterol levels. These are very tightly controlled investigations in which all individuals are fed exactly the same diet, the composition of which is known ounce-for-ounce and gram-for-gram each and every day.

One such study involved eight men given 100 grams of oat bran daily.[6] That's the equivalent of about one cup of cereal as it comes out of the box. They ate the bran in the form of muffins. Total cholesterol levels fell by 13 percent and LDL levels went down by 14 percent. More recently, Dr. Dennis Davidson at the University of California at Irvine gave first-year medical students either oat-bran or wheat muffins. Only the oat-bran muffins lowered cholesterol levels. The study was published in the *Western Journal of Medicine* in 1988.

In another controlled study, six men were admitted to the metabolic ward and fed control diets for seven days, then switched to diets supplemented with 100 grams of oat bran for twenty-one days.[7] Serum cholesterol levels were stable on the control diets and averaged 280 mg/dl. That put the men at significant risk of developing heart disease. With oat-bran supplements, average serum cholesterol dropped to 77.8 percent of the control values during the second week and were stable until the men went home after three weeks. At home, they ate a high-fiber diet containing 50 grams of oat bran daily, and were able to maintain a 23.5 percent decrease from their original cholesterol levels. These results are comparable to those obtained using drugs such as colestipol or cholestyramine.

Using other experimental conditions, Dr. Anderson showed that oat-bran feeding reduced serum LDL cholesterol concentrations by 36 percent while increasing HDL by 82 percent.[8] He notes that feeding other water-soluble fiber forms such as pectin or guar will lower serum cholesterol concentrations.

Most recently, Dr. Anderson showed that oat-bran diets decreased total serum cholesterol concentrations by 19 percent and LDL cholesterol by 23 percent.[9] Interestingly, even after the men went home, continuing to eat oat bran daily, their cholesterol levels fell even further, down a total of 24 percent. This indicates that the longer one stays on a diet including oat bran, the greater the effects. The men ate 50 grams of oat bran daily, the equivalent of three muffins.

The total diet fed the men in this recent study is also striking in that it is typical of the average American diet. Twenty percent of calories came in the form of protein, 43 percent as carbohydrates, 37 percent as fat, with approximately 430 milligrams of cholesterol each day. That diet, in other words, is not restricted at all. Note that the American Heart Association recommends keeping the cholesterol intake down to 300 milligrams daily for the entire population. For those with elevated cholesterol levels the AHA advises cutting down to as low as 150 milligrams daily. Bear in mind that one egg yolk contains about 250 milligrams of cholesterol. Even a very lean three-ounce serving of beef contains about 70 milligrams. Think of what the results might have been if Dr. Anderson had combined his oat-bran regimen with a more modified diet!

What do these findings and statistics mean to the average person? Simply stated, even without restricting the diet radically, one can expect considerable lowering of cholesterol by simply eating three oat-bran muffins a day. Assuming the same results Dr. Anderson found, some simple arithmetic shows that a person with a 265 mg/dl cholesterol level can anticipate dropping that number down to near the

200 mg level. Most authorities agree that keeping total serum cholesterol counts down under 200 greatly protects against heart disease. That encouragement makes those muffins taste even more delicious!

Can the same results be achieved with oatmeal? Since oat bran is one fraction of the oat flake, it would take more oatmeal than oat bran to achieve the same levels of lowering. There's no question, however, that oatmeal also exerts a cholesterol-lowering effect.

At Northwestern University in Chicago, Dr. Linda Van Horn studied the effects of oatmeal and oat bran as part of a low-fat diet versus a low-fat diet alone. She found that both oat bran and oatmeal provided an additional 3 percent reduction over the cholesterol lowering achieved by a low-fat diet alone. That low percentage of cholesterol reduction was due to the fact that the subjects in the study had normal cholesterol levels to begin with. People with elevated cholesterol counts can expect a greater percentage of improvement. And, at those higher cholesterol counts, it's generally recognized that oat bran will achieve better results than oatmeal.

How Does Oat Bran Work?

No one knows for certain how oat bran works. Most papers written on the subject point to the fact that, when oat bran is included in the diet, the excretion of bile acids increases.[7,8,9] What does that mean? Bile acids are formed by the liver from cholesterol. The more bile acids are excreted, the more the liver has to make. The more acids are made, the more cholesterol is drawn out of the blood, and eventually out of other parts of the body. Thus there is less chance of cholesterol being deposited in the arteries. This could very well be the reason oat bran reduces levels of cholesterol.

The general consensus in the medical community is that oat bran exerts its cholesterol-lowering effect by way of its soluble fiber. The specific kind of soluble fiber in oat bran is called beta-glucan. Researchers at the University of Wisconsin have found, for example, that when laboratory rats were given either oat bran or a special cereal with an even higher concentration of soluble fiber, cholesterol levels fell by an even greater degree for those animals getting the special cereal.[10] The researchers conclude that soluble fiber is the component of oat fiber probably responsible for the cholesterol-lowering effect. However, additional research is now under way to determine if the fat content of oats and other cereals such as barley may have a role also. Moreover, it appears that not all soluble fiber is created equal. The specific kinds found in oat bran and in dried beans and peas are chemically different from those in other foods, and those other foods may not have the same cholesterol-lowering capabilities, regardless of their soluble-fiber content.

A comparison of oat bran with drugs such as colestipol and cholestyramine is interesting and informative. Both of these drugs are resins which cling to bile acids in the intestine, causing them to be excreted and thus lowering the cholesterol level. This is not to suggest that oat bran is a drug but rather that the drugs seem to mimic the activity of this natural cereal food.

Does oat bran *really* work? One study said that it did not, and unfortunately that work got an enormous amount of publicity back in January of 1990. Harvard researchers compared oat bran and Cream of Wheat, a virtually fiber-free cereal, given to 20 women with perfectly normal cholesterol levels to begin with. In fact, they averaged a mere 172. So no one should have been surprised when the oat bran did not reduce cholesterol further. The study was like testing the efficacy of aspirin or Tylenol on those who didn't have a headache.

But because oat bran had become so popular, the seriously flawed study got lots of publicity. Many studies since that time have again and again demonstrated the effectiveness of soluble fiber in general and oat bran in particular.

While skeptical at first, the medical community has come to see the value of oat bran as part of a total cholesterol-reducing program. Dr. Bruce Kinosian at the University of Maryland's department of medicine compared the cost-effectiveness of oat bran versus the cholesterol-lowering prescription drugs colestipol and cholestyramine in treating patients with significantly elevated cholesterol levels. He found that, in terms of years of life saved by way of cholesterol reduction and thus lessened heart-disease mortality, oat bran was more cost-effective. He concluded in his report[11] in the *Journal of the American Medical Association* in 1988 that cholesterol reduction by way of diet and oat bran "may be preferred to a medically oriented campaign that focuses on drug therapy."

ADDITIONAL BENEFITS OF OAT BRAN

It shouldn't come as any surprise that oat bran has a number of benefits beyond the lowering of cholesterol levels. High-fiber diets such as those including oat bran actually lower insulin requirements for diabetic patients and help control blood sugar. Dr. Anderson's research has documented that high-fiber, high-carbohydrate diets brought insulin requirements down by 25 to 50 percent,[12] and also greatly helped those diabetic patients who previously required drugs other than insulin to control their disease. Using the high-fiber, high-carbohydrate diet, Dr. Anderson was able to discontinue drug therapy for 90 percent of non-insulin-dependent diabetic patients.

This same approach to the diet, with high intake of fiber such as oat bran, has been demonstrated to lower blood pressure by about 10 percent.[13] Additional studies are under way to further investigate this advantage.

There is a very special added benefit that may come as a pleasant surprise: eating a diet rich in oat-bran fiber virtually assures weight control. Some of the reasons for this are relatively obvious. First, eating a high-fiber apple is more satisfying than gulping a glass of apple juice. The simple act of chewing is more enjoyable than swallowing. Second, the fiber replaces other high-fat and high-calorie foods, resulting in a reduction of calories.

Most significantly, when one eats a lot of

oat bran, say three muffins a day, one just doesn't get hungry. This is more than a matter of simply filling the stomach and saying, "I'm full." Personally, after having my three muffins and a fruit-milk shake in the morning, I never even think about food until well past noon.

Oat bran keeps you satisfied. Compare this with the familiar story of being hungry an hour after eating a Chinese meal. There's a scientific reason for this. Chinese food typically is low in fat, especially true for Cantonese specialties. The vegetables and rice don't provide long-term satisfaction, so people get hungry faster than after a hamburger or steak dinner.

In addition to the fat content of food, satisfaction depends very largely on how quickly the food moves through the digestive tract. As it happens, oat bran slows down the rate of the so-called "gastric emptying," the time it takes to move out of the stomach. This adds to the feeling of fullness. Additionally, high-fiber foods provide more food mass in the small intestine and alter intestinal hormone secretion.

Certain nutrients such as carbohydrates are absorbed more slowly after high-fiber meals than after meals of low-fiber, refined foods. This slow absorption of nutrients for hours after fiber-rich meals contributes to that satisfied feeling.

Dr. Anderson reports three reasons as to why oat bran may help in weight reduction.[14] First, there is a certain amount of loss of calories directly through the feces. Second, carbohydrates are not fully metabolized. And third, fiber-rich foods such as oat bran require more energy to digest, thus actually increasing the rate at which calories are burned. Obviously, for those individuals who have a few pounds to lose, this is a tremendous benefit. For me personally, the diet plan including oat bran has meant that I can eat virtually as much food as I want. In fact, if there are a couple of days in a row when I don't make a point of eating as much as usual, I'll lose a pound or two. I actually have to eat more food, far more food, than I used to in order to maintain my weight.

Virtually every nutrition and medical authority has stated unequivocally that Americans should increase their fiber intake. The U.S. Department of Agriculture and the U.S. Department of Health, Education and Welfare jointly published the official "Dietary Guidelines for Americans" in 1980.[15] The advice given has been very well publicized in the media. In essence the guidelines call for eating a wide variety of foods, avoiding too much fat, saturated fat, and cholesterol, eating foods with adequate starch and fiber, and avoiding too much sugar and sodium. In 1988 Surgeon

General C. Everett Koop, M.D., issued his report on nutrition and health, in which he echoed the advice in an even stronger voice that the American public must reduce its consumption of fats, especially saturated fats, and cholesterol in order to decrease the incidence of coronary heart disease.[15]

To achieve those goals the authorities recommend eating more complex carbohydrates in place of simple starches and sugars. This can be done by selecting foods high in fiber such as whole-grain breads and cereals and fruits and vegetables. A logical choice would be oat-bran cereal, since in addition to the benefits usually associated with fiber there are a number of other highly significant health advantages, as we've seen.

Are there any reasons not to eat oat bran? Only one caution was ever expressed about eating a lot of fiber such as oat bran. Some authorities worried whether certain nutrients might be lost because of the effect on the intestine. I'm happy to report, however, that research has shown no such ill effects from oat bran and other high-fiber diets.[11] In one recent study fifteen patients were given a high-fiber diet for nearly two years. Their levels of nutrients, including calcium, phosphorus, iron, magnesium, vitamin B_{12}, folic acid, and vitamins A, D, and K, were studied and found to be absolutely unaffected. Follow-up studies showed similar results after more than four years.

The conclusion is simple: there are lots of good reasons to start eating oat bran and other fiber-rich foods, and no good reasons not to. If an apple a day keeps the doctor away, a few oat-bran muffins appear to do the same for cardiologists!

Will you notice any difference after you start eating oat bran regularly? Unless you're already eating quite a bit of fiber in your diet, oat bran will greatly improve your regularity. Constipation will never be a problem. In fact, you may even expect more than one bowel movement daily. Dr. Burkitt's original observations in Africa indicated that frequent bowel movements are, in fact, beneficial, and doctors no longer tell patients that it's perfectly normal not to move one's bowels daily.

While you're eating oat bran, the stools will be larger and softer. Not runny or unpleasant, but much softer and more easily passed. As might be expected, however, with the increased bowel activity comes a certain amount of flatulence. Rest assured, this does lessen over time, and it's perfectly normal. If gas presents a particularly difficult situation for you, try increasing the amount of oat bran you eat gradually over a longer period of time.

There's one recent development about soluble fiber certainly worth noting. In 1988 two studies, one at Texas A&M University and the other at UCLA, showed that soluble fiber might be a contributing factor in the development of colon cancer in rats. Let me assure you that this isn't anything to be concerned about, but it's worth explaining.

In these studies, rats were fed various diets containing different kinds of fibers and including a substance known to cause cancer of the colon called dimethyl hydrazine. In the presence of that chemical, cells in the colon begin to proliferate, which is the first step toward cancerous growth. While insoluble fibers protected against this proliferation, soluble fibers stimulated the cell growth. That's probably because soluble fibers slow down the passage of food through the digestive tract, while insoluble fibers speed up that passage.

Should humans be concerned? First, bear in mind that these were single-fiber diets. In other words, only one kind of fiber was given to the rats rather than a balance of fibers as one would expect in a typical diet. Second, there was the presence of the known carcinogen.

I spoke with Dr. Joanne Lupton at Texas A&M about her study. She still feels that those with high cholesterol levels would be well advised to seek soluble-fiber-rich foods such as oat bran, especially if there is a family history of heart disease. She also agreed that the soluble fiber in the oat bran should be balanced in the diet by other foods containing insoluble fiber. So, while rats consuming a single fiber in a diet also containing a known cancer causer should be concerned, humans seeking to lower their cholesterol levels by consuming reasonable quantities of oat bran as discussed in this book have nothing to worry about.

TAKING THAT FIRST BITE

Oat bran is now available in just about every supermarket and health-food store nationally. For the most part it comes packaged in one-pound boxes, and can be found in the hot-cereal sections of the store. While Quaker was the first to put oat bran on the market, a number of other companies have followed suit in the past few years. The package should list just one ingredient: oat bran. The amount that I advocate consuming daily is one-half cup, uncooked, as it comes out of the box. That's less than 2 ounces, or about 50 grams.

When the 1987 edition of this book first

popularized oat bran, a number of companies jumped on the bandwagon, trying to capitalize on the huge consumer demand. Unfortunately there wasn't enough oat bran to go around, and some unscrupulous manufacturers resorted to selling inferior products. Since there is no standard of identity for oat bran, one never knew what one was buying. In some cases the "oat bran" was likely to be ground-up oatmeal, which certainly wouldn't do any harm, but also wouldn't give the buyer the amount of soluble fiber he or she paid for. Although oat-bran supplies have now been expanded, you're still better off with the name brands. Take a look at the oat-bran and soluble-fiber contents of both hot and ready-to-eat cereals in Tables 12 and Table 13 on pages 174–77.

But cereal is just the beginning. On the side of the package you'll find a recipe for basic oat-bran muffins. Because the recipe calls for quite a bit of sugar and eggs, I began developing alternative recipes.

I found that, while oat bran is very different from other flours and cooking ingredients I had used before, it's really quite easy to work with. Since I'm not particularly fond of hot cereal, muffins seemed the logical way to go.

Personally I find myself on a tight schedule almost every day. I just don't have time to sit down and eat a nice little breakfast or brunch while reading the newspaper. Almost always it's a matter of eating on the run, often gulping my food right over the sink to save clean-up time. For me, and I think for millions of other busy men and women, muffins are the perfect fast food. That's not to say that such a fast-paced life is best. Sure, I prefer a relaxed breakfast with time to read the morning newspaper. But a somewhat rushed breakfast is far better than none at all. Frequently, also, I'll take the muffins with me in the car along with a commuter mug of decaffeinated coffee. You can't do that with bacon and eggs!

The beauty of muffins is that it's practically impossible to get tired of them. One day it's apple-cinnamon, the next day banana-date, the next day pineapple, with a shake to match. To make them even more delicious, I pop my muffins into the microwave oven for just 30 seconds to warm them. This is particularly useful since I store the muffins in the refrigerator to keep them from spoiling.

You can't eat too much oat bran when it's baked in muffins, breads, rolls, cakes, cookies, and other foods naturally suited to it. Try the recipes I've supplied in Chapter 18. Then think of your own favorites. Whenever a recipe calls for breadcrumbs or coatings, try oat bran instead.

If you happen to be a baker, or are lucky enough to live with one or have one as a good friend, oat bran offers a whole world of delicious possibilities. When I first began restricting my diet to things that were "good for me," I did rather miss the goodies. But as time has gone on, I've found so many alternatives that I don't feel a bit deprived. I eat cakes, brownies, coffee cakes, cookies, and all sorts of other treats. To make it all even better, I don't even have to worry about the calories. For once, the things you *should* eat taste as good as the things you *want* to eat.

To get started, buy a box of oat-bran cereal. This will be enough to make two dozen muffins. Sometime over the weekend, when you have about fifteen minutes, mix up a batch or two. Start out, perhaps, with twelve basic muffins and twelve apple-cinnamon. Figuring three muffins daily, that'll be more than enough to last for a full week. Even if you never baked a thing in your life, muffin making is simple and foolproof. Here's what you'll need to start:

- 12-cup metal muffin baking pan
- Paper muffin cup liners
- Measuring spoons
- Measuring cup
- Mixing bowls

In addition, take a look at the recipes to see what ingredients you'll need to start making the ones that sound best to you. Probably you already have most or all the ingredients you need already. And you'll find that practically any fresh, dried, frozen, or canned fruit makes a delicious variety of muffins.

If you have a blender, that's all the better for mixing the liquid ingredients. And it's lots faster to mash bananas, for example, in the blender than by hand. This is a small investment if you don't already have one.

The other thing that I would very highly recommend is an oven thermometer; you just can't trust the dial on your oven to set the temperature. Again, this is a very small investment, and one that you'll wonder how you ever got along without. Foods—all foods— come out a lot better when you follow the recipes to the letter, especially when it comes to cooking times and temperatures.

Oat bran is as effective eaten raw as it is cooked or baked. But you may experience some gastric upset, including a bloated feeling, from eating it raw. It is easier on the digestive tract when cooked. This is especially true for those not used to a high-fiber diet. On the other hand, some people have no problem at all with uncooked oat bran. Try it for yourself to see if you can tolerate it. Add some to a nonfat milkshake, or sprinkle it on other foods.

Since it was this book, in part, that spurred the healthful consumer interest in oat bran as an excellent way to control cholesterol levels, I'll have to take some of the responsibility for some of the more ridiculous ways in which some manufacturers have taken advantage of the situation. We now see oat bran touted in a wide array of products, many of them no more than gimmicks. If one were to rely on the oat-bran tablets now being sold, one would have to chew 100 of the typically terrible-tasting things in order to get the 50 grams I recommend—assuming that the oat bran is of high quality. But the most laughable product I've seen thus far is oat-bran potato chips!

Fortunately, a number of very good oat-bran products have appeared as well. Health Valley provides a nice variety of products that will give you substantial amounts of oat bran.

One brand-new product I'm particularly pleased with is the Health Beat oat-bran bar. This makes a terrific substitute for the typically high-fat granola bars sold in health food stores and elsewhere. Each bar contains 11 grams of oat bran and only 1 gram of fat. The Health Beat company also markets a high-quality oat-bran cereal. Their products are sold primarily in stores of the Jewel/Osco/SavOn chain nationally. (Health Beat also provides highly reliable fingerprick cholesterol testing.)

Before you put any food into your shopping cart, first read the label. Often you'll see that oat bran is one of the last ingredients listed, meaning that there just isn't much of it in these products. That goes for some of the top name-brand cereals. If oat bran isn't the number-one ingredient listed on the label, don't rely on that food as a major source of your soluble fiber. Oat flour contains little or no soluble fiber; remember that the flour is the fraction left over after milling for oat bran. And "oat fiber" may actually mean not oat bran but rather the nondigestible fiber from the hull of the grain, containing no soluble fiber whatever.

All this doesn't mean that the product in question isn't healthful and nutritious. It very well may be. But you have to know that it doesn't provide the amount of oat bran the maker would like you to think it has.

Be especially wary with regard to ready-to-eat oat-bran cereals. Cracklin' Oat Bran by Kellogg, for example, is heavy on fat and contains very little oat bran. Health Valley's oat Bran Flakes lists rolled oats first, indicating the largest quantity by weight; oat bran is next, with fruit juices, brown rice, rye flour, corn flour, and malted barley making up the rest.

That's a very nutritious product, but you'd have to eat twice as much of this cereal to get the amount of oat bran found in the pure cereal. New Morning Oatios have even less oat bran. The same is true for Cheerios; it's a nutritious cereal, but it's no replacement for pure oat bran. For the most part, the best source of oat bran is oat bran, although if you like to eat the other cereals for variety, by all means do so.

There's one stellar exception when it comes to ready-to-eat cereals. Remember that study at the University of Wisconsin in which researchers fed a special oat-bran cereal to rats? In that study the investigators found that the special cereal, fortified with an oat-bran concentrate and thus higher in soluble fiber than regular oat bran, provided even greater cholesterol-lowering effects.[10] That cereal is now available as Quaker Oat Bran High Fiber Cereal. Each one-ounce serving supplies 19 grams of oat bran, but a two-ounce serving or even more is more appropriate as a meal. It delivers 40 percent of its oat bran as soluble fiber, for a total of 7.6 grams per one-ounce serving. That's much higher than even the highest-quality pure oat bran. The best news about this new cereal is that it tastes wonderful. My family enjoys it regularly. A two-ounce bowl in the morning and an oat-bran muffin later on more than supply all the soluble fiber I need for the day. (Call 800-234-6281 for information.)

Table 13 on pages 176–77 shows the results of some research that was done to determine the amount of water-soluble fiber in a few foods. The numbers refer to the grams of fiber per 100-gram portion (3½ ounces). Following the recommendations in this book, you'll be eating two ounces (one-half cup) of uncooked oat bran cereal daily, which gives you almost four grams of water-soluble fiber. You can use that number when examining any other product on the market. Ask the salesperson or write the manufacturer to determine exactly how much water-soluble fiber the product contains, and therefore the amount of the product you'd have to eat.

Is it best to eat all the oat bran at once, say at breakfast, or would you be better off with some cereal and other soluble fiber-rich foods throughout the day? Remember that oat bran works in much the same way as the prescription cholesterol-lowering drugs colestipol and cholestyramine. Those are always prescribed in divided doses, to be taken two, three, or four times daily, depending on need. Both the soluble fiber of oat bran and the drugs work in the digestive tract by binding the bile acids, which are made from cholesterol. Those bile acids are made throughout the day. Thus by eating the oat-bran cereal, muffins, and other foods throughout the day, one has a better chance of cholesterol reduction.

Of course, the oat-bran cereal and muffins taste a lot better than the drugs, and for that reason as well as the significant cost differential, you'll be far more likely to stick with the oat-bran program. In another important way, oat bran can be more effective than drugs. That's because the oat bran becomes a food choice, replacing potential choices such as bacon and eggs. If you take drugs, you still have to decide what you're going to eat. With oat bran, it's a delicious, routine choice that benefits your overall health.

What about taking oat bran on the road when you travel? oat-bran muffins will last unrefrigerated in a hotel room for up to five days. To extend that life, you can place the bag of muffins on top of the air conditioning unit or fill a waste can with ice to form your own cooler. Or ask the hotel restaurant to place them in their refrigerator and take out a few each day or every other day.

You may wish to enjoy some oat-bran cereal on your trip. Place in individual plastic sandwich bags one-half cup of oat bran, one-quarter cup of raisins or other dried fruits, and some brown sugar or other sweetener. Make up as many bags as you'll need for the trip. If your hotel room has a mini-coffeemaker, you can use it to make hot water. Pour the cereal and fixings into a bowl, mix with 1 ⅓ cups of hot water, and let the mixture set for two minutes. Or take the bag with you into the restaurant, and order some hot water along with your coffee, juice, and fresh fruit. I travel extensively, and this has never been a problem for me.

When you get the results showing how much your own cholesterol level has fallen with this program, you won't mind going out of your way just a bit to stay on the program and eat some of that oat bran every day.

I was very pleased to learn from Dr. James Anderson, the man all are indebted to for discovering the benefits of oat bran, that the National Institutes of Health have given him a million-dollar research grant to compare the cholesterol-lowering potential of a diet with oat bran against the standard recommendations of the American Heart Association. I'd put my bet down that oat bran will come out the undisputed leader!

Bon appétit! Good health!

Table 12. Actual Oat Bran in Oat-Bran Products

BRAND	SERVING SIZE	OAT BRAN (GRAMS)
HOT CEREALS		
General Nutrition		
Stone Ground Oat Bran		
Hot Cereal	I ounce	28.0
Golden Temple Oat Bran	I ounce	28.0
Health Valley 100%		
Natural Hot Cereal	I ounce	20.0
Quaker Oat Bran	I ounce	28.0
Quaker Oatmeal	I ounce	9.0
READY-TO-EAT CEREALS		
Cheerios	I ounce	8.0
Common Sense		
Oat Bran	I ounce	13.0
Cracklin' Oat Bran	I ounce	9.0
Health Valley		
Oat Bran Flakes	I ounce	15.0
Oat Bran O's	I ounce	15.0
Kolln Oat Bran Krunch	I ounce	19.6
Oatios	I ounce	8.4

BRAND	SERVING SIZE	OAT BRAN (GRAMS)
Quaker Oat Bran High Fiber Oat Cereal*	1 ounce	19.0

BAKED GOODS

BRAND	SERVING SIZE	OAT BRAN (GRAMS)
Oatmeal Goodness Bread	1 slice	2.3
Health Valley Fancy Fruit Muffins	1 muffin	17.0
Oat Bran Jumbo Fruit Bars	1 bar	12.5
Oat Bran Graham Crackers	7 crackers	4.1
Oat Bran Fruit Jumbo Cookies	2 cookies	4.6
Health Beat Oat Bran Bar	1 bar	11.0

Contains a concentrated source of soluble fiber: soluble-fiber content greater than even pure oat bran.

Table 13. Fiber Content of Various Foods

FOOD	TOTAL DIETARY FIBER*	SOLUBLE FIBER*
GRAINS		
Barley, pearled	10.8	2.8
Cornmeal, whole grain	15.3	9.0
Oat bran, uncooked	18.6	7.2
Oatmeal, uncooked	12.1	4.9
Rice, brown, dry	7.2	0.7
Rice brain (Vita-Fiber brand Rice Germ & Rice Bran)	35.0	33.0
FRUITS		
Apple, raw	2.0	0.6
Apple fiber (Tastee Apple brand)	42.9	11.1
Prunes, dried	16.1	4.6
Raisins	6.8	1.7
DRIED BEANS & PEAS		
Beans, kidney, canned	6.2	2.7
Beans, kidney, raw	19.9	8.5
Beans, pinto, raw	18.7	7.0
Beans, white, raw	16.2	4.7
Lentils, raw	16.9	3.8
Peas, black-eyed, raw	25.0	11.0

Peas, chick, raw	15.0	7.6
Peas, split, raw	11.9	4.0

*Grams per 100 gram serving (3½ ounces). Taken from *Plant Fiber in Foods* by James W. Anderson, M.D., with permission from the Nutrition Research Foundation, Box 22124, Lexington, KY 40522.

6

The Amazing Story of Niacin

For many years I've been reading and writing about the needless and sometimes dangerous use of megadoses of vitamins. For the most part, a well-balanced diet appears to provide all the vitamins anyone needs. An "insurance policy" in the form of a multiple vitamin and mineral pill probably does lots more good than harm. This is especially true for the majority of people, whose diets are far from optimal in the first place, or for those who, because of their lifestyles, may require more than the Recommended Dietary Allowances set down by the National Academy of Sciences, National Research Council. But, when it comes to taking massive amounts of any one particular vitamin, there just doesn't seem to be any justification.

So, when I first heard about niacin and its effect on high cholesterol levels, I was, to say the least, skeptical. Then, coincidentally, I read an article by the Council on Scientific Affairs published in the *Journal of the American Medical Association*. This was an overview of what was generally accepted as effective dietary and drug therapy for heart-disease risk factors. Lo and behold, there it was in black and white: "Nicotinic acid in doses of three to twelve 500-mg tablets daily will also lower the plasma LDL level some 15% to 30%, and it is also effective in the reduction of VLDL levels. It also increases HDL levels."[1]

Amazing. Here was the medical community, the experts from the American Heart Association and the American Medical Association, actively advocating megadose vitamin therapy for a condition I was very personally interested in. This niacin or nicotinic-acid business deserved deeper investigation. So began my extensive search through medical literature, finding everything I could that had been written about the vitamin.

Niacin and nicotinic acid are interchangeable terms for the same water-soluble B vitamin. It was first discovered by a physician who found that diets deficient in some mysterious substance led to the condition known as pellagra. That was in 1917. It took another twenty years of research before niacin was identified, at the University of Wisconsin.

As with all vitamins, the amount recommended for the general population is based on the level needed to prevent a deficiency state. In the case of niacin, 20 milligrams daily will prevent pellagra, and this is the level set as the U.S. RDA for American men and women.

Even in multivitamin preparations in which other vitamins are doubled or tripled, niacin or its metabolic form, niacinamide, is kept to a minimum. Niacin is metabolized by the body to form niacinamide. It's the latter form that's useful in terms of the body's nutrient needs. But only the niacin, not the niacinamide, lowers cholesterol. *Niacinamide will have no effect in lowering cholesterol.* Perhaps this is due to the cholesterol-lowering action occurring at the time of metabolism from niacin to niacinamide in the liver.

The first discovery that niacin could reduce cholesterol levels was made in 1955 by Dr. R. Altschul and Dr. A. Hoffer. They gave patients three grams a day—hundreds of times the U.S. RDA—and the results were excellent.

But, for whatever reason, the scientific and medical communities didn't jump on the bandwagon. It wasn't until 1962 that two other researchers reported that niacin could not only reduce cholesterol levels, but also make triglyceride levels fall.[2]

Dozens of reports of research studies came to the same conclusions. Niacin very effectively lowers total cholesterol, LDL cholesterol, and triglycerides while actually elevating the protective HDL levels in the blood.[2] In fact, the results of the Coronary Drug Project in 1975 showed that niacin could be singled out as being responsible for a 29 percent reduction in nonfatal heart attacks. In 1980, a Swedish study revealed that risk factors for heart disease were significantly reduced in patients receiving niacin.

Just why this information hasn't been widely disseminated by the medical community to patients like me and millions of others who could profit by it, I don't know. For one thing, niacin does not have the profit margin of prescribed drugs. And, as we'll see, it has some unpleasant side effects that make taking it difficult in the beginning, but those side effects have been largely eliminated. But the facts are there, buried in dozens of rather obscure medical journals read by a handful of research scientists. I'm obviously delighted that I was able to discover the benefits of niacin for myself, and I'm equally pleased to share my findings with you.

How Does Niacin Work?

If you recall, cholesterol is manufactured by the liver. Happily, that's exactly where niacin exerts its unique action. Even the experts are uncertain as to the exact mechanisms, and probably more than one mode of action is involved. However, most authorities concur that niacin lowers VLDL (very-low-density lipoprotein) levels by decreasing the liver's production of it. And, since the worst offender, LDL (low-density lipoprotein), depends on VLDL for its production, the levels of LDL in the blood drop.[3]

This all makes sense when one realizes that the whole cholesterol problem probably comes down to a metabolic deficiency. That's why one person can gobble egg yolks and butter and keep his cholesterol level down while another has to watch every bite. An example of another metabolic deficiency would be diabetes, whereby the pancreas does not release enough insulin into the blood to break down sugars for the body's use. For years, researchers have been looking at the metabolic process of cholesterol manufacture by the liver to see if they could "short-circuit" the process. Niacin appears to do just that.

Niacin also appears to have a strong effect on the manufacture of the prostaglandins, minute amounts of hormone-like chemicals involved in practically every bodily function. In this case the prostaglandin in question is called PGI_2, and niacin stimulates the formation of PGI_2.

Why is that good? PGI_2 has been shown conclusively to be involved with platelet aggregation in the blood; without enough

PGI_2, the blood has more of a tendency to clot. And the larger the chance of clotting, the greater the risk of vascular occlusion. By increasing the body's PGI_2, niacin can inhibit the progression of the atherosclerotic processes.[2]

The next benefit of niacin is that it removes triglycerides from the blood through a process called "lipoprotein lipase activity."[3] Again, just how this happens is not clearly understood. But you will recall from Chapter 1 that when triglycerides are reduced in the blood, LDL levels are reduced as well.

And there's more. Those taking niacin at therapeutic levels have demonstrated increased HDL concentrations. By now you know that HDL has a strong protective influence, acting to draw cholesterol away from the lining of the arteries. This counters the effect of LDL, which draws cholesterol into the lining of the arteries, resulting in the atherosclerotic buildup of occluding plaque.

So there you have it. Niacin acts to lower LDL and VLDL production in the liver, to increase the amount of PGI_2, to decrease levels of triglycerides, and to increase the amount and proportions of the protective HDL in the blood.

RESEARCH RESULTS WITH NIACIN

The medical literature is filled with success stories in which cholesterol levels fall anywhere between 10 and 25 percent for those taking niacin alone or in combination with other approaches. Just taking niacin alone, without any changes in diet or lifestyle, is enough to produce a significant lowering of total cholesterol levels. And when taken along with a sensible, modified-fat diet niacin produces even more dramatic results.

Reporting from the University of Minnesota Medical School, Dr. Donald B. Hunninghake states that "Of all the lipid-lowering drugs, nicotinic acid probably produces the greatest elevations in high-density lipoprotein cholesterol levels, with many studies reporting rises of between 10 and 15 mg/dl. When given within the usual dosage range of 3 to 6 grams, most studies report between 20 and 30 percent reductions in low-density lipoprotein levels."[4]

In the book *Vitamins in Human Biology and Medicine*, Dr. Mark L. Wahlqvist writes that niacin achieves cholesterol-lowering results "at least comparable to those of the other principal lipid-lowering drugs clofibrate (Atromid-S), and the resin cholestyramine (Questran)."[3] He cites reduction of cholesterol concentration of 10 to 25 percent and, again, "consistent increase in high density lipoprotein."

Italian researchers reporting in the *American Journal of Cardiology* declare that "Treatment with large doses of nicotinic acid is generally associated with a marked reduction in both plasma cholesterol and triglyceride levels of about 15 to 20% and 45 to 50%, respectively."[5] Using a form of niacin, these doctors noted a 20 percent increase of the protective HDL levels.

But most of the reports deal with using niacin in combination with other drugs. Writing in the *New England Journal of Medicine*, Drs. John P. Kane and Mary J. Malloy give the results of long-term treatment of patients with high levels of cholesterol in their blood.[6] Their study was done in three phases. Phase I compared the effects of the drug colestipol and a placebo. Phase II looked at the effects of colestipol with another drug, clofibrate. Phase III investigated the use of colestipol with niacin. In all cases, patients followed a diet with no more than 200 milligrams of cholesterol per day and no more than 10 percent of calories as saturated fat. All patients had particularly high levels of cholesterol.

With colestipol alone, the average cholesterol levels decreased 16 to 25 percent. Addition of the drug clofibrate produced an average fall of only 28 percent. In bold comparison, serum cholesterol levels fell *45 percent* when colestipol was combined with niacin. Low-density lipoprotein cholesterol decreased 55 percent with colestipol and niacin and HDL increased.

More recently, medical researchers at the University of Southern California performed a controlled study with the combined therapy of niacin, colestipol, and a fat-controlled diet in men who had undergone coronary bypass.[7] Some men received the actual drugs while others got only a placebo. Both groups followed the modified diet.

The control group, those men with placebos but on a modified diet, showed no significant decrease in blood cholesterol levels. On the other hand, those receiving the colestipol and niacin demonstrated a 29 percent decrease in total cholesterol, a 41 percent decrease in triglycerides, and a 69 percent drop in LDL levels. The levels of HDL went up 33 percent. Much of this success can be ascribed to the niacin component.

Drs. Kane and Malloy also report an interesting phenomenon. "Some patients," they say, "maintained on the combined drug regimen (colestipol and niacin) have sustained decreases of LDL cholesterol levels whether they are consuming diets rich in cholesterol and saturated fats or the restricted diet."[8] However, they warn that other patients demonstrate an elevation in cholesterol levels when they go off the diet. They conclude that modified diet appears necessary for most individuals, and that colestipol and niacin, in their opinion, is the "most potent combined-drug regimen yet described."

We have already looked at how niacin achieves its cholesterol-lowering results. How about colestipol? This is a so-called "bile-acid binding resin." Colestipol and cholestyramine both act by binding the bile acids in the intestine. The drug is not absorbed by the body. Since cholesterol is necessary for the body to produce bile acids, the more bile acids are excreted the more cholesterol will be required and thus removed from the blood. Thus, by taking these resins three times daily, the cholesterol level drops.

Notice that colestipol and cholestyramine act in much the same way as we have seen that the naturally occurring, better-tasting, and much cheaper oat bran does. The logical conclusion, therefore, is that the ultimate idea for reducing cholesterol would be a modified diet with the combined therapy of oat bran and niacin.

Again, Drs. Kane and Malloy write that

"complementarity might be expected with drug combinations in which one agent (such as bile acid sequestrant) increases the catabolism (break-down) of LDL and the other agent (niacin) inhibits the secretion of the LDL-precursor lipoprotein VLDL . . . The complete normalization of LDL levels in compliant patients receiving colestipol with niacin indicates that the latter substance (niacin) has a potent complementary effect."[6] Similarly, the oat bran and niacin combination should be expected to produce significant and beneficial cholesterol lowering.

Depending on the individual, the combination of oat bran plus niacin could be sufficient to keep cholesterol levels well within or even below normal limits, even without changing the diet at all. This is particularly true for the millions of Americans who already have begun to cut back moderately on high-calorie fatty foods.

In January 1986 the *Journal of the American Medical Association* published a "Special Communication" to bring physicians up-to-date on the best approaches to lowering cholesterol levels.[9] The question of "whether to treat," the authors wrote, has been changed to "how best to treat." Written by doctors from the National Heart, Lung, and Blood Institute, the article stated unequivocally that "virtually all patients evaluated by a physician should be screened for hyperlipoproteinemia (high fat levels in the blood including cholesterol)."

How did these national experts advise physicians to help their patients? First, of course, the diet should be modified to cut back on fat and cholesterol. And to get individuals to "the target values of 180 to 200 mg/dl for total cholesterol" they recommended niacin.

With all the drugs at the physician's disposal, why did these doctors conclude that niacin is the way to go? First, they write, "niacin costs less than" the drugs. Second, niacin reduces LDL cholesterol levels. And third, "niacin also appears to reduce the risk of cardiovascular disease. In the Coronary Drug Project, a secondary intervention trial, niacin reduced the rate of nonfatal myocardial infarction by 21%."

When the government-sponsored panel of health specialists met in Washington, D.C., in October 1987 to "declare war on cholesterol," they pointed out that not everyone would be able to get his or her cholesterol level under the desired 200-mg limit by diet alone. Some may need to have drugs prescribed. They mentioned the bile-acid-binding drugs that I had discussed in the first edition of this book. And they also pointed out that niacin should be considered as a first line of treatment.[10]

Considering the effectiveness of niacin in lowering cholesterol, which had been reported just a little earlier, that recommendation was indeed warranted. On June 19, 1987, a landmark medical article published in the *Journal of the American Medical Association*[11] not only demonstrated the dramatic benefits of lowering cholesterol levels but for the very first time ever provided evidence that the atherosclerotic plaque buildup could actually be reversed!

Researchers at the University of Southern California worked with 162 male nonsmoking coronary-bypass patients for two years. Each was given an angiogram at the start of the study; the blockage in the arteries was carefully measured. Then the group was divided in two. The first group was given a fat-modified diet in which fat constituted about twenty percent of total calories, the bile-acid-binding drug colestipol, and niacin. The second group got a modified diet with placebos in place of the drug and niacin. At the end of the two-year period, in the first group there was a 26 percent reduction in total plasma cholesterol, a 43 percent reduction in LDL, and a 37 percent increase in HDL. Comparing angiograms done at the end of the study with those done two years earlier, the researchers found that not only was the progress of the disease stopped in those on the diet-colestipolniacin program, but also there was reversal of the atherosclerotic plaque buildup in more than 16 percent of patients.

The authors concluded that, in their opinion, virtually every person undergoing bypass surgery should be given aggressive cholesterol-lowering treatment. I was pleased to note that the program that demonstrated such powerful results was virtually identical to the one recommended in this book. Instead of colestipol, of course, I use oat bran and other foods rich in water-soluble fiber.

The USC researchers used doses of between 3 and 12 grams of niacin, with an average of 4.3 grams. I've found that far less than that can be extremely effective as part of the total program of *The 8-Week Cholesterol Cure*.

But what about taking niacin for a long period of time? The results of a long-term study of methods of treatment show the benefits of niacin not only in lowering cholesterol levels but, very importantly, in extending life! The paper was published in the *Journal of the American College of Cardiology* in December 1986.

The study was begun in early 1966 with men who had survived a previous heart attack.

After the initial study period of 6.2 years, patients given niacin showed a "significantly lower incidence of definite nonfatal myocardial infarction [heart attack] compared with patients in the placebo group." And as reported in the 1986 paper, after fifteen years the results were even more dramatic. There were sixty-nine fewer deaths in the niacin group, representing an 11 percent difference in mortality. Those receiving the niacin lived an average of 1.63 years longer than those not taking the vitamin.

The researchers also stated that "treatment with niacin proved to be the best lipid-lowering regimen among the five Coronary Drug Project treatment regimens."

Reporting at the First National Cholesterol Conference in Washington, D.C. in November 1988, Dr. Alan Wilson of the Robert Wood Johnson Medical School in New Brunswick, New Jersey, told of the long-term, eighteen-year treatment of patients with a combination of modified diet, colestipol, and niacin. He pointed to significant improvements in terms of both LDL lowering and HDL elevations. Of course, when combined with oat bran, as in *The 8-Week Cholesterol Cure,* the cholesterol-lowering effects of niacin are even stronger.

So there you have it. The program advocated in this book is the same recommended by some of the nation's most prestigious scientific and medical organizations. For some, diet, especially diet including oat bran and other water-soluble fibers, may be enough to get cholesterol levels down sufficiently. But, for many others niacin is the treatment of choice.

How to Take Niacin

Niacin has long been available in practically every health-food store, drugstore, and pharmacy. Most typically, tablets come in 50-milligram, 100-milligram, and 500-milligram strengths. Time-release formulations are also available. And there is a brand-new formulation that I'll tell you about shortly. Happily, the vitamin is quite inexpensive.

Up until just recently, there was only one safe way to begin taking niacin. The way I began, and the way I recommended to others for years, was to gradually increase the dosage. Most authorities in the past recommended starting with 100 milligrams three times daily, increasing the dose every third day until reaching a therapeutic level.[2,3,6]

Amounts of niacin prescribed by physicians in the past have varied from three to eight grams[6,7] and even up to twelve grams.[12] Most suggest a daily intake of three grams at first, with that level reached after a month's gradual buildup. If results are not adequate, patients can take more. I believe that for most individuals the maximum dosage needed with regular niacin is three grams; many individuals can successfully lower their cholesterol levels with even less. And, with the new formulation of time-release niacin, Endur-acin, which I discuss fully in this chapter, the maximum dosage is just 1.5 grams.

Some individuals on my program were able to maintain their reduced cholesterol levels even when they cut the niacin intake down to only two grams daily. And a report in *Family Practice News,* a physicians' newsletter, indicates that results can be obtained with as little as one gram of niacin.[13] Patients taking at least that amount each day for eight months experienced an 18 percent drop in total cholesterol, while protective HDL levels rose by 40 percent.

Researchers reported that even doses lower than one gram had effect, though not as much. This is particularly good news for those who might have adverse reactions, such as itching, with higher levels.

At the one-gram level, niacin had no side effects whatever. This means that everyone other than those with specific contraindication can benefit from this vitamin.

Noting that some patients had a difficult time taking large doses of niacin owing to the flushing and other unpleasant side effects that are frequently associated with regular types of niacin, Dr. Myron Luria tested the effectiveness of just one gram.[14] He began by giving patients 250 milligrams a day for the first week, gradually building to a total of one gram. He found that this dosage provided significant improvements in the ratio of total cholesterol to HDLs. In fifty-five patients given the one gram of niacin, average HDL levels rose by 31 percent after six months. Dr. Luria (then with Case Western Reserve University School of Medicine and now at the Department of Cardiology at Hadassah Hospital in Israel), noted that HDL levels increased after the first three months, and continued their rise through the sixth month.

How much will be right for you? If your cholesterol level is just a bit elevated, perhaps a modified diet including oat bran will be sufficient. Those with slightly higher levels may find one gram of niacin added to the diet daily will return cholesterol levels to safe values. And those with very high initial levels may need three grams of niacin daily. But thanks to the unique combination of diet, oat bran, and niacin, the vast majority of people will need no more than three grams of the vitamin. And, as I'll discuss in detail, with a new formulation the dosage can be much lower indeed, and without the side effects sometimes encountered with niacin.

The following table maps out the traditional manner of gradually building up dosages of niacin. This gradual step-up of dosage applies to both regular and most time-release niacin formulations. The dosage maximum of these types of niacin is 3000 mg (three grams). This dosage schedule does *not* apply to the niacin formulation. I now strongly advocate, Endur-acin, discussed in the coming pages.

Dosage Schedule for Initiating Niacin Therapy

First three days:
   one 100-mg tablet three times daily = 300 mg
Next three days:
   two 100-mg tablets three times daily = 600 mg
Next three days:
   three 100-mg tablets three times daily = 900 mg
Next three days:
   four 100-mg tablets three times daily = 1200 mg
Next three days:
   one 500-mg tablet three times daily = 1500 mg
Next three days:
   one 100-mg tablet plus one 500-mg tablet three
   times daily = 1800 mg

Next three days:

two 100-mg tablets plus one 500-mg tablet three times daily = 2100 mg

Next three days:

three 100-mg tablets plus one 500-mg tablet three times daily = 2400 mg

Next three days:

four 100-mg tablets plus 500-mg tablet three times daily = 2700 mg

From then on:

two 500-mg tablets three times daily = 3000 mg

A Revolutionary New Way to Take Niacin

When I first developed the program in this book, only the traditional formulations of niacin that I've discussed thus far were available. Then in 1987 I learned of a revolutionary new formulation being made by a small company in Oregon.

The product, known as Endur-acin, is a sustained-release niacin. The niacin very slowly trickles out of a wax matrix tablet, more smoothly than has ever been achieved before. Because of this smooth-release pattern, two wonderful things occur. First, there is no flush. Second, the dosage needed to achieve dramatic effects is drastically reduced.

Joseph Keenan, M.D., of the University of Minnesota, has done extensive research on both the safety and efficacy of Endur-acin. As he published in the July 1991 issue of the *Archives of Internal Medicine,* a dose of 1500 mg daily reduced levels of the "bad" LDL cholesterol by 19.3 percent. The ratio of total cholesterol to the "good" HDL cholesterol was improved by 19.4 percent.

His subjects took 500 mg of Endur-acin three times a day, typically with meals. Dr. Keenan found that doses at more than 1500 mg daily provided little if any additional benefit and were more likely to lead to liver enzyme increases. He feels that 1500 mg of Endur-acin is the dosage equivalent of 3000 mg of standard niacin.

While many people have difficulty taking standard niacin owing to side effects such as flushing, Dr. Keenan found that the drop-out rate due to such side effects in his study was only 3.4 percent.

Dr. Keenan subsequently collaborated with Russian physicians in Moscow and has published equally successful results. Endur-acin is now the "official" cholesterol-reducing agent in Russia.

Begin with one 500-milligram tablet taken at the evening meal. Assuming that you experience no difficulties or discomfort, after one week add another tablet with lunch. Then after a week taking the 1000-milligram total, go on to the three tablets, one 500-milligram tablet three times daily at lunch, dinner, and bedtime.

So, for those preferring to take this approach, the dosage schedule in this chapter can be completely ignored. And if you prefer to start with even a smaller dosage, 250-milligram tablets are available.

For most people this will be an unnecessary caution, but let me say that one should not chew the Endur-acin tablets, since this would spoil the sustained release effect.

I mentioned earlier that in the Endur-acin formulation niacin is incorporated into a wax matrix. Of course, this is not wax as in a candle but a particular type of pharmaceutical substance that is not absorbed by the body. In the process of passing through the digestive tract, niacin slowly trickles out. The wax matrix typically disintegrates and is passed out of the system. Some people, however, might see part or even all of the tablet matrix in the stool. Such individuals have a particularly fast rate of evacuation through the intestine. But there is no need for concern; although the matrix remains, the niacin has leached out.

The possibilities posed by this revolutionary new approach to taking niacin are enormous.

Needless to say, I was excited to hear of this development. I've asked a number of physicians here in Southern California to try the Endur-acin with their patients. One of those physicians, Dr. Charles Keenan of Santa Monica, was particularly enthusiastic. He was one of the subjects in my original research with this program, and subsequent to his own success in lowering his cholesterol level, he has put hundreds of his patients on the program. With the Endur-acin he was able to prescribe the program to many others. And, as a physician, he was pleased that the potentially confusing gradual buildup could be eliminated.

An interesting side note regarding the flush: While I personally have had little, if any, difficulty with the flush often associated with niacin, other people find this a major discomfort. Everyone's body is a bit different. My wife is a case in point. Several years ago she took a multivitamin preparation that contained a mere 50 milligrams of niacin, and she experienced, she recalls, a tremendous flush, turning her beet red. Although she has no problem with cholesterol, she took an Endur-acin tablet just out of curiosity. Sure enough, even though that 50 milligrams of niacin had caused a tremendous flush years ago, the 500-milligram tablet of Endur-acin brought on not even the tiniest blush or tingle. Many other people have reported the same experience. Endur-acin creates absolutely no flush for the majority of patients; however, a very few individuals may experience a slight flush. They are in the distinct minority.

And, of course, I wanted to try using Endur-acin myself. In order to put it to the best possible test, I waited until I was able to completely duplicate my first personal experiment—I wanted to very carefully compare the benefits of Endur-acin with the standard niacin tablets I had been taking.

For a full eight weeks, I monitored my diet closely to be certain I was eating the same amounts of fat and cholesterol as I had when I first began. Next, I consumed my half-cup of oat bran every day, either as muffins or as hot cereal in the mornings. And I took one gram of niacin with meals, three times daily, for a total of three grams a day. The results were very satisfying. I had a blood test done at Santa Monica Hospital Medical Center, where I had done the original research. My cholesterol level was a very respectable 161 mg/dl.

That day I switched over to Endur-acin, taking one 500-milligram tablet three times daily with meals, for a total of 1500 milligrams each day. And, of course, I continued with the same diet and with my daily breakfast of oat bran.

Another eight weeks passed, and I had another blood test. When the results came back, I felt there might have been some kind of laboratory error, even though I had the blood work done in the same hospital. My total cholesterol, the report said, was down to 137 mg/dl! To be certain that no error was involved, I repeated the test the following week. The report that time was 144 mg/dl—again, a spectacular response. (A small fluctuation in the numbers from week to week or even from day to day is to be expected.)

But the important thing here is that by taking *half* the amount of niacin I'd been taking for three years, I actually got *better* results! Physicians recommending Endur-acin for their patients have reported similar results. Although patients had achieved excellent success with three grams of standard niacin products, their response was even better with only 1500 milligrams of Endur-acin.

Combining a modified diet with oat bran, niacin dosage of three grams was effective in my own case and for the many individuals with greatly elevated cholesterol levels who participated in a clinical study, as reported in Chapter 14. With Endur-acin, the maximum dosage is 1.5 grams, not three grams.

Since original publication of *The 8-Week Cholesterol Cure,* thousands of men and women have used the program to lower their own cholesterol levels. Some were able to maintain reduced cholesterol levels even when they cut the niacin down to only two grams daily. Others, in keeping with the report mentioned earlier,[13] found that only one gram of niacin daily provided sufficient results. And, of course, one could expect even greater benefits from lower doses when using the new formulation Endur-acin. For many individuals one gram will be completely adequate.

For those with extremely high cholesterol levels, or, again, highly resistant levels that have not responded to diet alone, Endur-acin offers yet another benefit. If after taking 1500 mg of this sustained-release niacin, the cholesterol levels are still higher than desired, one can take another 500-milligram tablet. For such individuals the dosage pattern could be one 500-milligram tablet three times daily with meals, plus an extra 500-milligram tablet at bedtime. The total dosage of 2000 milligrams is still well under the 3000 milligrams I originally found effective, yet would be expected to produce far greater results. For the vast majority of people, 1500 mg is the maximum dosage of this form of niacin. Many people succeed beautiful with even less. But, regardless of dosage, be certain to discuss Endur-acin, or any kind of niacin, with your physician before taking it.

The dosages of Endur-acin I've just discussed have been used widely by patients
working with their physicians as well as in research conducted at the University of Minnesota. Dosage schedules for standard
formulations of niacin as seen on page 196
have been published widely in the medical literature. However, individual needs will vary
considerably, as will personal reactions to
niacin. Some will find that a total of 1000 milligrams of standard formulation niacin or 500
milligrams of Endur-acin will be enough. Others will need more. Some will experience adverse reactions to one extent or another from
a large dosage and will have to cut back to a
level at which cholesterol reduction can be
achieved without those reactions. Others will
experience virtually no reactions whatever.
This individual variance in response and needs
is yet another reason why one should embark
on niacin therapy in cooperation with his or
her personal physician.

Endur-acin can be ordered directly from
the manufacturer, the Endurance Products
Company in Oregon. They have made the
product available to the public through a separate company for mail-order sales. I'm particularly pleased that the cost for this very
high-quality product is extremely reasonable,
often cheaper than ordinary niacin found in

health-food stores. If you're interested in obtaining a supply of Endur-acin, you may write for order information to:

Endurance Products Co.
P.O. Box 230489
Portland, OR 97223
(800) 483-2532
www.endur.com

A few companies now claim that their product is actually Endur-acin—not similar to Endur-acin, but the real thing—packaged under their own label. Unfortunately, the only way you know you're taking Endur-acin is to buy it directly from Endurance Products Company. Some companies have actually been devious enough to buy a small quantity of Endur-acin from Endurance Products, and then imitate this product by forming look-alike tablets with cheaper, less-effective niacin. Such products may well cause a flush, and will not be effective at the reduced dosage of 1500 mg.

Because I so strongly advocate the use of Endur-acin over other kinds of niacin, including other time-release formulations, some have questioned whether I have a vested interest in the company. I want to state publicly that I have no financial interest in Endurance Products Company. To be honest, when I first saw how effective the product was, I wanted to buy some stock in the company, but I learned that it is a privately owned firm. I simply believe Endur-acin is the best type of niacin to use.

Possible Side Effects

Practically everyone taking standard formulations of niacin, and even sustained-release niacin tablets other than new Endur-acin, will experience a flush. This is a tingly, prickly sensation of the skin, primarily on the arms, shoulders, back, and chest. Often the skin will turn pink or red, as though one were blushing or had been in the sun. This flush is completely harmless.[23] Scientists say it has to do with release of prostaglandins. Some people become frightened by the first experience, thinking the flush is dangerous, even thinking it has something to do with the heart. Actually, it's limited strictly to the skin, and should be of no concern. Of course, those taking Endur-acin will experience no flush at all.

For those taking standard formulations of niacin according to the dosage schedule printed in this chapter, the flush is strongest when first taking niacin or when increasing the dosage level. After a few days of taking niacin at a given dose on a regular basis, the flush tends to diminish. Most people find that after a while even three grams daily, one gram with each meal, produces little if any flush.

In the past, people who had difficulty with the flush could reduce it significantly by taking half an aspirin tablet either with the niacin or thirty minutes beforehand. This will decrease the flush without influencing the effectiveness of cholesterol lowering.[2]

Some people react to the flushing experience more strongly than others. My printer, for example, started taking the tablets after we talked about the program and his flushing was quite pronounced. In fact, after each dose he looked as though he had been in the sun for a couple of hours. He found that a sustained-release niacin helped to cut back on the flush. That was several years ago, when I was first beginning to develop the program. Today, of course, I'd simply advise him to take Endur-acin.

Certain individuals—very few in my experience—have a bit of gastric upset when taking niacin or other vitamin preparations. Some of the older sustained-release niacin formulations did cause some gastric upset. Happily, the Endur-acin causes no such problems at the lower dosage needed for effectiveness. To best ensure avoiding stomach problems, scientists recommend taking niacin with meals. This makes sense, since most of us eat three meals a day, and this would fit the niacin dosage schedule perfectly.

The most troublesome side effect reported in the literature, one that cropped up during the research reported later, has been an itching rash. There is no way to predict who will develop this adverse reaction. If it occurs at all, it will be during the early period of niacin intake. Unlike the flush, the rash does not go away and it is the reason some people cannot take three grams of niacin. Don't confuse some initial itching with this rash, however. The itching as part of the flush passes, but the rash does not. Those who do develop the rash find that after discontinuing niacin the rash disappears within a few days. No such rash appeared in those taking one gram of niacin or less. And one would expect little, if any, incidence of rash with Endur-acin.

Another side effect that has been reported with high doses of niacin is blurred vision. Again, this disappears without residual ill effect after discontinuing the niacin. This, too, would not be a problem with the Endur-acin.

Since I first began to use niacin, and since my book was first published, scientists have learned that the body makes most of its cholesterol in the evening and nighttime hours. That's why it's best to take the niacin later in the day. Ideally, if you're taking three 500-milligram tablets of Endur-acin, the best times to take them would be at lunch, dinner, and bedtime. A tablet in the morning with breakfast would have the least effect. Do not take more than one tablet at a time.

Niacin is metabolized in the liver, where cholesterol is manufactured, and some people are unable to tolerate the added burden on that organ. Symptoms of nausea and vomiting may develop. As noted later in this chapter, everyone taking niacin should have a liver function test two to three months after beginning, just to be sure the liver is, in fact, tolerating the niacin.

Remember that no two of us are alike; we respond to different things in different ways. Most people will be able to take niacin, especially the Endur-acin, with no problems at all. A few will develop reactions of one sort or another. That's why it's best to take the niacin only under the supervision of your doctor, who will be able to answer any questions you may have.

CONTRAINDICATIONS TO NIACIN

As is the case for many, if not all, substances, certain people should not take niacin at all.

Contraindications for taking this vitamin in large doses include active peptic ulcer, liver disease, severe heart arrhythmias, diabetes, and gout. Interestingly, however, physicians have told me they have given Endur-acin to patients with diabetes and even mild cases of gout without difficulty. Certainly though, such patients should be closely monitored by their physicians.

If you're a heavy drinker, or were a heavy drinker in the past, be sure to have a liver test before taking niacin to be sure your liver is still up to it. This is recommended because niacin is metabolized by the liver, the same organ that breaks down alcohol, and sometimes the liver has been compromised by long-term, heavy alcohol use. (It's interesting to note that heavy drinkers are sometimes referred to as "high livers" and are the very people who can wind up with bad livers.)

If you do take niacin, keep alcohol consumption under control; otherwise you'll be asking your liver to do double duty.

You'll note that severe arrhythmias are one of the contraindications to niacin use. It has also been reported that some individuals, although very few, will develop heartbeat abnormalities after taking niacin. While this is very infrequent, you should at least be aware of the possibility. If this happens to you, discuss it with your doctor. He or she can decide to modify the dosage or to take you off niacin completely.

SAFETY OF TAKING NIACIN

The majority of people will be able to take even three grams of niacin without side effects. All but those for whom niacin is contraindicated will experience no side effects at the one-gram level. And few if any side effects would be anticipated with 1500 milligrams of Endur-acin. The safety of taking niacin has been long documented.

The Coronary Drug Project showed that niacin can be taken for prolonged periods of time with only the minor side effects described above.[15] This study involved more than 8000 individuals from 1969 through 1975.

Many physicians have been using niacin to treat patients with elevated cholesterol and triglyceride levels for years. Dr. Louis Cohen, professor of medicine at the University of Chicago Medical Center, has been prescribing niacin in conjunction with the drug probucol for the past twenty years.[12] He has had dozens of patients taking the vitamin for six years and more without any difficulties, and feels that niacin can be used for a lifetime.

As stated on the previous page, if you have been drinking heavily for many years, your liver may have been compromised and not be functioning as well as it should. Similarly, if one has had a disease such as hepatitis or cirrhosis, the liver has been damaged and may not be able to accommodate the niacin being taken, even at lower dosages. (Hepatitis can be cured but frequently results in liver damage. Cirrhosis cannot be cured, and by its definition results in damage to the liver.)

That's why I recommend that after taking niacin for a period of time—say, two months or so—one should have a blood test to check the function of the liver. Actually, this is not at all inconvenient since one will want to check the cholesterol level to determine progress by that time anyway.

The tests will show how well the liver is metabolizing the niacin. For the vast majority of people, there will be no problem at all. In fact, physicians, including those at Harvard, point out that a slight fluctuation in those liver function tests simply shows that the niacin is doing its job. But for those people whose livers have been damaged previously, the test might show that they should not take the niacin.

The value of having this liver function test is another example of why it's important to work with your physician in your efforts to lower cholesterol levels.

Don't let my recommendation for having the liver function test done frighten you. First, it's a very simple test. Second, the vast majority of men and women will show no problems whatsoever. Third, especially if you're using the Endur-acin, the low dosages are expected to pose no difficulties, as shown in research done at Harvard. Fourth, the test need be done once after taking the niacin for two to three months, and once a year thereafter to establish positively your body's ability to metabolize niacin properly. And fifth, compare the recommendation for one liver test with the suggestions of the manufacturers of the much-publicized new cholesterol-lowering drug.

Mevacor is the brand-name for lovastatin made by the Merck, Sharp & Dohme pharmaceutical company. It received Food and Drug Administration approval in September 1987 for prescription by physicians for lowering cholesterol levels. The drug has been much touted in the press, and stock in the company soared when approval was granted.

But while the drug probably will have a legitimate role in lowering cholesterol levels for those patients needing it, there are a number of other considerations. First, there is absolutely no track record of use with the substance. Many authorities are concerned that long-term side effects will show up years down the road. Second, consider the company's recommendations regarding liver function tests for patients taking Mevacor: "It is recommended that liver function tests be performed every 4 to 6 weeks during the first 15 months of therapy and periodically thereafter in all patients."[16]

That's quite a difference: one liver test annually for niacin versus a liver test every four to six weeks for Mevacor. The reasons for suggesting such frequent liver testing for the new drug are enough to make many medical authorities very cautious about the use of the drug. Such authorities have frequently stated that they are concerned that the drug will be over-prescribed before attempts have been made to lower cholesterol levels by dietary means and through the use of more proven substances, such as niacin.

As a side note, you may be interested to know that the cost of Mevacor will be as much as $3000 annually. Compare that with the cost of some breakfast cereal and a few bottles of vitamins!

Many people trying to control their cholesterol levels also take a variety of prescription drugs. Fortunately, niacin does not have any adverse interactions with such drugs. In fact, it can and has been used very successfully in combination with prescription drugs, including drugs designed to lower cholesterol levels.

NIACIN AS PART OF A COMPLETE PROGRAM

Niacin can be an important part of your program to reduce serum cholesterol. Along with a modified diet including oat bran, niacin has been shown to be safe and effective. I've been particularly edified that in the past years since this book was originally published an increasing number of physicians have begun to write the words "8-Week Cholesterol Cure" on their prescription pads and to instruct their patients to follow the program and to come back in eight weeks. While my program continues to have its critics, the number of doctors who have seen the program's safety and efficacy continues to grow.

Niacin has advantages beyond cholesterol reduction. In fact, no prescription drug can match its benefit profile. Niacin alone can slash the levels of the newly identified lipid risk factor termed Lp (a); it does so by up to 50 percent. It changes the structure of cholesterol molecules from the dangerous small, dense form to the more benign larger, looser configuration. Niacin improves the ability of your body to break down blood clots that could cause a heart attack. And it improves the ratio of substances called prostaglandins, reducing the risk of heart disease.

If you decide to include niacin in your program to lower serum cholesterol levels, be sure to inform your personal physician. Perhaps he or she would also like to read this book. By sharing the book with your doctor, you'll help bring the information about this effective program to even more people.

A Few Words of Caution

While niacin has been demonstrated to be quite safe for most people and is available in any health-food store or pharmacy, or through mail order, a few words of caution are in order. First of all, niacin should not be viewed as a substitute for good, healthful eating habits. Remember that the basis of any healthful diet is the reduction of fats and cholesterol and the increased consumption of complex carbohydrates.

Second, niacin should be considered part of the program for those with quite elevated cholesterol levels. Does your serum level put you at risk? For those with moderately elevated cholesterol counts, say just twenty points over the desired level, modified diet alone, especially combined with oat bran, will probably be effective.

Third, there are definite medical contraindications for niacin. Some people should not attempt to take the vitamin at all. Those contraindications include gout and/or elevated levels of uric acid, ulcer, diabetes, and liver abnormalities. If you have any doubts at all, talk with your doctor. He or she is your best source of medical advice and supervision.

Fourth, niacin causes occasional minor side effects in some individuals. In addition to the flushing at the beginning of niacin consumption, some people develop a rash, skin itch, and possibly blurred vision. These effects disappear after one stops taking the niacin, within three to five days. There have been no reported long-term adverse reactions. As mentioned before, some people will not be able to tolerate niacin. For those men and women, diet and oat bran are still the best ways to control cholesterol levels. For those unable to take niacin, but whose cholesterol levels remain quite elevated even after following a good diet including oat bran, you and your physician may wish to consider prescription drugs as a last resort. I've discussed the cholesterol-lowering drugs in Chapter 15.

For the vast majority, niacin can be taken for years and years to reduce and maintain lowered cholesterol levels. Together, diet, oat bran, and niacin form the most effective answer to the problem of elevated cholesterol and heart-disease risk available for the general population.

As stated above, **if you decide to include niacin in your program to lower serum cholesterol levels, be sure to inform your personal physician.** He or she will want to include that bit of information in your personal records. If you have any questions about using this vitamin, by all means discuss them with your doctor.

Is Niacin a Vitamin or a Drug?

Since the publication of the first edition, my book has been criticized by some reviewers for calling niacin a vitamin. They point out that niacin taken in megadoses acts pharmacologically; that is, it acts like a drug. Therefore, they argue, it must be called a drug.

Certainly, niacin is commonly considered to be a vitamin. While it does lower cholesterol better than many prescription drugs, oat bran does this also. Does that make oat bran a drug?

Any vitamin taken in large doses should be

used carefully and under the supervision of a physician. That's why I have consistently recommended that every person who follows this program should consult with his or her physician about it.

Is niacin a vitamin or a drug? Call it what you will, niacin has helped control my cholesterol level and those of thousands and thousands of others. It has been shown to prolong the lives of heart patients. And I strongly believe that niacin will help keep me alive for years and years to come. Call it what you will. I call it a lifesaver.

7

Other Marvels and Fabulous Foods

In terms of cholesterol, one could classify foods into three groups: those that raise cholesterol levels, such as eggs and butter; those that have no effect on blood fats, such as carrots, lettuce, breads, and so on; and those that can actually lower lipid levels, such as oat bran. The really good news is that there are other marvels throughout the supermarket in that third cholesterol-lowering category.

Oat bran has beneficial effects because it contains a large percentage of water-soluble fiber termed "gum." There is more gum, ounce for ounce, in oat bran than in oatmeal, and that's why the bran works better. It makes sense then to think that other gums would work as well. And the medical literature indicates that, in fact, they do.

One such substance is guar gum, a type of carbohydrate found in cluster beans. Unfortunately, there is not enough in the beans. While isolated guar gum found as a powder has been shown to be effective in lowering cholesterol, it's difficult to incorporate into the diet as such. (First, cluster beans are not available as food. Second, guar gum content is low and must be extracted.) When mixed into foods such as soups and stews guar gum makes them extremely thick and heavy—five to eight times thicker than cornstarch. To see if they could get around this, scientists gave patients capsules containing guar gum rather than mixing it with foods. Patients lost no weight and followed normal eating patterns. After four weeks, guar gum lowered total serum cholesterol by an average of 16.6 percent. Neither triglycerides nor HDLs were affected. But to achieve this effect patients had to consume five capsules at breakfast, lunch, and dinner, for a total of fifteen capsules containing nine grams of guar gum.

Unfortunately, guar gum is no longer available commercially.

But we can all get similar effects by regularly consuming a variety of dry beans or legumes. Pinto beans, Great Northern beans, lima beans, lentils, red beans, navy beans, and many others all over the world contain large amounts of water-soluble fiber. The same man who investigated the cholesterol-lowering effects of oat bran also looked into the possibilities of beans.

Dr. James Anderson fed subjects a daily bean diet containing 115 grams of dried beans, based on dry weight before cooking, for three weeks. The participants in this study were given all their meals in the hospital so the researchers could determine exactly what was eaten. Pinto beans and navy beans were served as cooked beans or bean soup. Cholesterol levels fell by an average of 19 percent.

Now, granted, that's a lot of beans to eat each day. In fact, the study participants ate only 88 percent of the beans served. It would be difficult to expect anyone to eat this amount of beans daily for the rest of his or her life. But there's no reason why one couldn't include dry beans as a regular part of the diet. See Table 13 in Chapter 5 for a listing of soluble fiber in various kinds of beans. Even though the soluble-fiber content is lower than in oat bran, beans are remarkably effective in cholesterol reduction, indicating that something other than the fiber—scientists don't yet know what—works to cut cholesterol.

The possibilities are infinitely varied. In addition to soups and cooked beans, bean dips are a delicious and healthful alternative to high-fat snack dips. Try the bean recipes included in the recipe section and you'll soon turn into a real bean addict. One of my favorites is the dish called *hummus,* which is a staple food of people throughout the Middle East. I keep a supply in the refrigerator and use it as a snack along with pita bread.

According to a survey conducted at the Baltimore Gerontology Research Center, in subjects of all age groups, from thirty to seventy-nine, each gram of dietary fruit fiber consumed corresponded with a mean 1.5 mg/dl decrease in serum cholesterol. Fruit-fiber intake among the 556 men in the study ranged from less than 1 gram to about 11 grams. There was a difference in cholesterol levels of about 14 mg/dl between the lowest and the highest fiber-intake groups. Isn't that a good reason to eat more apples and oranges?

Another excellent source of the water-soluble fiber that can lower cholesterol levels is rice bran. Just as oat bran is a part of the whole oat grain, so rice bran is a portion of the whole rice grain. While available in some health food stores, rice fiber is hard to find. But you can order it by calling Ener-G Foods at (800) 331–5222.

The product is 36 percent fiber, of which fully 94 percent is soluble. That means, without your having to do the calculations, that you can get as much soluble fiber from two tablespoons of rice fiber as you can from one-half cup of oat bran.

You can use rice bran to sprinkle over cereals, as a topping for yogurt and other foods that might need a bit of a crunchy texture, and as an ingredient in muffins and other baked goods. It is every bit as good as oat bran for lowering cholesterol, and so it is one more food to consider and to use in the diet. You'll find that rice bran isn't quite as versatile as oat bran in its cooking and baking potentials, but it's nice to have for variety.

Did your mother or grandmother ever make barley soup? For some reason, we don't use as much of this grain anymore, and it's time to get it back into our diets. First, the kind of barley you're likely to buy to be cooked into soups and stews contains about 5 grams of water-soluble fiber in a 100-gram (3½-ounce) serving. Sure, you're not going to eat it daily, but barley is yet one more source of water-soluble fiber to include in your diet.

But there's more to the barley story, according to researchers at the University of Wisconsin's Cereal Institute. Dr. David Peterson, the Institute's director, reports that they have isolated two compounds in barley's protein-rich outer portion, which is normally discarded in processing, that appear to have a potent cholesterol-lowering effect. And that effect is different from the bile acid-binding effect of water-soluble fiber. Instead, those barley-derived substances work on the activity of the enzyme HMG Co-A reductase, which determines the amount of cholesterol made by the liver. These substances are called tocotrienols, and are the chemical cousins of vitamin E. They finally came on the market in 1997 under the brand Evolve which you can find in most drug and health food stores. Evolve has a three-way mode of action including cholesterol reduction, antioxidant activity even stronger than vitamin E, and protection of the lining of the walls of arteries to prevent formation of blockage.

The old saying that "an apple a day keeps the doctor away" may be closer to the truth than we ever imagined. But change that to "keeps the cardiac surgeon away." Apples contain pectin, another soluble fiber proved to have a cholesterol-lowering effect. While an individual apple has just a little bit of that pectin, we can get a lot more of it with a new product called Tastee Apple Fiber. This is made by removing the juice from the apple, resulting in a light reddish-tan-colored flour-like powder with a pleasant, mild flavor. You can use it in making delicious muffins and cookies, as well as in sauces. Don't confuse this apple fiber with apple pectin itself. You can also buy apple pectin, but its use is limited to traditional applications, including jelly making. Look for Tastee Apple Fiber in supermarkets and health-food stores. If you can't find it, call the company at (800) 262-7733 in Newcomerstown, Ohio.

Since Dr. Anderson first did his research with the water-soluble fiber in oat bran, people have been looking for other ways to work the substance into the diet. Surely rice bran and barley are excellent, natural sources. But there's another approach you might want to consider.

Metamucil is the best known of a group of laxatives—made from psyllium seeds—that have been on the market for many years. Recent research has shown that these products are rich in soluble fiber and have a cholesterol-lowering effect. In fact, Dr. Anderson himself did some investigation and found that three teaspoonfuls daily are both safe and effective.

I hasten to point out that although they are "natural," these products should not be confused in any way with food. I certainly would not recommend that people use laxatives rather than good, wholesome cereals. But there may be times, such as during travel, when they might be used.

There's no question that we'll be seeing more and more research done in the years to come into new and exciting approaches to cholesterol control. One very novel effort involved the use of activated charcoal.

An article that appeared in the British journal *Lancet* in 1986 continues to attract attention because of the finding that activated charcoal reduced cholesterol levels by an average of 41 percent in seven patients. But don't rush out to the store to buy some just yet. Here are a few things to consider.

First, to equal the amount given to those volunteer patients—eight grams three times daily in a water suspension—you'd have to swallow ninety-two charcoal capsules. Personally, I don't think I'd enjoy gulping all that charcoal every day of my life.

Second, the long-term effects of such a radical idea haven't begun to be explored. The study lasted only four weeks. Charcoal works by adhering to insoluble particles and excreting them through the colon. But we don't know whether the charcoal might also grab onto and get rid of vitamins and minerals.

A longer study with a larger group of subjects will be done to see if there might be some merit to the charcoal concept. In the meantime, it's nice to know that oat bran achieves the same goal of binding onto bile acids formed of cholesterol, thereby reducing the body's total supply of the culprit.

I first wrote about artificial fat way back in 1989. It took nearly 10 years to get to the supermarkets but olestra is now available in potato chips and other crunchy snacks. Made by Proctor & Gamble company, olestra, also called Olean, is a specially designed oil that contributes absolutely no fat to the diet.

Food scientists begin with a molecule of sucrose, ordinary table sugar, and then add fatty acid particles until the resulting molecule is so large that it cannot pass through the walls of the digestive tract. It passes, undigested, out with the bowel movement.

The good news is that chips made with Olean are very tasty; in fact, most people can't tell them apart from the regular chips. And unlike the regular chips that pack 10 grams of fat per ounce, about 18 chips, the WOW! brand chips have none of the fat and half the calories.

The bad news is that olestra can cause gastric upset including diarrhea in some persons. Even worse, it carries away fat-soluble vitamins including vitamin E and beta-carotene.

Although the Food and Drug Administration has given approval for marketing, I advise strict moderation. To enjoy a few WOW! Chips or fat-free Doritos with a sandwich now and then is probably harmless. My family and I all do so. But remember that a serving size is just one ounce. Don't go overboard on olestra until we have more complete research data.

Another area of product development to keep an eye on is pectin. A soluble fiber, pectin has been shown to lower cholesterol levels.

But common food sources contain little of the substance, and artificial sources have produced some ill effects. But work continues.

Researchers at the University of Florida in Gainesville have found that patients taking about three tablespoons of grapefruit pectin either as capsules or as a food additive experienced cholesterol reductions on average of 7.2 percent. The substance given was specifically derived from the rind and flesh of the grapefruit, rather than the grapefruit itself. This was a well-controlled study, with groups receiving first the pectin and later crossing over and receiving a placebo. Some of the twenty-seven volunteer subjects achieved up to a 19 percent lowering of their cholesterol level. Grapefruit fiber, pectin, along with guar gum is now commercially available in a product called Pro-Fibe, developed by the physician who did the original research. You can order Pro-Fibe by calling (800) 756-3999.

Some interesting research now being conducted indicates there may be another lipid-lowering vegetable category for us to consider. Some dietitians now believe that cruciferous vegetables, notably broccoli and cauliflower, can help lower cholesterol levels. These are preliminary observations; however, there are no reasons *not* to eat more of those vegetables. If they do help to lower cholesterol, that's wonderful. If not, they still provide fiber in the diet as well as vitamins.

The Fish Story

Next on the cholesterol-lowering food shopping list should be plenty of fish. Years ago people thought fish was brain food. Now, thanks to advances in nutrition, we know it's great for the heart.

Not too many years ago, dietitians and nutritionists placed certain seafood dishes on the list of foods to limit or avoid. Salmon, they said, was a fatter-than-average fish. The same went for mackerel. Shellfish, the common wisdom advised, was high in cholesterol. Avoid these if possible, the helpful manuals said. But times and techniques have changed and improved.

As for those fatty fishes, it turns out that the particular fat in salmon and mackerel is a tongue-twister called eicosapentaenoic acid, a polyunsaturated variety of fat found in most cold-water fish. This particular fish oil, termed EPA for short, has the remarkable ability to reduce both triglyceride and cholesterol levels.

For many years medical scientists were confounded by the seemingly contradictory facts that Eskimos ate a great deal of meat in the form of whale blubber, seal, and fish, and yet their rate of heart disease was remarkably low. In the early 1970s we learned that one possible explanation was that the flesh of those marine animals was rich in polyunsaturated rather than saturated fat.

The first definitive research was published in 1976; it showed unequivocally that Eskimos' heart-disease incidence was one-tenth that of Danes or North Americans. In fact, as Eskimos emigrated from Greenland to Denmark, their rates of heart disease rose rapidly to become equal to those of Danes. This was remarkable since the diets were similar in terms of fat and cholesterol. The big difference was in the composition of the fat. The Danish diet contained twice as much saturated fat and more polyunsaturated fats from vegetable origin. Conversely, the Eskimos consumed a great deal of polyunsaturated fat of animal origin.

To digress for a moment to clarify this matter, the polyunsaturated fats from plants are chemically designated omega-6 fatty acid class. While one can find some omega-3 fatty acids in certain vegetable oils, notably canola and safflower oils, principally they come from fish and marine mammals. Some fish oils have more EPA than others. Salmon, mackerel, and menhaden store this fat in their flesh, while cod and shark store it in their livers.

The difference, then, between the Eskimo and Danish diets was the amount of omega-3 fatty acids or EPA fish oils. Eskimos eat an average of one pound of flesh (fish, whale blubber, and seal meat) daily. Studying the Eskimos further, researchers found that cholesterol levels in their blood were not all that much lower than those in Danes or North Americans. This indicates that fish oil protects against heart disease in some way other than by lowering cholesterol levels. We've seen the benefits of fish consumption in other populations as well.

German researchers fed healthy adult volunteers two eight-ounce cans of mackerel in addition to their other daily foods each day. They gave another group the same amount of herring, a fish without EPA in its fat content. After two weeks of the fishy diets, the mackerel group showed a 7 percent drop in cholesterol and a 47 percent dip in triglycerides. Blood pressure also fell, by about 10 percent. No such benefits for the herring eaters, though.

In fact, a very recent study reported in the *New England Journal of Medicine* indicated that the death rate from heart disease was more than 50 percent lower among men who ate at least 30 grams—that's one ounce—of fish daily as compared with men who ate no fish at all. Just one or two fish dishes a week, the researchers wrote, may offer significant protection against heart disease.

A great number of studies on this issue have been conducted in recent years. Japanese living in coastal fishing villages were compared with those dwelling in inland farming areas. For those near the water fish consumption was, understandably, higher and the rate of coronary heart disease and strokes was significantly lower. That study helped to confirm the findings on Eskimos.

In a Dutch study, 852 middle-aged men who did not have coronary heart disease at the outset were followed for 20 years. The more fish they ate, the less the incidence of heart disease. That's when we learned that as little as two ounces of fish daily, on average, resulted in about a 50 percent reduction in mortality from heart disease.

In America, data were analyzed from a study of Western Electric workers in Illinois. Similarly researchers found that fish protected the workers from heart disease. But a very small amount of fish was actually eaten.

By now you may be wondering how it can be that the Eskimos are protected from heart disease by extremely large quantities of fish oils by way of their intake of fish, seal, and whale, while the Dutch and Americans apparently received protection from relatively small amounts. In fact, Eskimos consume up to fourteen grams of EPA daily. A four-ounce piece of fish provides only one to two grams of EPA; even the very fatty chinook salmon supplies not that much more. And to duplicate the EPA levels in Eskimo diets, researchers have fed patients a handful of EPA fish-oil capsules daily. So why the discrepancy?

Many experts who have looked at the data have come to the conclusion that the benefits from eating fish are cumulative. When one is given a dozen or more fish-oil capsules daily, the investigation lasts only a few weeks or months. But those who have been shown to receive protection against heart disease have been eating fish all their lives.

Virtually everyone who has been involved with this kind of research has come to the same conclusion I have reached. People are lots better off eating more fish than swallowing fish-oil capsules. We'll look at some of the reasoning for *not* taking those capsules shortly.

A number of physicians in the country have been recommending that their patients take fish-oil capsules to lower their cholesterol levels. Ironically, the fact is that fish oil does little if anything to lower those numbers. Remember that the Eskimos' cholesterol levels were not much different from those of Americans, yet they were protected from heart disease.

What fish-oil capsules *can* do, and quite efficiently, is to reduce levels of triglycerides. And, in some cases of patients with elevated triglycerides, there will be a simultaneous lowering of cholesterol. That's because the abundance of triglycerides leads to elevated levels of VLDLs, the very-low-density-lipoprotein carriers of cholesterol. But for individuals who do not have simultaneously high triglycerides, cholesterol levels are not affected. In fact, the levels of LDL may actually be raised by EPA capsules. Researchers at the University of Kansas Medical Center found that the equivalent of only about one tablespoon of fish oil per day significantly raised LDL cholesterol in the blood. On the other hand, some have wondered whether or not this is actually offset by beneficial effects on clotting. Since we don't understand entirely how fish oil exerts its protective benefits, it's best not to take fish-oil capsules at this time.

Animal studies have shown in the past that rather large doses of fish oil can prevent the atherosclerotic process from occurring. Now we have evidence that, in very special cases, fish-oil capsules can be useful in humans as well. A well-controlled study was conducted to determine whether fish oil could prevent reclogging in arteries which had been opened by way of angioplasty.

Typically one-third of arteries dilated with the balloon technique are closed six months later. Researchers at George Washington University and the Washington (D.C.) Hospital Center studied 194 angioplasty patients. One half received nine fish-oil capsules containing a total of 4.5 grams of EPA daily for six months after their angioplasties; the other group did not. Both groups received counseling and advice to consume a low-fat diet.

By the end of six months, 35.4 percent of those not taking fish oil showed signs that their dilated coronary arteries had become narrowed again, while the recurrence rate was only 19 percent in the fish-oil group. But the director of the study, Dr. Mark Milner, said he does not recommend taking fish-oil capsules for anyone other than those undergoing angioplasty.

In his study eleven patients stopped taking the fish-oil capsules within the first week because of disagreeable but not dangerous side effects. The large doses resulted in flatulence and other slight digestive problems in some patients. Many patients complained about the persistent taste of fish oil in their mouths.

A similar study was conducted at the Dallas

Veterans Administration Medical Center. There patients received either 3.2 grams of EPA daily of an aspirin tablet along with the drug Persantine (dipyridamole). That drug combination is most often used following both angioplasty and bypass surgery. Treatment began seven days before angioplasty and continued six months after.

In those receiving fish-oil capsules, renarrowing of the arteries developed in 16 percent of patients. Those getting the drugs showed artery closure in 36 percent.

There's no doubt that those who anticipate having an angioplasty performed should seriously discuss these findings with their physicians in order to benefit potentially from fish-oil capsules. Unfortunately, however, no such data have shown any benefit for those taking fish-oil capsules to either prevent future atherosclerosis or to slow down the process.

Perhaps by now you're wondering why one shouldn't take fish-oil capsules "just to be on the safe side." If there could be some potential benefit, some protection against heart disease, why not do so? I can only offer my own opinion, backed by the opinions of the many investigators whose work I've read and with whom I've spoken. They and I agree that the best possible advice would be to increase the amount of fish in the diet rather than to take the fish-oil capsules. I personally do not take those capsules, and I don't intend to do so until I see some definitive clinical proof of benefit. At this point we have more questions than answers when it comes to fish-oil supplements. But we do know the benefits of eating more fish. Table 14 will help you choose the fish to include in your diet for their omega-3 fatty-acid content.

All cold-water fish supply some EPA. And all fish, both salt-and fresh-water varieties, have far less saturated fat than beef. When you look at Table 11 (see page 139), you see that some fish contain higher amounts of fat and cholesterol than others. In those fish with higher-than-average levels of cholesterol the fat content is often quite low. The conclusion reached by the medical authorities, then, is to eat a wide variety of many kinds of fish. There's no need to avoid any of them.

And what about those much-maligned shellfish? Well it turns out that, through no fault of their own, the original compilers of cholesterol data were in error on this one. Cholesterol is just one of a large family of chemical substances collectively termed the sterols. Other sterols include, for example, vitamin E (alphatocopherol) and precursors of vitamin D (ergosterol). The original testing methods could not distinguish among all the sterols. So the shellfish earned the undeserved reputation of having high cholesterol levels. Actually, scallops contain a mere 35 milligrams per 3½-ounce servings. That Alaskan delicacy king crab has only 60 milligrams. Clams, oysters, and mussels are particularly low in cholesterol. Lobster, once a distinct no-no for even those who could afford it, has a bit less than 100 milligrams. In fact, the only food from the sea that has a considerable amount of cholesterol is shrimp, which contains more than 100 milligrams per serving. Even so, when planning a 250-milligram-per-day program, a serving of shrimp should be no problem.

Shellfish have the added benefit of being particularly low in fat. Scallops have only 0.2 grams of fat per serving. Shrimp contains only 0.8 grams. And lobster provides just 1.9 grams. All those contributions are practically negligible. So while your selection of a given shellfish may provide the daily limits of cholesterol, the dish won't even be counted in terms of fat. As Dr. William Castelli of the famed Framingham Heart Study in Massachussets puts it, if you can't be a vegetarian, eat a vegetarian of the sea. Enjoy lots of shellfish and watch your cholesterol level fall.

Is there anything to watch out for in the fish market? Yes, there are exceptions which probably won't bother too many people. Caviar, that costly curiosity, tips the scales both for cholesterol and fat content. But consider the amounts you may actually eat and the frequency of having a nibble, and most of us won't have to worry. The other is squid, also known as calamari. While low in fat, this seafood has as much cholesterol in a 3½-ounce serving as an egg yolk.

As I've often complained, when I ate little or no fish and lots of beef, the prices of fish were low and those of beef were high. Now the reverse is true. We can buy good steaks for much less than salmon or swordfish. But smart shoppers can enjoy seafood frequently without bending the budget at all.

First of all, all food prices are based on supply and demand. Many fish are in lesser demand. Try some of the less popular varieties such as monkfish, sand dabs, catfish, tilefish, rockfish, and many others. Talk with the person behind the counter to find out some tasty treats you wouldn't have considered otherwise. "Go with the flow" for fish that are in season and thus priced inexpensively.

Next, find some very acceptable alternatives. Swordfish can be replaced with shark steaks. Shark is especially delicious when broiled over the charcoal grill. Try it marinated in a teriyaki sauce made with low-sodium soy sauce, freshly grated ginger, cooking sherry, and just a little bit of garlic and brown sugar. Delicious!

Leave it to the Japanese to imitate some of the best things in life and bring them to those of us with champagne tastes and beer budgets. Their latest innovation is called *surimi*, an imitation crab product made from white fish such as pallock. Try it in salads and main dishes. And look for the soon-to-be-introduced imitation shrimp and scallops. These foods provide great nutrition with low fat and low cholesterol. Even if you're not a real fish lover, there must be some fish you can enjoy, at least two times each week. If you like tuna salad, try making it with canned salmon instead. Try a Caesar salad with bits of anchovies in the dressing. Moreover, you might find you like fish a whole lot more if you try it cooked a bit less; like any other meat, all the flavor and juiciness disappear when fish is overcooked.

GETTING THE LOWDOWN ON FATS AND OILS

By now you've probably heard that polyunsaturates and olive oil are good for your cholesterol levels, but we're also told to cut down on fats altogether. Does it really make any difference which oil we use to cook with? The answer is yes. But, when in comes to fats and oils, information and misinformation abound, leaving many consumers utterly confused. It's time to put fats and oils into perspective.

First, I'll get a pet peeve off my chest. *No* vegetable oil of any kind has any cholesterol at all. Period. Cholesterol comes from animal sources only. Thus, when a manufacturer claims that a brand of vegetable oil "has no cholesterol" it makes about as much sense as saying that water is wet. So much for that. Only those cooking fats from animal sources, such as bacon grease, butter, and lard, contain cholesterol. Avoid these as you would poison. So it is the fat, not the cholesterol, that we are concerned about in cooking oils.

Fats are one of three sources of energy in the diet, along with protein and carbohydrates. We need all three to remain healthy; but as discussed in Chapter 12, on nutrition, it's a matter of balance. Protein and carbohydrates provide four calories per gram, while fat supplies nine (and some researchers believe that the number may actually be as high as twelve). That's because the body uses fat far more efficiently than ever thought before. Needless to say, then, fat in the diet is a major source of calories and, very often, the reason why so many men and women are overweight. Cut back on fat and you won't be fat.

Just as protein is made up of a series of amino acids, fats and oils are composed of a variety of fatty acids. Each of those fatty acids is a molecule of carbon atoms with hydrogen atoms attached. The more hydrogen atoms attached to the carbons, the more the fatty acid is said to be saturated. In practical terms, if a fat remains in a liquid state at room temperature, it is unsaturated, while saturated fats are solid. The more saturated the fat, the harder it is.

Every fat and oil consists of a combination of saturated, polyunsaturated, and monounsaturated fatty acids. When we refer to a fat as saturated, that really means that the fat contains more saturated fatty acids than it does polyunsaturated or monounsaturated. Olive oil is referred to as monounsaturated because it contains a great proportion of monounsaturated fatty acids. Corn oil has more polyunsaturated fatty acids than olive oil, and we refer to it as being polyunsaturated. This can be confusing, especially when we hear that saturated fats such as coconut oil are more saturated than lard or beef fat, which we know have mostly saturated fat. This simply means that coconut oil contains a greater proportion of saturated fatty acids than do either lard or beef fat. I've listed a wide variety of fats and oils in Table 15 so you can compare the percentages of saturated, monounsaturated, and polyunsaturated fatty acids in each.

Many years ago, scientists learned that saturated, monounsaturated, and polyunsaturated fats have different effects on cholesterol levels.

The first significant information along these lines has by now become almost gospel throughout the land because we've heard it said so often. *Saturated fatty acids tend to raise cholesterol levels in the body.* That, in turn, results in the process of clogging of the arteries we call atherosclerosis.

The obvious recommendation, therefore, is to cut way back on saturated fats in the diet. To do so, many of us have reduced the amount of beef we eat, and have substituted margarine for butter. But we don't realize that a great amount of saturated fat we eat is hidden in foods we don't even think about.

Here's where reading the labels on the foods we buy in the supermarket becomes vitally important. Foods may be advertised as being cholesterol-free or made entirely with vegetable oils, but a closer inspection of the ingredient listing may reveal that those vegetable oils are in fact coconut oil, palm oil, or palm kernel oil. As you can see in Table 15, those contain a vast amount of saturated fatty acids and are, therefore, saturated fats.

Manufacturers like to use these tropical oils for a few reasons. They are very inexpensive imports, which are readily available at all times. They give foods made with them a long shelf life, since the saturated fats do not go rancid easily. And frequently they give food a good flavor. But there has been a tremendous public clamor recently to urge manufacturers to stop using those oils owing to their adverse effects on health, and many companies have responded favorably.

Responding to the tremendous public reaction against tropical oils, palm oil producers have placed ads in newspapers supporting the use of palm oil. They call palm oil a "balanced" oil with "only" 50 percent saturated fat. Now that you understand the chemistry you can see through such nonsensical claims easily. And therefore you'll want to avoid palm oil as well as palm kernel and coconut oils.

Frequently manufacturers of such polyunsaturated oils as corn, soybean, and cottonseed oil will "hydrogenate" or "partially hydrogenate" the oils, especially for use in baked goods. This prolongs the shelf life of the product and gives it a better taste and texture, but it also makes the fat more saturated. For this reason, in the earlier edition of this book, I recommended strictly limiting consumption of these products. But my opinion has changed considerably. To understand why, let's look at some recent research.

Dr. Scott Grundy at the University of Texas Health Sciences Center in Dallas has found that stearic acid, one of the saturated fats found in beef and chocolate, does not elevate cholesterol levels in the same way that other saturated fatty acids such as palmitic acid do. Does that mean that we're free to enjoy beef and chocolate in unlimited amounts? Not at all. Stearic acid is just one of a whole profile of fatty acids in those foods, and there's even more palmitic acid, which is really artery clogging. But his study does have important implications regarding hydrogenation. When manufacturers hydrogenate soybean oil and corn oil, the process leads to an increase in the percentage of monounsaturated fats and of stearic acid. Therefore, yes, the product does contain more saturated fat. However, since the specific hydrogenated fat created is stearic acid does not raise cholesterol levels any more than polyunsaturated acids, we don't have to worry about it.

Does this mean that we can eat unlimited amounts of such foods? Of course not. Even polyunsaturates and monounsaturates should be consumed in moderation.

We've known for some time that the higher the ratio of polyunsaturated fat to saturated fat, the greater the cholesterol-lowering effect. The opposite, of course, is also true. Therefore, medical authorities began advising us to consume more polyunsaturated fats and oils, and less of the saturated types. This made good sense and was proved effective in test after test.

The only problem that showed up was that a diet high in polyunsaturated fats, that is, one having a high P/S ratio, tends to also lower the level of the protective HDL. It was one of those damned if you do and damned if you don't situations.

Then along came some more information from research headed up by Dr. Grundy.

For years it has been known that there was little or no heart disease in the Mediterranean countries, and the cholesterol levels of Mediterranean people are traditionally low. The foods there are low in fat and cholesterol. The cooking oil used is primarily olive oil, a monounsaturated oil.

Interestingly, however, when one looks at the complete lipid profile of Mediterranean people, one finds that while the total cholesterol levels remain low, the HDL levels stay high. Therefore it appears that, by using olive oil instead of the polyunsaturated types such as corn oil, one can lower total cholesterol while preserving HDLs.

How does the lowering effect compare between the two oils? Dr. Grundy studied 20 patients who were fed either monounsaturated oils or the polyunsaturated type. Both were equally effective in reducing total blood cholesterol levels. Importantly, the levels of protective HDL did not drop with diets high in monounsaturated fats as they did with high-polyunsaturated-fat diets.

A number of studies have been done since then. We've seen that olive oil, when used to replace saturated fats, can be as effective as replacing the saturates with carbohydrates in terms of lowering cholesterol levels.

The consensus in the medical community today is that we should make an active effort to replace saturated fats with monounsaturates. Some go so far as to say that the saturated fats are the most important element in the cholesterol-raising equation, and that simply by replacing them with monounsaturates and polyunsaturates many individuals could consume a high percentage of calories as fat and still see significant cholesterol reductions.

I take a far more cautious approach. I believe that the general population would benefit from consuming more olive oil in place of, say, butter. We also know that no ill effect could come from this advice since we have a track record of centuries in the Mediterranean populations. But, for those with an already elevated cholesterol level, I believe the total fat in the diet should also be controlled.

As stated before, I think the ideal is 20 percent fat for those of us trying to get those cholesterol levels down significantly. And to reiterate what I've covered in Chapter 16, on regression, we need to see total cholesterol fall to well under 200 in order to see the disease process stopped or even reversed. Of that 20 percent, I believe the best approach is to reduce saturated fats to as low a level as possible on a long-term basis. Make up those fat calories with monunsaturated fats.

The best known of the monounsaturates is olive oil. I enjoy the flavor of olive oil in salads, used to sauté main courses, or on pasta, but sometimes the flavor of a particularly strong olive oil can get in the way of other ingredients in a recipe. To avoid this one can use one of the so-called "light" olive oils, which are no lighter in oil or fat content, but rather are light in flavor.

When it comes to choosing a vegetable oil for all-round cooking and baking purposes, I opt for canola oil. You'll see in Table 15 that this has the highest percentage of monounsaturated fats other than olive oil and is the oil lowest in saturated fatty acids. Canola oil is a new name for rapeseed oil. Since much of it is imported from Canada, it has been renamed canola. The best-selling brand in the super-market is Puritan.

Peanut oil is also high in monounsaturates, but contains more saturated fat than olive oil. We use peanut oil for our Chinese cooking.

Another oil to consider is a newcomer to the market. Dr. Shinjiro Suzuki, head of Japan's National Institute of Nutrition, has found that rice-bran oil can significantly lower cholesterol levels. After comparing the effects of several oils alone and in combination, Dr. Suzuki determined that a combination of 30 percent safflower oil and 70 percent rice-bran oil has the most potent effect. When he gave about one-half cup of the oil daily to a group of female volunteers, cholesterol levels fell by an average 26 percent. Watch for this oil in your health food stores and supermarkets.

You may have heard that we need a certain amount of polyunsaturated fat daily in order to provide a supply of the essential fatty acids oleic and linoleic. These cannot be made in the body from other fatty acids, and must come from the diet. That is absolutely true; however, we don't have to go out of our way to get them. As you can see in Table 15, all the fats and oils contain some polyunsaturated fats. Moreover, whole-grain breads and cereals are another source of these essential fatty acids. Don't worry about not getting enough.

The bottom line, then, is to avoid as much saturated fat as you can. Enjoy the foods that provide monounsaturated and polyunsaturated fats instead. Rest easy with the knowledge that you don't have to worry excessively about foods listing partially hydrogenated corn or soybean oil. Just limit your fat consumption to 20 percent of calories, and keep track by way of your personal formula for calculating your daily grams of fat. See page 113 for that equation.

Well, before sitting down to that meal of fish sautéed in olive oil, bean soup, and perhaps some oat-bran muffins or rolls, how about a cocktail?

IS ALCOHOL GOOD FOR CHOLESTEROL LEVELS?

For some time now, researchers have observed that moderate alcohol intake is associated with a lowered rate of heart disease. At first no one knew why this was the case, but a closer look demonstrated that a little daily drink raises the protective HDL level. Actually, to be precise, alcohol tends to raise the so-called apolipoprotein component of HDL.

How much is enough and how much is too much? Moderation is the key word. Moderate alcohol intake has been defined as about 1½ ounces of alcohol in the drink of choice. Having that martini before dinner, or a glass of wine or beer with dinner, or a nightcap snifter of brandy seems to be perfectly acceptable. But doctors hurry to say that they do *not* suggest that previous teetotalers start to tipple. These data merely indicate the safety of moderation in alcohol consumption for those who do choose to imbibe.

Bear in mind, however, that recent studies have been completed which show the toxic effects of immoderate alcohol usage. Cardiologists at the University of Chicago have shown that three drinks of 90-proof scotch at one sitting have a definite negative effect on heart function.

To my mind, it's nice to know that we have some very interesting choices to make when shopping in the supermarket. Scientists have provided the knowledge we need to avoid the foods that are harmful and to choose those with excellent nutrient contributions and cholesterol-lowering potentials.

AND NOW A WORD ABOUT SODIUM . . .

Just as cholesterol has been positively associated with heart disease in as much as half the population, sodium is associated with hypertension, or high blood pressure. To explain very briefly, sodium is essential in the diet in small quantities in order to preserve blood volume and pressure by attracting and holding water in the blood vessels. But for many individuals too much sodium brings the blood pressure too high. Actually, two things happen. First, the sodium results in the body's inability to excrete water properly. That's why doctors often prescribe diuretics for hypertensive patients. Second, there is a long physiological process by which the kidney produces chemical substances that directly elevate pressure in the arteries.

Thirty million men and women have frank hypertension, and another 30 million are "borderline" hypertensives. The problem is that no one knows who will develop high blood pressure. Many people have the disease without even knowing it. That's why health authorities have recommended that all of us should reduce our sodium intake.

How much is too much? The National Research Council indicates that a "safe and adequate" daily sodium intake is about 1,100 to

3,300 milligrams for adults. To put that into perspective, one teaspoon of salt contains about 2,000 milligrams of sodium. And estimates place sodium consumption by adults in the U.S. at from 2,300 to 6,900 milligrams daily.

Salt is the principal source of sodium in our diets. But one must also consider the input of sodium from food preservatives and curatives such as sodium nitrite, sodium nitrate, and sodium benzoate. In addition, many Oriental foods contain a large amount of the flavor enhancer MSG, monosodium glutamate. Soy sauce is another source.

Some authorities estimate that as much as one-third of our sodium comes from salt added either during cooking or at the table. How significant is that shake of the salt shaker? Try this for yourself. Shake out some salt over an empty plate as though you were seasoning food. Then collect the salt and measure it. If you used about ⅛ teaspoon, that amounts to 250 milligrams of sodium.

You've probably heard this before, but it's worth repeating. Salt is an acquired taste and habit. Absolutely *no* added salt is needed in the diet. Sodium is naturally occurring in many, many foods throughout the diet, and levels consumed in normal eating habits provide more than enough. Many of us salt our food before even tasting it. Weaning ourselves from the shaker may be difficult at first, but after not too long a time our taste perceptions begin to change. Soon the natural flavors of foods predominate, and, at the very least, we need to add less salt. The first step is to take the salt shaker off the table. There are a wide variety of seasonings that can easily replace salt. Try some garlic powder, a pinch of pepper, or a squeeze of lemon.

Next, start to pay more attention to the labels on foods in the supermarket. All prepared and processed foods today have a prominent nutrient label that states the sodium content. And because so many of us are trying to limit the sodium in our diets, manufacturers are now offering low-sodium and reduced-sodium alternatives. One can even buy low-sodium soy sauce.

Cheese is a major source of sodium in many diets. One ounce of American cheese contains 406 milligrams. And that same slice of cheese also comes loaded with nearly 9 grams of fat, practically all saturated. The best advice about cheese is to avoid it completely.

As with cholesterol, knowledge of content levels is an important step in controlling sodium intake. Table 11 included in Chapter 4, "Winning by the Numbers," also lists the sodium content of foods.

If you are already under a doctor's supervision for hypertension, by all means follow his or her advice and recommendations. If you don't know your blood pressure, make the small effort to find out.

High blood pressure has no symptoms. You cannot "know" when the pressure inside your arteries rises. This is truly a silent killer, resulting in strokes and heart attacks often without warning.

Even if you find that your blood pressure is currently normal, it's wise to consider a sodium-limited diet. Simply enough, you cannot know whether you are prone to developing the disease later in life. Why take the chance for the sake of a seasoning?

While you're limiting your sodium, think about yet another bit of very interesting research data done by Dr. David McCarron at the Oregon Health Sciences University. In studying patients with hypertension, he found that the disease correlated not only with high sodium intake but also with low calcium intake. Dr. McCarron speculates that the two minerals may be involved in a balance; if one is out of balance, blood pressure can be affected. His suggestion is to increase the calcium intake in the diet.

Although this theory remains controversial, and certainly it should not be construed as a denial of the importance of sodium moderation, increasing calcium in the diet can do no harm but can do much good, for we all need calcium throughout our lives. Certainly there has been considerable publicity given to the problem of osteoporosis for women, whose bones slowly demineralize with the passage of time.

There are a number of calcium-rich dairy foods that are also low in fat and cholesterol. Two servings of nonfat milk or low-fat yogurt a day provide much of the calcium needed for good health. Women, especially, may also require a calcium supplement.

Ultimately, the most marvelous word in nutrition is moderation. We are blessed today with an abundance and variety of foods never before imagined. We can have strawberries in the winter and squash in the summer. Fish from oceans and streams across the country and around the world can be on our tables every night of the week if we choose. Many of those foods in our supermarkets can control and even improve our blood lipid profiles. Let's enjoy them all in moderation, with a toast to good health and well-being!

Table 14. **Omega-3 Fatty-Acid Content of 3¹/₂-Ounce Servings of Fish**

	GRAMS		GRAMS
Sardines (Norwegian)	5.1	Bluefish	1.2
Sockeye salmon	2.7	Pacific mackerel	1.1
Atlantic mackerel	2.5	Striped bass	0.8
King salmon	1.9	Yellowfin tuna	0.6
Herring	1.7	Pollock	0.5
Lake trout	1.4	Brook trout	0.4
Albacore tuna	1.3	Yellow perch	0.3
Halibut	1.3	Catfish	0.2

Table 15. **Comparison of Dietary Fats and Oils**

Type	SATURATED FATTY ACIDS (% OF TOTAL)*	MONOUNSATURATED FATTY ACIDS (% OF TOTAL)*	POLYUNSATURATED FATTY ACIDS (% OF TOTAL)*
Canola oil	6	62	32
Walnut oil	9	23	64
Safflower oil	10	13	77
Sunflower oil	11	20	69
Corn oil	13	25	62
Olive oil	14	77	9
Soybean oil	15	24	61
Peanut oil	18	49	33
Margarine (tub)	18	47	31
Cottonseed oil	27	19	54

Tuna fat	27	26	21
Chicken fat	30	45	11
Margarine (stick)	31	47	22
Shortening (can)	31	51	14
Lard	40	45	11
Mutton fat	47	41	8
Palm oil	49	37	9
Beef fat	50	42	4
Butterfat	62	29	4
Palm kernel oil	81	11	2
Coconut oil	86	6	2

*Percentages are averaged and thus may not total exactly 100 percent.

8

Winning by Losing

Following the nutrition advice in this book will ensure that you can eat all you want of the right foods, with no feelings of hunger, and never gain a single pound. Simply enough, you'll be eating the foods that are lower in calories and, especially, lower in fat content. If you're a few pounds overweight now, that weight will slowly disappear. In our research, those who were compliant with the program lost weight in just weeks—and while eating a wide variety of satisfying foods.

But, if you have a significant amount of weight to lose, more than fifteen pounds or so, it will be worth your while to pay special attention to your diet. Again, you can do this without ever feeling hungry or deprived. It's just a matter of tipping your eating patterns more in favor of those foods that will help you lose those pounds.

It's worth the effort. You'll see the immediate benefits in the mirror, and you'll love the compliments you'll get—not to speak of the added confidence you'll feel, and the increased vitality. But there are even more important reasons to attain and maintain your ideal weight.

First of all, just reducing down to the ideal weight for your size will automatically reduce your cholesterol level. How this happens is not fully known, but as weight falls, cholesterol levels fall. It may have something to do with the sequence of blood fat storage. Blood pressure is also greatly affected by weight. If you have diabetes, your need for drugs will decrease. And you'll vastly improve your shot at longevity.

These are not idle promises. They're backed up by the findings of the nation's most recognized authorities in the medical and scientific communities. In an article published in 1984 in the *Annals of Internal Medicine*, Drs. Artemis Simopoulos and Theodore Van Itallie, writing for the Nutrition Coordinating Committee of the National Institutes of Health, concluded that the weight associated with the "greatest longevity tends to be below the average weight of the population." Speaking even more strongly, they say that "overweight persons tend to die sooner than average-weight persons."

The fourteen-member panel of the NIH concluded in 1985 that the 34 million Americans who are more than 20 percent overweight should be treated for obesity. The panel chairman, Jules Hirsch, M.D., said that "Fat is not just a cosmetic affair—a concern of especially vain Americans. At surprisingly low levels, it's a biologic hazard." He estimated that half the medical problems seen in overweight patients in doctors' offices are obesity related.

The evidence has been building for a long time. The Provident Mutual Life Insurance Company studied male policyholders from 1947 to 1964. In every group, the mortality rate increased with weight. The more overweight, the more likely to die prematurely.

Investigators involved in the famous Framingham Heart Study showed a linear relationship between obesity and coronary heart disease. That study also demonstrated a direct link between obesity and total mortality.

Dr. Hirsch went so far as to say that "Obesity is a killer. It is a killer just as smoking is." Another panel member, Dr. Harriet P. Dustan, Professor of Medicine at the University of Alabama in Birmingham, said that about 40 percent of new cases of hypertension in whites and 28 percent in blacks could be prevented if weight were to be controlled.

The American Cancer Society concluded after a long-term study that the lowest mortality rates occurred in persons weighing 80 to 89 percent of the average weight. And literally every national and international medical and health organization has stated again and again that overweight individuals are at the greatest health risk.

What is ideal weight? Certainly a man who is six feet tall can weigh 180 to 190 pounds without being overweight—and we've all heard the joke about the doctor who tells the patient that he or she isn't too heavy, just too short! Various tables and charts have been devised to determine and identify ideal or desirable weights. Most authorities prefer the guidelines developed by the Metropolitan Life Insurance Company in 1959. Table 16 lists weights according to body-frame type for men and women. But, if you're seriously overweight, you really don't need a table or chart to tell you.

There is no "magic" about weight control. It's all a matter of proven, hard-nosed science. Weight gain is one of the laws of nature. You just can't break those laws. No matter how many times you drop an apple from a tree, it's going to fall to the ground. That's the law of gravity. You can't break it. And the same thing goes for weight gain. Or weight loss.

Here's a simple fact. Not much fun, but a good, solid example. If you watch every calorie you eat every single day, go through the ritual of dry toast and skim milk for breakfast, cottage cheese and tomatoes for lunch, and a nice nutritious, low-fat dinner for supper, you may be just fine.

But let's say you keep eating those good foods, exercising the same amount, sleeping the same hours, and keeping everything else equal. Only now you start having just one doughnut for your coffee break. Not a big one, just a medium-sized doughnut. Not covered with chocolate, just plain. That's 100 calories. In thirty-five days, about a month, you'll take in an extra 3500 calories. And you'll gain a pound. After a year you'll gain over ten pounds. Just because of that one little doughnut. That's the "Doughnut Law."

Actually, scientists have another name for it. They call this a law of thermodynamics. If you take in calories, a measure of energy, you will either expend them as energy or the body will store them as fat.

No matter how much we learn about nutrition, the basics still apply. All food can be measured in terms of the energy supplied. Protein and carbohydrates provide 4 calories per gram. Fat yields 9 calories per gram. Alcohol supplies 7 calories per gram. Obviously, then, those eating less fat and more complex carbohydrates—starches rather than sugars—will take in fewer calories.

For the average adult male, it takes 15 calories per day per pound of body weight to maintain the same weight. Let's say that hypothetical man weighs 150 pounds. That means he must consume 2250 calories daily in order not to lose or gain any weight. But let's take another hypothetical case of the man who wants to weigh 150 pounds, but currently tips the scales at 180. If he, too, eats at the 2250-calorie-per-day level, eventually he'll weigh 150. The food eaten still maintains the 150 pounds, and the rest gradually disappears. And he can speed up the process by cutting his calories back even further.

Of course, every situation differs. If one is far more active than the average person, more calories will be needed to maintain weight. Completely sedentary individuals need fewer calories. As one gets older, the need for caloric energy decreases. And, unfortunately, the needs for women are less than those for men. An average, moderately active adult woman needs not 15 but only 12 calories per pound of ideal body weight.

The sad truth is that most people who try to lose weight fail. And most people who do lose weight gain it back almost immediately. In one study done in 1983, 43 percent of all Americans went on diets; 53 percent of all women did so. Of those, 35 percent started their diets six times or more that year alone.

Physicians often consider treating obesity one of the least rewarding efforts because of the high failure rate. Weight loss has become one of the biggest health related industries.

In the long run, diets simply do not work. Going on a diet normally implies eventually going off that diet. In the meantime, nothing has happened to change the poor eating habits that led to obesity in the first place. The only way to lose weight permanently is to completely change one's attitudes and approaches toward food. Certainly that's not easy. Nor is it easy to quit smoking cigarettes. But both are necessary for anyone who really wants good health and long life.

The first step is to take a really close look at your current eating habits. Do this by starting today to keep a daily log of everything you eat and drink. Keep track for two weeks. I recommend carrying a little note pad in your pocket or purse. Don't trust your memory. Jot down even the tiniest nibble.

Then look at your diary with objective eyes. What foods can be completely eliminated? What foods can be replaced? What foods can you cut down on? Buy one of those little calorie counters. What foods have the most calories?

At the same time, follow the recommendations in Chapter 4 to cut out much of the fat in your diet. Keeping the diet diary will also help you watch the fat and cholesterol.

For the next week or two, make the adjustments in your eating patterns. Continue to keep a diary. See how much you've improved. Ask yourself whether there are foods that really don't belong on your table anymore.

Don't delude yourself that for you it is completely impossible to lose weight. Cruel as it may sound, if you stopped eating completely you would eventually starve to death. But at some point between now and then you would be at your ideal weight.

That's not to say that fasting is the way to go. Although some doctors have used this approach under careful supervision, it can be dangerous. Moreover, the basic eating patterns do not change because, after all, eventually one must begin eating again. Ultimately, any type of calorie-restricted diet will achieve weight loss. The fewer calories consumed, the faster the weight loss. Whenever you follow a highly restricted diet, it's best to take a complete vitamin/mineral supplement.

For a short period of time, not more than seven days, you can take a "break" from normal eating. You may, for example, decide to limit your daily intake to just the three oat-bran muffins. Eat one for breakfast, lunch, and dinner. Wash each one down with a glass of skim milk. Drink lots and lots of water throughout the day.

Each muffin has about 150 calories when made with lots of fruit and sweetened with apple-juice concentrate. You can cut the calories down a bit by making them plainer. An eight-ounce glass of skim milk has about 100 calories. So the daily calorie intake on such a program would be about 675 calories. At that rate, you would lose weight quickly.

If that sounds too difficult, try adding some fruit juice to the diet, and an apple for the mid-morning snack. And a big salad with a squeeze of lemon or lime juice in the evening. You'll still be at about 1000 calories.

Interestingly, if you take this approach you can gradually build your diet up from the basic three-muffin-a-day plan to the total calories you will eventually need to maintain your ideal weight. For the hypothetical 150-pound man we spoke of earlier, this means that he can add another 1250 calories to the 1000 calories above. Those 1250 calories can come from breads, cereals, fruits, vegetables, and, of course, some meats, poultry, and fish. All that food for a reasonable amount of caloric intake.

The best part of having oat-bran muffins as the basic foundation of your diet is that they are incredibly satisfying. The reason is that oat bran absorbs a lot of water in the digestive tract. As it soaks up the water, it expands, filling the stomach and giving one that satisfied "full" feeling.

Because of this property of oat bran, it's best to drink a lot of water. Eight eight-ounce glasses a day would be best for everyone, regardless of other dietary considerations. The advice from your school nurse back in elementary school still holds today: you just can't drink too many fluids. If you don't like water, club soda with a squeeze of lime also counts. As do coffee, tea, and all other beverages. Make your selections wisely. Choose low-sodium club soda. Pick decaffeinated coffee and tea. Limit the number of high-calorie beverages. A six-ounce serving of apple juice contains more than 90 calories. And, while beer and other alcoholic beverages do contain water, they also provide a lot of calories.

Many people today take diuretics on their doctors' orders to help control blood pressure. Often those men and women make the mistake of thinking that, since the pills help drain water from the body, they shouldn't drink extra water because it would defeat the purpose of the pills. Not true at all. The pills control the amount of water stored in the tissues. The water taken daily as beverages will be naturally excreted in the urine by the kidneys. Ask your doctor if you have any doubts or questions. He or she will agree that more water in your diet is not only acceptable, it is advisable.

No matter what you weigh or how many calories you are consuming, it's important to keep the metabolic rate up. A frustrating physiological phenomenon that occurs when people try to diet is that the body compensates for reduced food intake by burning calories more slowly. Actually this is the body's natural way to deal with times of famine and starvation. When there is less food available, less energy is consumed and burned by the tissues.

To get around this, one must become more active, to reach the next level of calorie burning. For most people this can be done merely by taking a walk once a day. If you haven't already done so this would be a good time to begin a regular exercise program as described in Chapter 9, "Exercise Your Options for Long Life."

In a study done at Stanford University, fourteen sedentary middle-aged men were asked to run as much as they could and to eat as much as they wanted. Over a two-year period of time, they ran an average of twelve miles a week. That also happens to be just right for cardiovascular fitness. They increased their calorie intake by 15 percent. In the process, however, their proportion of body fat fell from 21.6 percent to 18 percent. In addition, the levels of their blood lipids dropped significantly.

Take a good look at the foods you're eating. Go into the supermarket and look for good alternatives. Think of all the fruits and vegetables grown all over the world that you've never tried before. If you were on a luxurious vacation on some tropical island and went to a buffet dinner, the table wouldn't be laden with Twinkies and cupcakes, would it? You'd find fruits of all kinds, shapes, and colors and you'd think it was delicious. So go to that supermarket and pretend you're on a tropical island!

Another food that works well for those trying to lose weight is soup. First of all, soup is an excellent way to get more vegetables into your diet. It's a nice alternative to having salad all the time. Pick the types that are not loaded with cream and butter, of course. And soup takes time to eat—one spoonful at a time. You'll eat less that way, and set a slower pace for the other foods you'll eat at that meal.

A study done with soup eaters showed that they ate an average of 5 percent fewer calories for the day. Now 5 percent may not sound like much, but keep adding it up and it becomes significant. Just as having an extra doughnut a day puts the weight on, soup can help take it off.

While we're talking about how fast one eats food, remember that it takes about twenty minutes from the time you eat a morsel of food to the time the body absorbs it into the blood to give that satisfied feeling. So give yourself time before reaching for that second helping.

Speaking of timing, remember how your mother always told you never to eat before dinner because you'd spoil your appetite? Well, this is the time to disobey your mother, and get your daily dose of oat bran at the same time. Twenty minutes before each meal, eat an oat-bran muffin. You'll find that one muffin, washed down with a glass of water or a cup of coffee (preferably the decaffeinated type) will effectively cut down your appetite and you'll eat less food during the meal to come.

If you prefer to eat your muffins at breakfast, try having a piece of bread or a small piece of fruit before meals. The same principle applies.

When it's time to sit down for that meal, think of the behavior-modification techniques you've probably heard many times before. This time, actually start to practice these techniques. They really work.

Start by using a smaller plate to make your meals look larger. Eat at the same times each day. When you eat, concentrate on your food, not the TV or a magazine. Always sit down to eat; never nibble away at the counter. In general, these techniques help you focus on how much you actually are eating.

You'll find that you'll enjoy your foods more when you take the time to taste them rather than gulping them down. Take small pieces. Put down your fork between bites. Chew each mouthful fully before the next bite.

Many overweight individuals have no idea how many calories they take in each day while snacking. Keep that diet diary and see for yourself. Is the midnight snack your downfall? Do you destroy all your good intentions with a candy bar in the evening?

Here are a couple of ways to think about snacks. Instead of having an ordinary candy bar, treat yourself royally: have strawberries skewered on fancy toothpicks. Or arrange orange slices on a nice platter with a maraschino cherry for color. Now and then splurge on something special like raspberries, or melon out of season. You're saving money not buying fat foods, so you have the extra grocery money.

The experts refer to the next step in changing our behaviors and attitudes "cognitive restructuring." In simpler English that simply means learning to think positively rather than negatively about our diets—and everything else in our lives.

Interestingly, most of us at one time or another start to see things in a gloomy, negative way. Just by becoming aware of it we can change the way we think. How does this apply to eating habits and staying at ideal weight? Let's look at some examples.

Negative: It takes *forever* to lose weight.
Positive: I *am* losing weight and I *will* be slender.

Negative: I've tried all sorts of things that failed.
Positive: This is *the* answer I've been looking for.

Negative: I hate giving up snacking.
Positive: I love these beautiful strawberries.

Negative: I keep thinking about chocolates and cheese.
Positive: I keep thinking about my weight falling.

Negative: This is so hard for me to change.

Positive: I'm so glad to be headed in
                  the right direction!

If any of those negative statements sounds
like something you might have thought, it's
time to start some "cognitive restructuring."
Think positive!

While you're thinking along positive lines,
try a simple mental exercise. Each day spend a
bit of time, perhaps five to ten minutes, completely alone in a darkened, quiet place. Close
your eyes. Relax. Let your body loosen up.
Concentrate on slow, regular, deep breathing.
Then picture yourself when you've lost
twenty, twenty-five, thirty pounds or whatever. Imagine how your friends and loved ones
will react.

Each day, picture yourself thin. What will
you do? Will you buy some new clothes? How
will you reward yourself with something other
than food?

Start thinking also about your levels of cholesterol. Close your eyes and picture the blood
actually becoming "cleansed" of those dangerous lipids.

Those who succeed in any of life's ventures
have a very positive outlook. They think of
themselves as successes and never doubt that
they'll succeed. Our research has proven without a doubt that cholesterol levels *can* be re-

duced to completely normal levels. And thousands of people have successfully lost weight and kept it off. You can too!

You certainly don't need any of the well-advertised fads for losing weight. Most of the things you hear about don't work, except to make money for those selling the books or the pills. What's really behind the promises?

Let's start with the major diets, usually promoted in order to sell books written by people who have terrific smiles and winning ways on TV talk shows.

Dr. Atkins' Diet Revolution is one of the latest of the high-fat, high-protein, low-carbohydrate diets. You can eat all the rich meats, cheeses, and ice creams you want . . . just give up breads and rolls. A "revolution"? Not at all. This idea first came up in the nineteenth century, called the Banting Diet. Then it was the Drinking Man's Diet, the Air Force Diet, the Mayo Clinic Diet, and the Calories Don't Count Diet. Does it work? Well, yes, for a while. You'll excrete a lot of water. Does the weight stay off? No, it comes right back when you return to normal eating patterns. Is it safe? Because it includes excessive amounts of fat and protein it can result in higher blood cholesterol levels as well as the short-term problem of the development of ketosis, a condition similar to diabetic shock. The American

Medical Association has roundly condemned this as a truly dangerous toxin-producing diet, which can result in permanent damage to the body and heart.

Dr. Stillman's Quick Inches Off Diet and other low-protein, high-carbohydrate diets are reissues of a 1948 fad called the Rice Diet. Once again, you *can* lose weight temporarily by water loss. But you'll put it right back on when you return to previous habits and endanger yourself in the process by following a nutritionally deficient diet plan.

The *Scarsdale Diet* is dangerous to use without medical supervision. Even the author said to use it for only fourteen days. It's one of the so-called "ketogenic" diets, which supposedly burn off fat directly into the urine. Again, you have a lot of water loss, you lose protein tissue, and you expose yourself to some of the same dangers faced by diabetics whose bodies have unbalanced metabolisms. How can you control your weight for the rest of your life with a diet designed for fourteen days? You can't.

The *Last Chance Diet* was literally the last diet for nearly sixty women who dieted with a liquid protein formula. They died as a result. Needless to say, authorities have cautioned the public against using this approach.

Fasting Is a Way of Life can also mean the end of *your* life if followed faithfully. A one-day fast is perhaps not dangerous, but fasting as a way of life can result in very serious problems if followed for prolonged periods. But probably you'll never get that far since, like most of these diets, this is so boring and difficult that you'll be back to your old ways soon. And that means regaining all the weight you painfully shed.

The *Cambridge Diet* is a powder that one mixes to form a beverage as part of a diet program. (There is no book that accompanies the program.) While the diet can result in weight loss, it doesn't teach how to handle regular foods properly, so when returning to the use of these foods, the weight all too frequently returns. First you buy the book. Then you buy the formula. Then you lose a little weight. Then you get bored with the same dull pattern of drinking every meal. Then you start to cheat. Then you drop the diet completely. And gain back all your weight.

The *Beverly Hills Diet* tells you that certain combinations of fruits "magically melt" fat. Hogwash. Everyone with the slightest knowledge of nutrition and physiology got a good laugh reading this book. Any weight loss is due to the diarrhea you're likely to get from eating inordinate amounts of fruit and excluding other foods. The same applies to the *Fit for Life* diet.

The *Dolly Parton Diet* limits you to certain foods on certain days. This is difficult if not impossible to follow for life, and can lead to serious medical problems. On day four of the diet you eat nothing but bananas and skim milk. Sound like fun?

The *Zen Macrobiotic Diet* was popular a few years ago and comes back on the scene now and then. Gradually you limit your total diet to only grains. Nothing else. Many fanatic religious followers of the developer of this diet have died as a result. This is nothing to count on as a way of permanent weight control.

The *Pritikin Program* is a severely restricted diet. While it can be effective both for weight control and for reducing cholesterol levels, most individuals are unable to follow the program for prolonged periods of time. Strict adherents to the diet develop sallow skin and lackluster hair. HDL levels are also compromised by ultra-low-fat diets.

So much for the books and the special diet plans. How about those heavily advertised diet aids?

Human Chorionic Gonadotropin (HCG) was first proposed by a Dr. Simeons in 1954. You still see clinics advertising regular, expensive injections of hormones extracted from the urine of pregnant women. And you have to follow a 500-calorie diet. The diet works, but research has shown no difference between the diet alone and the diet with shots. The reason for effectiveness, if any, is that people get motivated to stay on the diet when they've spent so much money for the injections.

Herbal Body Wraps make you feel pampered and relaxed. Some are done for "spot" reducing, some for the entire body. Weight loss? Sure, just like after sitting in a sauna. You lose fluids. You lose weight. You drink water. You gain the weight back.

Starch Blockers are sold as a food that acts as a drug. The Food and Drug Administration of the U.S. would like to put all its promoters out of business. Users of the product have complained of nausea, vomiting, diarrhea, and stomach pains. Supposedly these starch blockers inhibit enzyme production and foods pass through undigested. A very unhealthy idea even if they did work. Our goal should be to *improve* digestion of foods!

Glucomannan has been heavily advertised as the secret from the Orient. It is a food in Japan, which the promoters say keeps Asians slim. The FDA is trying to shut down this operation, claiming that the product as it's being sold is really a drug prepared from the konjac root, not a food. But does it work? Preliminary studies seem to reveal that by eating the glucomannan people eat less other food. But in and of itself, the product is not effective.

Amphetamines are prescription drugs that have been used for years to curb the appetite. As with many of the over-the-counter imitations that have sprung up, the effectiveness of these drugs lasts for only days—two weeks at most. Yes, you'll eat less for that period. But, unless you change your dietary habits, you'll slip right back into your weight-gaining mode when you stop taking the pills. Side effects include extreme nervousness, speeding up of the heart rate, sleeplessness, and, if abused, death. The Food and Drug Administration has publicly stated the desire to remove these products from the marketplace and is moving in that direction. The most frequently encountered ingredient in over-the-counter weight loss preparations is phenylpropanolamine.

What about the various professional services you see advertised? Those spas and salons and centers? Read the ads carefully and you'll soon find out that no miracles are being sold. What frequently is sold is prepackaged food. You buy a week's supply at a time, with portions already determined. You may not like the choices they offer in terms of the fat and cholesterol levels. And you'll probably stop buying all your food at the center. And that means going back to the old ways, which led to the problem in the first place.

Other salons offer "professional" guidance to help you stay on a very-low-calorie diet. Not bad for an idea, if you feel you really need the help and don't have the willpower yourself. But brace yourself for some big expenses.

On the other hand, there are many self-help groups that offer worthwhile, genuine assistance. Some of these can be found in YMCA and YWCA groups. Weight Watchers is an effective program that stresses the notion of life-long habit changes. The same applies to the TOPS (Take Off Pounds Sensibly) program. These are also fine in terms of limiting fats and cholesterol. They have helped thousands of men and women over the years.

Essential to any approach to weight loss and weight control is a moderate intake of calories equal to the expenditure of calories in your life. Moderation can be delicious when one considers all the marvelous foods available to us. This is one time that when you lose you're the real winner!

Table 16. Desirable Weights for Men and Women

HEIGHT (WITH SHOES)	WEIGHT (IN INDOOR CLOTHING)		
	SMALL FRAME	MEDIUM FRAME	LARGE FRAME
men			
5 ft. 2 in.	112–120 lbs.	118–129 lbs.	126–141 lbs.
5 ft. 3 in.	115–123 lbs.	121–133 lbs.	129–144 lbs.
5 ft. 4 in.	118–126 lbs.	124–136 lbs.	132–148 lbs.
5 ft. 5 in.	121–129 lbs.	127–139 lbs.	135–152 lbs.
5 ft. 6 in.	124–133 lbs.	130–143 lbs.	138–156 lbs.
5 ft. 7 in.	128–137 lbs.	134–147 lbs.	142–161 lbs.
5 ft. 8 in.	132–141 lbs.	138–152 lbs.	147–166 lbs.
5 ft. 9 in.	136–145 lbs.	142–156 lbs.	151–170 lbs.
5 ft. 10 in.	140–150 lbs.	146–160 lbs.	155–174 lbs.
5 ft. 11 in.	144–154 lbs.	150–165 lbs.	159–179 lbs.
6 ft. 0 in.	148–158 lbs.	154–170 lbs.	164–184 lbs.
6 ft. 1 in.	152–162 lbs.	158–175 lbs.	168–189 lbs.
6 ft. 3 in.	156–167 lbs.	162–180 lbs.	173–194 lbs.
6 ft. 3 in.	160–171 lbs.	167–185 lbs.	178–199 lbs.
6 ft. 4 in.	164–175 lbs.	172–190 lbs.	182–204 lbs.
women			
4 ft. 10 in.	92–98 lbs.	96–107 lbs.	104–119 lbs.
4 ft. 11 in.	94–101 lbs.	98–110 lbs.	106–122 lbs.
5 ft. 0 in.	96–104 lbs.	101–113 lbs.	109–125 lbs.
5 ft. 1 in.	99–107 lbs.	104–116 lbs.	112–128 lbs.
5 ft. 2 in.	102–110 lbs.	107–119 lbs.	115–131 lbs.
5 ft. 3 in.	105–113 lbs.	110–122 lbs.	118–134 lbs.
5 ft. 4 in.	108–116 lbs.	113–126 lbs.	121–138 lbs.

5 ft. 5 in.	111–119 lbs.	116–130 lbs.	125–142 lbs.
5 ft. 6 in.	114–123 lbs.	120–135 lbs.	129–146 lbs.
5 ft. 7 in.	118–127 lbs.	124–139 lbs.	133–150 lbs.
5 ft. 8 in.	122–131 lbs.	128–143 lbs.	137–154 lbs.
5 ft. 9 in.	126–135 lbs.	132–147 lbs.	141–158 lbs.
5 ft. 10 in.	130–140 lbs.	136–151 lbs.	145–163 lbs.
5 ft. 11 in.	134–144 lbs.	140–155 lbs.	149–168 lbs.
6 ft. 0 in.	138–148 lbs.	144–159 lbs.	153–173 lbs.

SOURCE: Prepared by the Metropolitan Life Insurance Company. Derived primarily from data of the *Build and Blood Pressure Study, 1959*, Society of Actuaries.

9

Exercise Your Options
for Long Life

To exercise or not to exercise. For an ever-increasing number of people of all ages that is no longer the question. When the Gallup Organization did a survey they found 66 percent in the 18-to-29 age group exercising regularly. A full 54 percent of the entire population now does some kind of workout.

Those sweating masses appear to be on the right track. Dr. Ralph Paffenbarger, speaking of his research published in the March 6, 1986, *New England Journal of Medicine,* said those who regularly exercise throughout their lives add from one to more than two years to their lives. Those are average numbers, with some individuals expected to tack on ten or even twenty years of living. Put another way, Dr. Paffenbarger said that every hour spent exercising will be returned in added life, with an extra hour as a dividend. You just can't beat that kind of investment.

Three separate studies have now provided definitive proof that regular aerobic exercise improves the health of the heart. These research studies used animals rather than people for the very simple reason that animals could be sacrificed so their hearts could be examined.

One study at the University of California used pigs, whose hearts and circulatory systems are similar to ours. A coronary artery was artificially blocked in each of eighteen animals. Nine were then strenuously exercised on a treadmill for five months; the other nine did no exercise. At autopsy, the hearts of the exercised pigs showed twice the development of collateral vessels. That's important because, when an artery is blocked, no blood can get through. Collateral vessels can form a kind of natural bypass around the blockage, providing the needed blood flow. A good system of collateral vessels can sometimes prevent a heart attack and can lessen the likelihood of death should a heart attack occur.

For many years, advocates of regular exercise have cited the development of collateral circulation as a major benefit. Now we have the proof.

In a second study, physical exercise was shown to protect against sudden cardiac death. This work was conducted at the University of Oklahoma, using dogs that had had previous heart attacks. Some were given exercise and others were not. After just six weeks of training, all the dogs were put on the treadmill for testing. None of the exercising dogs showed any cardiac arrhythmia or ventricular fibrillation, signs of weakened or malfunctioning hearts, while seven of eight nonexercising dogs showed those signs.

A third study showed the benefits of exercise for those with high blood pressure. At Montefiore Hospital in New York ten rats were put on a program of regular swimming while another ten remained sedentary. All had high blood pressure. Cardiac function returned to normal in all the rat swimmers.

For those of us concerned about the risk factor of cholesterol, there is more heartening news. It appears that strenuous exercise on a regular basis can elevate the protective levels of HDL. A study reported in the *Journal of the American Medical Association* indicates that's even true for older men and women. Participants in that study showed an HDL increase from 52 ± 5 to 58 ± 6, enough to strongly affect the total cholesterol/HDL ratio, indicating protection from coronary heart disease.

Writing in *Circulation* in July 1988, researchers reported that eight to eleven months of exercise training in previously sedentary men boosted HDL levels by an average of 5 mg/dl. Some men experienced as much as an 8 mg/dl rise, while others gained only

2 mg/dl. But even a little improvement in HDL levels can mean a significant change in the very important ratio of total cholesterol to HDL. In this particular study, body fat and body weight didn't change. The men exercised on stationary bicycles at 80 percent of their maximum heart rate for one hour a day, five days a week for the first fourteen weeks of the program and four days weekly thereafter. The average 13 percent increase of HDL levels significantly improved the cholesterol ratios and thus provided additional protection against heart disease. The authors discussed the fact that elite athletes have been shown to have HDL levels 10 to 20 mg/dl higher than sedentary individuals.

Researchers at Stanford University studied the influence of dieting and exercise by way of running on weight and blood lipids in a one-year project and reported their results in the November 3, 1988, issue of the *New England Journal of Medicine.* Both dieters and exercisers showed significant weight loss and improvements in their HDL levels. These were not big gains, average increases being a bit more than 0.4 mg/dl. No doubt one requires fairly serious exercise to show significant HDL improvements, but every little bit helps.

It appears that so-called resistive training, that is, the use of weights or machinery such as Nautilus equipment, can also increase HDL levels. Reporting in *Medicine and Science in Sports and Exercise,* researchers described a study in which eleven volunteers underwent a sixteen-week course of supervised Nautilus training three to four times a week, while ten men acted as untrained controls. The average age of the men was forty-four years. HDL levels in exercisers rose by 10 percent, while control-group men showed no such increase.

While these data are promising, few studies have been done with resistive exercise as opposed to aerobic exercise. We don't know the long-term effects of such training on HDLs, and whether one type of training is better than another. But the interest in HDL cholesterol is fairly new, so we can expect additional information in the years to come. In the meantime, all indications are that all forms of exercise appear to have a beneficial effect on HDL levels.

Writing in the *Journal of the American Medical Association,* in May 1988, Dr. James Rippe recommended walking for health and fitness. He noted that even low-to-moderate levels of exercise, when done regularly, provide important cardiovascular health benefits. Brisk walking provides strenuous enough exercise, he says, for cardiovascular training in most adults. Walking has been shown to reduce anxiety and tension and to aid in weight loss. And done regularly, walking can improve cholesterol ratios by elevating HDL levels.

One of the biggest studies yet undertaken to investigate the risks of heart disease is the Multiple Risk Factor Intervention Trial, known as the MR. FIT program. In one report that came out of that study, published in the *Journal of the American Medical Association* (JAMA) in November 1987, Dr. Arthur Leon showed that the choice of leisure-time physical activity plays a significant role in the incidence of heart disease. When the activities of more than 12,000 middle-aged men were studied after seven years of follow-up, moderate leisure-time physical activity was associated with 37 percent fewer fatal heart attacks and sudden deaths than light activity.

Also writing in JAMA, in November 1988, researchers found that physical fitness was a valid predictor of cardiovascular mortality in American men with no heart-disease symptoms. They looked at more than 4000 men aged thirty to sixty-nine years. A lower level of physical fitness was associated with a higher risk of death from cardiovascular and coronary heart disease even after adjusting for age and other cardiovascular risk factors. Fitness was determined by the ability to perform well on a treadmill test.

Documentation on the importance of exercise continues to build. One such report came from the Centers for Disease Control. Researchers there said flaws in earlier studies kept authorities from making a firm connection between inactivity and heart disease. The CDC did a comprehensive two-year analysis of all studies published in English dealing with exercise and heart disease. Their conclusion was that the least active people were almost twice as likely to have heart disease as those who were most active.

The importance of inactivity is becoming more apparent because so many men and women do not do enough aerobic exercise. Yes, smoking is probably a more significant risk factor—but only 18 percent of our population currently smokes cigarettes. Yes, hypertension is probably a more significant risk factor—but only 10 percent of adults have a systolic blood pressure level above 150. The bottom line is that 80 to 90 percent of our population still do not do sufficient cardiovascular exercise.

An interesting side effect of exercise is that those who get actively engaged in such activities as swimming and jogging tend to quit smoking cigarettes. This is true even for those who have smoked for years and who have tried to quit before.

Then, of course, there's weight loss. Exercise should be an integral part of any weight-loss program. It appears that exercise speeds up the metabolism in such a way that calories are burned more efficiently for hours afterward. The result is pounds lost even when one is eating the same amount of food.

A final benefit also involves cholesterol, but in an indirect way. Stress raises cholesterol levels and has been considered a significant risk factor in heart disease. For more details, see Chapter 10, "Defusing the Stress Bomb." Exercise, it turns out, can effectively reduce stress, and, in turn, cholesterol.

One measure of heart-healthy physical fitness is the rate at which your heart beats at rest, that is, when you are not exercising. The average heart rate is about 72 beats per minute. Well-trained athletes get their rates well below 60, and often under 50.

The easiest way to check your own rate is to hold a finger to the carotid artery in your neck. You can feel it pulsing next to the windpipe. Count the beats per minute with a sweep-second watch or clock. Then you can use that figure to see how you progress. As you become more fit, your resting rate will fall.

Once you've gotten your doctor's approval to begin a program of cardiovascular fitness, you'll want to do some exercise that will increase your heart rate. But how much is enough and how much is too much?

First you can determine the maximum heart rate for your age simply by subtracting your age from the number 220. That will give you, in practical terms, the absolute capability of your heart to beat. Of course you don't want to exercise at that maximum rate since that would severely strain your heart, perhaps even to the point of death.

Instead, multiply that number by 65 percent; this is the level at which you want to exercise in the beginning, occasionally checking your heart rate as you do your workout. Gradually work your ability up to 70 percent, then to 75 percent, and finally on to 80 percent. You don't want to exceed 80 percent of your maximum heart-rate potential; that's your training rate.

To reap the benefit of exercise, do it a minimum of three days weekly at your desired training rate for at least thirty minutes. First do a bit of warmup, perhaps some stretching exercises, and then on to thirty minutes at your training rate. It's best to do such exercise four or five times per week. In fact, the rule of thumb is that you need four to five days per week to gain, and three days per week to maintain, fitness.

I've frequently been asked about my own

fitness regimen. Monday through Friday, I like to start off each day with a strenuous cardio-vascular workout at a health club. I begin with five minutes of stretches, followed by twenty minutes on the Schwinn Airdyne stationary bicycle, fifteen minutes on the rowing machine, and thirty minutes on the treadmill. After a brisk shower I'm ready to face anything the day has in store for me. I just don't feel right without my workout.

When traveling, I try to select hotels based on the availability of a health club or a pool for lap swimming. If no such facility exists, then I put on my sweatsuit and walking shoes and head out for a really brisk thirty- to forty-minute walk. And sometimes, in a high-rise hotel, I'll do thirty minutes of stairwalking. I refuse to accept any excuses not to exercise. My health and my life depend on it.

At the time of this writing I've been exercising for five years, and I'm pleased to report that my resting heart rate is now forty-six to fifty beats per minute.

What kind of exercise is best? Basically any kind of strenuous workout—jogging, energetic walking, swimming, various sports—you may enjoy is fine. The important thing is to make a commitment to exercise regularly, three to five days each and every week.

If you haven't done any physical exercise in

quite a while, be certain to start off slowly and gradually increase your tolerance. Especially if there has been any family history of heart disease or if you are over the age of thirty-five it's best to check with your physician before starting off on an exercise program.

The consensus now is that regular exercise will have both long-term and short-term benefits for all. So exercise your options for a long and healthy life.

"All parts of the body which have a function, if used in moderation and exercised in labours in which each is accustomed, become thereby healthy, well-developed and age more slowly, but if unused and left idle they become liable to disease, defective in growth, and age quickly."—Hippocrates

10

Defusing the Stress Bomb

Although it is only recently that stress has been given a great deal of attention, it is by no means a purely modern phenomenon. Back before history began, our ancestors the cavemen experienced stress; even they had their problems. Finding food. Fighting off a saber-toothed tiger. Getting out of the way of a mastodon stampede. But, when measuring stress, the cavemen had it a lot easier than we do today. After that battle with the tiger, he could sit back and rest for a while. Once the stampede passed by, he could contemplate his navel. Stress was an intermittent thing that came and went.

Today, on the other hand, for many people stress never lets up. Or at least people don't give it a chance to let up. It's one crisis on top of another, from traffic jams to irate customers to family arguments—all superimposed over our ongoing anxiety about money, careers, and any number of things.

It's enough to give one a headache. Even worse, it's enough to contribute to heart disease. That's why this chapter is necessary in a book about cholesterol. So let's start at the beginning and see what stress is, how it affects our health, and what we can do about it.

Stress can be defined as any unpleasant emotion; be it anxiety, worry, anger, hostility, or pressures of many kinds. There's no way to eliminate all stress from our lives. Besides, we really wouldn't want to do so. A bit of stress has been shown to enhance performance, whether on an athletic field or during a college exam. Waiting for the winning ticket to be drawn in a lottery has its own excitement. But there's a point where constructive stress gives way to a far more destructive form.

The first man to study this was the famous Canadian medical researcher Hans Selye. His detailed observations of both animals and humans led to dozens of articles and books on the subject. One of his classic studies involved a population of house mice allowed to grow to overcrowded conditions. As their numbers grew and interactions and confrontations increased, the mice developed a number of physical reactions. Hostility and aggression increased. Food intake was affected. Even reproduction was decreased. Sadly, the conditions are those found today in our overcrowded, bustling cities.

For many years, medical authorities have felt that stress can be both counterproductive and destructive. In their book *Type A Behav-*

ior and Your Heart Drs. Meyer Friedman and Ray Rosenman discussed the time-conscious, driven individual whose lifestyle differs so much from that of his more laid-back Type B counterpart. The Type A person is always in a hurry, so much so that he often completes your sentences before you can do so. There's never enough time for him to finish his business, and no time at all for him to relax.

Invariably, the Type A considers the Type B as either flat-out lazy or at least not working at his fullest potential. But, as Drs. Friedman and Rosenman point out, that's not at all the case. In fact, many Type A individuals are so flustered all the time that they are working inefficiently. And in some closer looks at success there seems to be no correlation to stress type. The Type B has just as much or even more chance to succeed. And he's much more likely to enjoy his success.

As with just about everything having to do with heart disease, there's been a bit of controversy regarding the Type A personality theory. At the heart of it were a few studies that did not support the concept, showing no difference in incidence of heart disease between Type As and Type Bs. In one report, published in the *New England Journal of Medicine,* researchers at the St. Luke's–Roosevelt Hospital Center in New York found that Type

A patients were actually more successful in recovering from heart attacks than were Type B individuals. That report in the March 1985 issue created a furor within the medical community, generating a bit of media attention and a number of letters from professionals and laypeople arguing one side of the issue or the other.

Dr. Redford Williams, Jr., reported in *Psychosomatic Medicine* in 1988 that in a study of more than 2200 patients treated at Duke University, Type A personality was associated with more severe arterial blockages, but only in younger patients. In older patients, Type B individuals were those with more severe disease. Keep in mind, though, that we would expect older persons to have more advanced illness owing to the progressive nature of the disease. And by age 55 many of the susceptible Type As are no longer alive. Yet, even among the younger patients, Type A behavior wasn't as strong a predictor of heart disease as the "big three," cholesterol, smoking, and high blood pressure. But, as Dr. Williams put it, "something" about Type A was associated with more severe coronary disease in his younger patients.

Originally, Drs. Friedman and Rosenman gave the term Type A to those exhibiting a wide range of characteristics. Yet those characteristics didn't fit all the individuals having heart attacks. So investigators began to look at those characteristics individually rather than as a group. Today the evidence points primarily to two of those traits, namely anger and hostility.

Interestingly, many of the other characteristics of the Type A individual can often be explained by the traits of anger and hostility themselves. For example, if one becomes very time conscious, upset when someone is late or when waiting on a long line, that time consciousness really is a type of anger. The same can be applied to ambition. Certainly every successful person has a degree of ambition, but not all of them die of heart disease. The difference is whether one becomes hostile to those on the same career path.

Duke's Dr. Williams is a major proponent of the idea that anger and hostility contribute to the development of heart disease, and I happen to agree with him. He used the Minnesota Multiphasic Personality Inventory (MMPI) to test for the characteristics of anger and hostility, which are collectively termed the "Ho" scale. Dr. Williams found that scores on the Ho scale correlated strongly with the severity of arteriosclerotic blockages in the coronary arteries of patients treated at Duke.

Looking at groups of 255 male physicians

and 1877 men employed by a large industrial firm, Dr. Williams found a death rate of 14 percent over a twenty-five-year follow-up period among the doctors whose Ho scores had been high when they took the MMPI in medical school. In comparison, the death rate for those who had low Ho scores was 2 percent. Similar findings applied to the industrial workers.

In a recent study Dr. Williams published in *Psychosomatic Medicine*, the traits of 118 lawyers who took the MMPI while in law school twenty-five years earlier were analyzed. Those with higher Ho scores died of heart disease at a rate 4.2 times higher than those with lower scores.

How do anger and hostility damage us? When persons with high Ho scores are subjected to experimental conditions that arouse their mistrust of others and that anger them, they show larger blood pressure responses than those with low Ho scores. At a science writers' conference held in January 1989 by the American Heart Association, Dr. Williams explained another biological rationale, involving the effect of anger and hostility on the nervous system.

As he put it, the autonomic part of our nervous system works automatically to maintain basic bodily functions without our even thinking about them. The sympathetic branch serves the emergency function of preparing our body for fight or flight in a surge of adrenaline flow. The parasympathetic branch exerts a more calming effect, slowing the heart and generally countering the aggressive messages sent by the sympathetic branch.

Dr. Williams studied the effects on the heart of a drug that mimics the actions of the sympathetic branch. He found evidence that the parasympathetic branch of nonhostile Type B men kicks in sooner to blunt those actions than it does in hostile Type A men. This blunting of the sympathetic branch effects on the heart could also help explain the lower disease risk found in nonhostile Type B persons.

Does this mean that the earlier beliefs in the classic Type A personality are without basis? I think the two theories are perfectly compatible; the recent work by Dr. Williams and others merely refines the earlier impressions.

Thus one can be career-oriented, conscious of time constraints, and ambitious without necessarily doing damage, as long as one is not angry or hostile. Can it be done? I think all the work now on record showing that the Type A person can think in a more Type B mode indicates that the elements of anger and hostility can be tempered. And all of the techniques of relaxation and stress reduction apply to toning down that anger and hostility.

Stress takes its toll by contributing to a number of physical ailments including ulcers, headaches, stomach aches, colitis, and high blood pressure. It can make asthma and arthritis worse. Stress can even be traced to sexual dysfunction. And, it seems certain to say today, stress kills.

While many authorities have believed that for some time, today we have documented proof. We now have a physiologic explanation for what happens, and we can see the effects of stress on the heart with various modern diagnostic techniques.

For our friend the caveman, when those saber-toothed tigers jumped out of the woods, his body's chemistry changed. The sympathetic nervous system produced chemical agents known as catecholamines. The best known of these is adrenaline, the so-called "fight or flight" hormone. It served the caveman well for his encounters with dangerous animals.

Not only was Neanderthal man ready to do battle mentally, his body also reacted to protect him from any injuries. In case of cuts blood was drawn from the limbs. And the blood became enriched with platelets that facilitated the clotting process.

As man evolved, he kept those protective devices. Except today there are no saber-toothed tigers. And for many of us there are no rests in between fights. But the stress encountered still causes the clotting process to accelerate. The problem with this is that those clots can lead to deposits in the arteries and can actually precipitate a heart attack.

And, unfortunately, there's even more. The coronary arteries, which supply the blood to the heart, have a muscular layer that gets its supply of nerves from the same sympathetic nervous system that produces those fight or flight hormones. Stress, it turns out, causes the nerves to react in such a way that the muscle tissue of the arteries constricts. Doctors call this a "spasm."

In an individual with no blockage in the arteries, the potential problems with spasm are great enough. But, when the arteries are occluded by deposits of plaque formed from cholesterol deposits, the spasm may completely shut down the flow of blood to the heart. The result is a heart attack. In less severe cases of spasm brought on by stress, an individual may experience the chest pain known as angina, signaling that the heart isn't getting enough blood supply. The pain felt is really very similar to that experienced when other muscles cramp or have a spasm, say, for example, after extensive exercise or when one develops a so-called "charlie horse."

Interestingly, some people can take a stress test on a treadmill in a doctor's office and show no blockage whatever. Yet in times of stress they feel chest discomfort. Modern diagnostic techniques show why.

One such test is called Holter monitoring. The patient has electrodes attached to the chest, which lead into a kind of tape recorder worn at the waist. The machine runs for a full twenty-four hours, during which time the patient keeps a diary of what's happened and how he or she has felt. Then the doctor can compare the recorded tracings with the diary. Often the periods of discomfort as written down by the patient coincide with indications on the recording of insufficient blood supply to the heart.

Insufficient blood supply results in insufficient oxygen, given the term "ischemia." When the person relaxes, and the blood flow increases with its supply of oxygen, the discomfort passes.

How much stress can cause such reactions? Of course it depends on the individual. The British journal *The Lancet* reported a study in which fourteen very sick patients were hooked up for EKG readings and asked to perform relatively simple arithmetic problems. Even though they experienced no pain, the EKGs showed the telltale signs of cardiac insufficiency. While a simple arithmetic problem may not be enough to precipitate stressful oxygen deprivation in healthy individuals, the frenetic pace of modern society may be just as destructive.

The case has often been cited of the accountants whose cholesterol levels were tested just before the April 15 tax deadline and two weeks afterward. There was a significant drop after the deadline. The same thing happened when medical students were tested before and after examinations.

There we have the stress-cholesterol link. As much as we try to control the amount of cholesterol in our blood through the dietary aspects of this program, stress may be thwarting our good intentions. The answer is to do something about reducing the effects of that stress.

There are three things to shoot for in dealing with stress: (1) reduce the number of stressful incidents, (2) reduce the intensity of those episodes, and (3) find ways to rest and relax in between. While it may be difficult, taking those three steps is not impossible.

The first thing to do is to become aware of your own stressors, the things that lead to your personal feelings of pressure and stress.

Just as it is a good idea to keep a diary of what you eat and drink when trying to modify the diet, it is very helpful to keep a log of daily stresses.

Let's say that you record stress while driving to an appointment for which you might be late. Perhaps a way to deal with that is to leave ten or fifteen minutes earlier the next time. Maybe you can make the drive more pleasant by bringing along a cool drink and turning to a soothing music station on the car radio.

Your daily log may also show that you're going from one stressful episode right into another without having a chance to rest and recuperate in between. The body is a truly resilient machine, but such abuse can't go on for long without ill effect. If you think honestly about it, there must be a way to give yourself a "breather" when one stress ends and before another begins.

The next step is more difficult for the vast majority of fast-paced Americans. Learn to relax during those breathing spaces between stresses. For most people, that time is spent simply stewing about what made them anxious or angry in the first place, making matters even worse as the mind allows the episode to gain even greater proportions.

There is no best prescription for relaxation. For some lucky men and women, it's enough to simply remind themselves to stop and smell the roses. For others, the old prescription of counting to ten really helps. But for most of us special efforts are needed.

Fortunately, professionals have come up with a number of techniques to help defuse the stress bomb. Practically every YMCA offers courses in yoga, meditation, and other relaxation methods. Such courses are also given at community hospitals and clinics, often at very low cost. A number of self-help books and tapes are available. And, for those who need special assistance along these lines, professionals can help with such techniques as biofeedback training or group sessions of self-analysis.

There are tremendous relaxation benefits from regular exercise workouts. Ask runners or swimmers and they will tell you about the blissful feeling they get. Scientists explain that feeling as the result of a chemical substance called a beta-endorphin, which is released into the blood during heavy-duty exercise.

Even if you don't become a marathon runner, regular exercise pays off in a number of dividends. The late President Eisenhower's personal physician and famous cardiologist Paul Dudley White lived to a ripe old age, attributing much of his vim and vigor to regular exercise, including bicycle riding. For others a nice long walk at the end of the day is a veritable tonic.

Just as with the type of exercise you do, the trick is to find a relaxation technique that's right for you. It has to be something that fits your own lifestyle, and that you find actually enjoyable. Don't let your efforts to relax become yet another source of stress.

Diet and alcohol play important roles in terms of stress, since many people use both food and drink as ways of dealing with their emotions. That heavy meal or enormous snack at midnight eaten as consolation for a miserable day will only lead to a miserable, sleepless night. Ironically, the same thing applies to alcohol. While liquor in moderation can be an enjoyable part of living, it's not meant to be used as a general anesthetic. Instead of leading to a good night's sleep, excessive alcohol intake results in poor rest and a terrible feeling in the morning.

Drinking coffee with caffeine is like pouring gasoline on a fire. The last thing one needs is jittery "coffee nerves." Try some of the new brewed decaffeinated coffees. The water-process types sold in specialty shops are particularly good since they avoid the use of chemicals.

A great way to cope with daily stress is to do something nice for yourself—like taking that long walk. We often don't treat ourselves well out of a misguided sense of guilt, living as we do in a society where hard work is praised and "play" gets short shrift. For my own personal treat, about every two weeks or so, I indulge in a full hour of massage. The person I go to has arranged a room as a "sanctuary" with plants growing, water trickling, and music playing. I lie down on that table and allow those fingers to whisk me away from daily pressures and gently ease away tensions and anxieties. Yet, as much as I enjoy those sessions, I frequently find myself coming up with excuses to cancel out for the day. Then I have to remind myself that this is just as important as exercise or even diet in terms of maintaining good health.

Think of something that would be equally enjoyable for you. Perhaps a facial. Or a manicure. Or a steambath or sauna. Maybe something as simple as a cup of decaffeinated coffee in a snackshop with the morning paper or a crossword puzzle. If you're not good to yourself, how can you expect the world to be any better?

Which brings up the next step in learning to deal with stress. The problem, of course, is in those six inches between the ears. The way we think about things is the way those things will be. The self-fulfilling prophecy, as it were—an old adage, but true nonetheless. One man looks at a glass of water as half full while another views it as half empty. The result is that the first man is happy and contented while the other is sad and disappointed. If you wake up in the morning thinking that everything bad will happen, it probably will. Instead, try getting up after a good night's rest and vow to think of something good in everything that you experience that day. Turn those lemons into lemonade. Someone's late for an appointment with you? Great: a good time to read a magazine! Your spouse is in a lousy mood in the evening and can't face up to fixing dinner? Terrific: a wonderful opportunity to try that new Japanese restaurant down the street. No parking place close to where you need to go? Marvelous: another chance to take a stroll down the sidewalk and do a little window shopping. Don't scoff: it can be done and you know it can. We all know someone who is virtually unflappable. Try to be more like that person.

This leads into the next step in the anti-stress program. Drs. Friedman and Rosenman have demonstrated that the Type A person can gradually turn into a Type B personality. And that can be done without any loss of ambition or chance at success. Take another look at that daily stress diary you've been keeping.

Compare your notes about your stressful episodes with those of a personality Type A. You're a Type A person if you overly stress certain words during conversations—driving the points home in case your listener doesn't catch them to your satisfaction. You do everything rapidly, both working and playing—never taking the time to savor the moment. You're impatient with how slowly everything takes place and you want to speed things along. You find it difficult to enjoy a conversation that doesn't have anything to do with your own interests or current lifestyle. You feel somewhat guilty about relaxing, thinking of work that could be done instead. You judge your own efforts in terms of numbers and you gauge progress by the clock and calendar, and somehow there's never enough time. You're more interested in things to have than enjoyable things to do. You find yourself doing or redoing the work of others because your standards so far exceed theirs. And you're certain that everything you've ever achieved is the result of your hard-driving personality. In short you're the kind of person the world needs more of to be a better place!

If you're nodding your head "yes" to even a few of those traits, it's time to start thinking about how to reverse the process. Face the hard, cruel facts of life: if you died today, the world would go on without you. No man or woman is indispensable. *Yes* you have time to go on vacation. *Yes* that appointment can be postponed until later. *Yes* your children will love you if you don't bring home as much bacon. *Yes* it doesn't really matter if the appointment starts ten minutes late.

You're not a horse with blinders leading your vision. You're a thinking human being who is smart enough to realize that, if you don't come to grips with the stresses around you, those stresses will come to grip you—around the heart.

11

Dining Out:
To Your Health!

Salut! L'Chaim! Na Zdrowya! All over the world, diners raise their glasses to each other and toast "To your health!" There couldn't be a better wish to make. And there isn't a better time or place to pursue a healthful diet than in a fine restaurant. "To health!" "To life!"

Some health writers have given eating out an unjustified bad name. Nathan Pritikin actually calls restaurants "the enemy camp," and advises against going out to eat at all. When forced to do so, he advocates, order steamed vegetables and rice. That's rather a gloomy future for most of us who truly enjoy the pleasures of restaurant dining.

Now, by this time in your reading of this book, it must be perfectly clear that I don't recommend the fatty and cholesterol-laden foods that may be on the menu. Fast-food spots, for example, have little to offer anyone seeking a healthful meal. Just take a look at the calorie, fat, cholesterol, and sodium content of fast foods listed in Table 11 in Chapter 4, "Winning by the Numbers," and you'll see what I mean.

On the other end of the spectrum, the old-fashioned cuisine of traditional French restaurants can be equally unhealthful. Interestingly, however, even some of the great French chefs have gravitated to a lighter version of cooking called *nouvelle cuisine.* Those dishes get away from rich butter-and-cream sauces and emphasize the fresh tastes of fish and vegetables prepared in novel and delicious ways.

Somewhere in between the fast-food restaurants and the traditional French restaurants, however, are a wide variety of dining experiences that are not only delicious but also healthful, and they can be found all over the world. In fact, a great way to decide on a place to eat out is to spin the globe, close your eyes, and point your finger. Ethnic cooking offers a never-ending variety of tastes and textures, from the sauces of Thailand to the ratatouille of the Mediterranean.

Like Marco Polo, you can explore the Orient. The cuisines of China as well as Korea, Japan, Thailand, and Vietnam can be a dieter's delight. Deciding on Chinese isn't specific enough. There are Cantonese restaurants, serving the traditional chop suey dishes as well as chow mein, won ton soup, mu shu, and moo goo gai pan; or, if you prefer, the spicy Szechwan cuisine, offering da-chien chicken made with hot peppers, yu-shong scallops, hot braised fish, and tongue-twisting listings with black mushrooms, ginger, and oyster sauce.

When I eat Chinese with friends, we always enjoy ordering a number of dishes. For four persons, for example, we'll get a fish dish, a chicken dish, a vegetable dish, and plenty of steaming rice. Those vegetable dishes are anything but boring. Try yu-shong eggplant, cooked with hot garlic, ginger root, and green onion, or a dish called imperial jade with garden-fresh snow pea pods sautéed with crunchy and tasty water chestnuts. Or a medley of American and Chinese vegetables done in the inimitable manner of the stir-fry wok.

Fried? Yes, I did say fried. But notice some important differences between typical "American" frying and Chinese frying. First, the Asians use no butter. They prefer the very healthful (monounsaturated) peanut oil, which imparts a unique flavor. Second, the amount of oil used is very small indeed. Third, the wok, a large bowl-like cooking utensil, is heated so hot that foods are cooked before they have a chance to absorb much oil. To be even more cautious, as I am in unfamiliar restaurants, I request that the chef use very little oil, and no MSG—monosodium glutamate. Many restaurants, in fact, now advertise that they use no MSG at all, since so many people are becoming sodium conscious.

Can you eat anything at all on the Chinese menu? No, of course not. Avoid the typical appetizer dishes such as egg rolls and spring rolls. These are deep-fried and often contain eggs. Second, duck dishes are absolutely out. That delicacy Peking duck is primarily skin, and a 3½-ounce serving contains nearly 30 grams of fat. Choose chicken or seafood dishes over those containing either lamb or pork to avoid fat. The nice thing about Chinese restaurants is that the same dish can be ordered with any meat, so one need not be deprived of a specific flavor sensation just because it is listed on the menu as containing pork.

If you've had enough Chinese food for a while, it's time to turn the corner and try one of the many Thai or Vietnamese restaurants opening up all over the country. The dishes are flavored in ways you may never have tried before. Salads, a great way to start, come with dressings made with peanut butter and cilantro. One local restaurant lists "pla lard plick," which is a sweet white fish specially imported from the China Sea, prepared with a light red curry sauce with bamboo shoots. Or how about "goong nai som," which turns out to be boiled prawns in a fresh orange shell with orange sauce. If there's something about the dish that you don't want, chopped egg yolks, for example, simply have them eliminated. Everything is made to order, so you get to design your own meals.

And don't forget the wonderful meals waiting at any Japanese restaurant. Many Americans have come to love the fresh tastes and textures of sashimi and sushi, specially prepared raw fish delicacies, sliced before your eyes by chefs wielding razor-sharp knives. Not ready for that yet? Then consider yosenabe, a Japanese-style bouillabaisse made with a variety of seafoods and vegetables. Then there are always the teriyaki chicken and sukiyaki. But don't forget to inform your waitress that you don't want eggs in your dishes. You'll never miss them in your sukiyaki. The only other advice is to avoid the soy-sauce container on the table. While the Japanese have almost no heart disease, thanks to their low-fat, low-cholesterol foods, they have a considerable amount of high blood pressure because of the high levels of sodium in their diet.

Moving west, we come to the foods of India. Again, practically every city has at least one Indian restaurant. And most offer that delicacy known as tandoori chicken, specially marinated and baked in an Indian clay oven. There is no way to precisely describe the flavor and texture—it's like no other chicken you've ever had. To go with it there are a variety of vegetarian side dishes. The only warnings for eating Indian style are to avoid the breads made with butter between the layers, and to stay away from the lamb dishes, which unfortunately are brimming with fat. Actually, though, Indian cooking tastes much better with chicken than lamb. Two other dishes worth mentioning are "murg jalfraize," chicken flavored with fresh spices and sautéed (ask for no butter) with tomatoes, onions, and bell peppers, and "saag" chicken prepared with spinach and Indian spices. Then, of course, there are the traditional curries, as hot as you want them to be, washed down with lots of tea or cold beer.

The foods of other countries also offer taste treats. Consider the whole culinary experience of Mexico. While it's true that many of the dishes contain a great deal of cheese, which is high in fat and cholesterol, most can be ordered without it. And the sauces created to go with seafood are excellent.

Our own country has contributed a large number of excellent, healthful dishes. This is the time to discover the variety of American foods, including New England seafoods, New Orleans Creole, and Cajun gumbos and jambalayas. Then there's the Western-style mesquite-broiling technique that's taken over like wildfire. Somehow foods taste so much better when cooked over the coals in this manner.

Another particularly American phenomenon of late is the salad bar. We're not talking here about a few leaves of wilted lettuce and a limp piece or two of radish. Instead, experience a salad bar that extends over an entire wall of a restaurant, laden with twenty or thirty or more different ingredients to build your own creations.

One of the nicest parts about salad-bar eating, in my opinion, is the opportunity to go back again and again. And the sheer beauty of it is that you can do so without guilt, as long as you avoid the egg yolks, limit the avocado, and make wise decisions about the salad dressings.

Most people, speaking of salad dressings, think that the best bet in terms of calories and fat content is oil and vinegar. Wrong. Actually, a creamy dressing such as Green Goddess or Ranch is lower in both fat and calories. Ask the waiter or manager about the ingredients used. Ask the server to bring the dressing on the side so your salad won't be drenched. Then sprinkle the dressing on with a fork, not a spoon, to distribute it evenly over the greens. You'll be surprised at how far a little will go.

Notice that one or more times I've mentioned asking the waiter or waitress about the foods served in a restaurant. I find it almost incredible that people can be shy when it comes to speaking up about the foods they're about to order and eat and pay for. When you're in a restaurant, you're the boss!

If an item is listed as being sautéed, simply ask that the dish be prepared without butter. The chef can sauté in either a bit of broth or a dash of vegetable oil. If you're not sure of a certain offering, ask how it's prepared. Then, if there's an offending ingredient, request that something else be substituted or that it be eliminated. If you find yourself in a restaurant that balks at your requests, you're in the wrong restaurant. The best ones have no problem with such requests.

Often restaurants serve extra-large helpings of foods. There are a number of ways of getting around this. If you're with other people, why not consider ordering a number of appetizers, then splitting an entrée? Or try getting two entrées for three people. Or any combination you can think of. This not only cuts down on the amount of food eaten but also gives you a chance to taste more than one dish.

When your meal comes, mentally divide what you really need to and should eat. Then eat only that amount. If you've ordered a piece of meat and they give you, say, twelve ounces, cut it in half. Your waiter or waitress will know how many ounces are in every entrée—that's a major consideration for every restaurant.

What to do with the amount not eaten? Ask for a "doggie bag" to take the leftover food home. This is accepted practice, and nothing to be ashamed of at all. Everyone does it, in even the very finest restaurants.

A word of explanation is in order. Restaurants today must keep prices up in order to pay for the ever-escalating operating costs. To justify those costs, they offer more food than you want. It's impossible for the restaurants to reduce costs by giving you less food. So simply take that extra food home. It'll make an excellent lunch or even another dinner.

Obviously, not everyone is concerned about limiting fat and cholesterol in his or her diet. My brother, as I've mentioned before, views the baked potato as a vehicle for butter and sour cream, and maintains a cholesterol level of just 170. But, if you're not that lucky, you'll want to order your baked potato plain.

Now that can be pretty dull and boring. So here are a few suggestions. Try some spicy salsa. Or ask the waitress if she has any sauces in the kitchen that would be appropriately low in fat and cholesterol. My next suggestion may at first make you feel uncomfortable, but after you've done it once or twice, you'll agree that it's a terrific idea. Bring along your own packet of Butter Buds. This is the brand name of a no-cholesterol, nonfat butter-flavored powder. Sprinkle some over the steaming baked potato. Delicious!

Being prepared is the best defense against your own lack of willpower. It's a lot easier to have that baked potato with the Butter Buds than to eat it plain. Otherwise you just might break down and have a dollop of sour cream. Next it'll be some butter on the rolls. And before you know it you've completely blown it.

Does that mean you can never have the sour cream? Or the butter? Or the dessert? Of course not. Remember the advice in Chapter 4, "Winning by the Numbers." The important thing is the total amount of fat and cholesterol you consume during the entire day.

So, if you order a low-fat broiled fish, it's perfectly O.K. to enjoy some sour cream on your potato. Or you may prefer to have a nice dessert. Remember that it's your choice and the only thing that counts is keeping the total number of grams of fat and milligrams of cholesterol under your own personal limit.

Personally, I have the greatest difficulty not with elaborate sauces and fancy desserts, but with junk foods. So, if I've watched my intake during the day, I permit myself some guacamole and tortilla chips, even though I know they're loaded with fat. Or I may have been craving a dip of Häagen Dazs. After a day of salad for lunch, fish for dinner, and, of course, my oat-bran muffins, I feel no guilt about having that special ice-cream treat later in the evening.

It's important to realize that just because you've decided to lower your cholesterol levels you don't have to enter a monastery and give up all the taste treats in the world. In fact, those who try to follow such a spartan regimen typically fail in the long run.

Let's get back to the restaurants for a moment. If you've been used to a lifetime of eating in Italian places, it's ridiculous to think that you can simply stop going to them. Instead, compromise a bit. Order your veal dish with tomatoes and basil instead of a cheese sauce. Have linguine and clam sauce instead of fettuccine Alfredo.

The worst thing to have happen in a restaurant is to be surprised by a menu that offers nothing appealing that satisfies your needs. If you find yourself in a restaurant with nothing but fried foods, you're going to eat a lot of fat and there's practically nothing you can do about it. So be prepared by first knowing the restaurants you go to. If in doubt, call them and ask about the menu. You may have to suggest an alternative to your friends if you find that the menu doesn't permit you to order enjoyable food without a lot of fat.

One way to choose restaurants is by reading the restaurant review sections of newspapers and magazines. Reviewers typically describe the ingredients of a number of dishes in detail, so you'll know in advance what you're getting. Another way is to purchase a book of discount coupons. My wife and I frequently use these books to find restaurants that we would otherwise never consider. One book, *Entertainment '89* (or whatever year it happens to be), sold through charitable institutions, prints the menus from a large number of restaurants. With the coupon, one gets the lesser-priced entrée free along with one purchased at the regular price. We often plan our meals well in advance, and there are no unpleasant surprises.

Mention fast food and most people think first of the artery-clogging fare served up at McDonald's and Kentucky Fried Chicken. But there's a very healthy trend in fast food, and it's now quite possible to eat heart-healthy even when in a hurry.

The Subway stores springing up all over the country offer submarine sandwiches of all sorts. Choices include tuna, turkey breast, crab/seafood, and vegetarian, which you can order on either white or whole-wheat buns. Ask the server to pile your sub high with all the available vegetables, but hold the mayo and the oil and vinegar, or at least go easy on the fats.

Sizzler Steak, Salad, and Seafood Restaurants continue to offer a delightful salad bar for lunch or dinner. They now include soup and pasta, so you can make a very satisfying meal, or you can order an entrée of broiled fish or chicken on the side. Just watch out for the fatty premade salads, the taco chips, the fried potato skins, and the like. And limit the amount of salad dressings you ladle onto your greens.

El Pollo Loco, Pollo Pollo, and Chicken on Fire restaurants specialize in the Mexican-style broiled chicken that is coming into vogue on the West Coast and elsewhere throughout the country. Marinated in fruit juices, with no added oil, the chicken is absolutely delicious. Enjoy it with a side order of rice, some corn tortillas and salsa, and a fresh green salad.

You can also find a number of fast-food places nowadays serving up broiled-chicken-breast sandwiches. Many such restaurants also serve baked potato, which I like with salsa in place of sour cream. Avoid the deep-fried chicken sandwiches.

No matter where I travel in the country, I know I can get a heart-healthy quick meal at Denny's. For breakfast they offer Egg Beaters omelets, scrambled eggs, or French toast. Low-fat, low-cholesterol sandwiches and entrées are marked with a heart. I order hash-brown potatoes done with little or no oil, and nonfat milk is always available.

If it's pizza you want, you have a number of options. You can order the pizza without any cheese at all, but with extra vegetables, including sliced tomatoes, onions, green peppers, olives, and even anchovies if you like them. Or you can ask that the chef prepare the pizza with half the regular amount of cheese. Finally, and I think this is the best option, you can bring along your own cheese. Just put a few ounces of low-fat mozzarella cheese into a plastic sandwich bag, and hand it to the server for the chef to use to prepare your pizza. That way you'll get all the delicious flavor, without the cholesterol and the saturated fat. If it's inconvenient to bring your own cheese along, simply ask to have your pizza prepared with half the normal amount of cheese.

You don't have to abandon your healthy eating habits when you go on the road. Knowing my hectic travel schedule, people often ask whether I have a tough time sticking to my diet. Actually I find that it's easy. Many hotels today recognize that business-people are very health conscious, and so they offer low-fat, low-cholesterol meals in their coffeeshops and restaurants. Marriott and Hyatt, for example, offer Egg Beaters omelets for breakfast. And I can always count on a piece of fresh fish for dinner. I've never been refused in my request to have olive oil used instead of butter for sautéing.

But eating heart-healthy begins when I step aboard the plane. Every airline now offers low-cholesterol meals, as well as seafood platters, fruit plates, or vegetarian meals, which you can order when you make your flight reservations, at least twenty-four hours in advance. Let's face it, airline cuisine is not known for its excellence, but the special meals are almost always better than the standard fare.

And, of course, I never leave home without my oat bran. I bring some muffins for breakfast in my room and I keep two or three muffins along with a banana in my attaché case in case of delays at the airport; they can be a lifesaver.

Do you prefer your oat bran as cereal? Before leaving home, measure out individual servings of a half cup of oat bran, a tablespoon or so of brown sugar, and some raisins into Ziploc sandwich bags. In restaurants, just order some boiling water and a bowl along with your coffee and juice. In your room, you can use one of those portable water-heating coils to heat up a half cup of water. Pour it over the oat bran and flavorings in a plastic bowl you bring from home. (To make breakfast more pleasant, and far less expensive than room service, I now bring along a one-cup coffeemaker. That way I can heat up the water for cereal and then a cup of fresh-brewed decaf. If you travel at all frequently, this is a terrific investment.)

But no discussion of dining out would be complete without considering the problems (if you want to think of them as such) of eating at friends' homes. Again, this is a simple matter of communication. First, remember that these are your friends. Friends care about each other. For you, eating a cheese omelet can actually be an unpleasant experience when thinking about what it's doing to the lining of your arteries. So talk to your friends about it.

The time to start, actually, is before a luncheon or dinner invitation. Let people know how excited you are that you've discovered a way to control your cholesterol and that you've cut down the risk of coronary heart disease. Let them know that there are certain foods you prefer to avoid or at least limit. Then when it comes time to go to their homes, it'll be almost an afterthought to mention that you're still not eating butter or egg yolks, and that you keep your cheese intake low. No surprises.

You'll find—at least I've found—that most people who know you're watching what you eat will ask about the foods you'd rather have.

Today more people than ever before are aware of the impact food has on their health. In any given group of men and women, one will be cutting down on calories, another will have gone vegetarian, another will have found that he or she is allergic to certain foods, and still another will have developed intolerance over the years to, say, dairy foods. And almost everyone today knows the relationship between fat and heart disease and cancer.

That's why more and more restaurants are catering to health-conscious individuals. Many use the little heart symbol to indicate dishes that are low in fat and cholesterol. Others advertise that they limit the amount of salt in their foods. Occasionally you'll even find whole special sections on menus that feature particularly healthful dishes.

If you'd like to learn which restaurants in your area are making a special effort to serve heart-healthy food, call your local chapter of the American Heart Association and ask for their publication "Dine Out to Your Heart's Content." They'll give you a list of many food establishments in your home town offering low-fat, low-cholesterol meals.

Restaurants not only can provide the kinds of foods you need to reduce your total intake of fats and cholesterol, but also offer ideas for cooking in your own home. Ask about certain recipes you find enjoyable. Or invest in a cookbook featuring the foods you relished.

But by all means don't limit the pleasures of dining out. Next time, just raise your glass in that worldwide and traditional toast: To your health!

12

Painless Primer on Proper Nutrition

The problem with most attempts to teach an overview of nutrition, I believe, is that writers get carried away. People don't have to become nutritionists in order to select foods wisely for themselves and their families. What everyone does need, however, is an understanding of the basic principles that should affect food choices. This is particularly true when we make a concerted effort to alter the diet, in this case to reduce the amount of fat and cholesterol we plan to eat.

Ultimately the whole science of nutrition comes down to this: Nutrition is the process by which food and everything else we consume becomes a part of our bodies and affects out total health and growth. Food allows us to function. It's as simple as that.

The next concept to grasp is that food consists of various chemicals working together in interaction with the chemicals of our bodies. Certain foods have certain nutrients while other foods have other nutrients. By eating a wide variety of foods, as we'll see, we ensure that we get a full spectrum of those nutrients.

Everyone, regardless of age, sex, or other physical or medical characteristics, needs the same nutrients. Some need more and some require less food. But throughout our lives we continue to need the basic nutrients offered in the foods we eat.

Food plays important roles in life. The feast has long been a part of ceremony, whether on a jungle island or in a lavish Manhattan reception room. When guests arrive in our homes we offer food. Gatherings and celebrations of all sorts frequently involve meals, often on a grand scale. Yet, regardless of what, when, how, where, or why we eat, food supplies those basic nutrients. Those nutrients provide materials to build, repair, and maintain body tissues. They supply the chemicals we need for regulating our bodily functions. And they furnish fuel needed for energy.

As a broad classification, there are six classes of nutrients: protein, carbohydrates, fat, vitamins, minerals, and water. (Yes, water is a distinct nutrient we just can't live without.) Each nutrient has its own particular function, but many of them work together. For example, to build bones vitamin D, calcium, and phosphorus interact. In this case, bone will not form efficiently when one of those nutrients is inadequate or deficient. Within the broad classification of six classes of

nutrients, there are about fifty specific nutrients.

Does that mean we have to be aware of fifty
different nutrients in the foods we eat daily?
That would take a lot of effort and calculation.
Instead, nutritionists have designated just ten
as what they call the "leader" nutrients. Those
ten are protein, carbohydrates, fat, vitamin A,
vitamin C, thiamin, riboflavin, niacin, calcium,
and iron. The generally accepted belief is that,
if one consumes those nutrients in sufficient
amounts, the foods containing them will also
provide the other forty. With that in mind,
let's look at those ten leader nutrients.

Protein

Throughout our lives we need protein to
maintain and build body tissues, which are
constantly being replaced; to make hemoglobin in the blood to carry oxygen to the
body's cells; to form antibodies in the process
of immunity, which protects our bodies from
infection; and to produce enzymes and hormones that regulate bodily functions. Excess
protein may also be used, though inefficiently,
as an energy source. While we can store
some nutrients, protein cannot be stock-
piled for later use. That's why we need to eat

protein on a regular basis. Happily, that's easy to do.

The fact of the matter is that most Americans consume far more protein than they actually need. There are a number of reasons for this. First, we live in a land of plenty. Second, protein is found in a wide variety of both animal and plant foods. Third, our tastes lead us to choose foods with high protein levels.

What we really need are the eight or nine indispensable or essential amino acids, which are the "building blocks" of protein. When we get those eight, our bodies can construct complete molecules of the total twenty-two amino acids in our bodies. Protein from animal sources contains all the amino acids we need in one place. Proteins from a variety of plant sources can also provide that complete amino-acid profile. For example, beans and rice work together beautifully, and are part of many Latin diets. Unless one is a strict vegetarian, however, it's not terribly important to worry about balancing those amino acids. Again, we actually consume more—far more—protein than we require.

How much is enough? Scientists studying the needs of Americans offer their recommendations every five years in the form of the Recommended Dietary Allowances. The RDA for protein is 45 grams. To put that into perspective, an 8-ounce glass of skim milk contains 9 grams of protein. A 4-ounce portion of white-meat chicken gives you about 37 grams. Even a matzo cracker has more than 3 grams. So you can see that it's no problem at all to consume enough protein. Even following a strict vegetarian diet, it's not difficult to get all the protein one needs.

This is important to remember when reducing fat and cholesterol. Since the majority of that fat and cholesterol comes from meat and eggs, there's no need to worry that by cutting back on the amounts we eat we'll have protein deficiencies. Actually, cutting down on protein saves wear and tear on the kidneys, which metabolize the nitrogen byproducts.

If you wish to do so, you can very easily determine how much protein you're consuming on a daily basis. Keep a little diary for a few days. Look at the nutrient labels on various packaged foods and add up the grams of protein you're eating on a per-serving basis. Next count on 30 grams average per serving to calculate the protein you're getting from animal foods. You'll probably find you're far beyond the basic RDA of 45 grams.

Vitamins

Most nutritionists feel that the foods we typically eat contain enough of the thirteen known vitamins. Many people, however, feel that swallowing a multivitamin tablet or pill daily provides extra insurance. I've never heard anyone say this could do any harm, and many authorities, especially in private, say it's probably a good idea.

There are basically two types of vitamins, the fat-soluble and the water-soluble kinds. Fat-soluble vitamins are stored in the body and include vitamins A, D, E, and K. Water-soluble vitamins are not stored in the body and include vitamin C and the whole series of B vitamins. Water-soluble vitamins are excreted in the urine when the body receives an excess amount, whether from foods or pills. The fat-soluble vitamins are stored, and toxicity can result if excess amounts are consumed.

Let's take a moment to very briefly review the thirteen known vitamins. RDAs for each are listed in Table 17 (see pages 352–53).

Vitamin A helps to build cells in the body, is necessary for seeing in dim light, and prevents certain eye diseases. We get this nutrient in vegetables, including carrots, sweet potatoes, and green, leafy vegetables as well as in enriched foods such as milk and cereals. Is it difficult to get enough? Just one-half cup of sweet potatoes contains 150 percent of the RDA.

Vitamin D aids in building bone tissue and in absorbing calcium from the digestive tract. We get all we need from fish oils, fortified milk and other dairy foods, and sunshine. Vitamin D deficiencies are simply unknown in this day and age.

Vitamin E protects vitamin A and unsaturated fatty acids from destruction by oxidation. While deficiencies can lead to sexual dysfunction, excessive amounts cannot promote sexuality. Claims for the role of vitamin E in preventing heart disease have never been substantiated. Foods containing vitamin E include vegetable oils, green leafy vegetables, whole-grain cereals, wheat germ, butterfat, and egg yolks.

Vitamin K is the last of the fat-soluble vitamins and is essential in the clotting of blood. There is virtually no chance of deficiency here, since in addition to the vitamin K contained in vegetables and elsewhere, the body produces its own supply in the intestine.

Vitamin C forms the substances that literally hold the cells and body together, hastens the healing of wounds, and increases resistance to infection. Found in a variety of fruits and vegetables, vitamin C is also added to a number of foods and beverages. No one to date has been able to prove the benefits of *very* large doses.

Vitamin B$_1$ (thiamin) contributes to the functioning of the nervous system, promotes a normal appetite, and aids in the use of energy by the body. This nutrient is found in nuts, fortified cereal products, and lean pork. Just a little is all we need.

Vitamin B$_2$ (riboflavin) promotes healthy skin and eyes, and also aids in the utilization of energy. Milk, yogurt, and cottage cheese are excellent sources of this nutrient.

Niacin is a B vitamin without a number. It promotes healthy skin, nerves, and digestive tract, and also is a part of energy utilization. Natural sources of niacin include meats, fish, and poultry as well as peanuts and fortified cereal products. In large doses niacin has the effect of lowering levels of LDL cholesterol and triglycerides while raising those of HDL cholesterol. The niacin metabolite, niacinamide, does not have this property although it does perform the functions listed above.

Vitamin B$_6$ assists in red-blood-cell regeneration and helps to regulate the use of protein, fat, and carbohydrates. It's found in various meats, soybeans, lima beans, bananas, and whole-grain cereals.

Vitamin B$_{12}$ assists in the maintenance of

nerve tissues and normal blood formation. Only animal foods supply this nutrient. Sources include fish, shellfish, milk, and other dairy foods. Vegetarians must take vitamin B_{12} supplements if they are strict practitioners.

Folic Acid/Folacin assists in maintaining nerve tissues and blood cells. It is mainly found in green leafy vegetables, nuts, and legumes. You'll need 400–800 micrograms (mcg) daily to reduce levels of the amino acid homocysteine, a newly recognized heart disease risk factor, in the blood.

Biotin is another B vitamin but does not have a specified RDA. Found in most fresh vegetables and in milk and meats, this nutrient helps regulate carbohydrate metabolism. There is no problem with deficiencies.

Pantothenic Acid is another vitamin without an RDA. Found in whole-grain cereals and legumes, this nutrient aids in general nutrient metabolism.

MINERALS

Daily recommended allowances have been established for six minerals, including calcium, phosphorus, iodine, iron, magnesium, and zinc. In addition to these, there are nine other minerals that are needed in lesser amounts and that are considered to be supplied by the same foods offering the six major minerals. Minerals in general are required for body building and regulatory functions.

Calcium requirements continue throughout life to ensure sufficient amounts of this mineral for bone health and for regulatory functions in the blood serum. The major sources of calcium are milk and other dairy foods. While it is possible to get calcium from sardines and canned salmon by eating the bones, this is not a practical source on a daily basis for most people. Vegetable sources are also not practical both in terms of frequency of consumption and poorer availability of the nutrient. Dairy foods also provide the vitamin D and phosphorus necessary for formation of bone tissue.

Two eight-ounce servings of milk or their equivalent in other dairy foods provide most of the calcium needed for an adult according to the RDA. Happily, there is as much or more calcium in skim or low-fat milk as in whole milk. There is no dietary reason to consume whole milk. To get the amount of calcium found in an eight-ounce glass of milk from cheese, a one-or one-and-a-half-ounce serving will do. Cottage cheese is a poor choice for calcium. Imitation or so-called filled cheeses contain calcium without cholesterol in the large quantities found in real cheese. If one prefers yogurt, bear in mind that fat content varies greatly. Choose the low-fat or nonfat varieties. Other dietary sources of calcium, including sardines and various vegetables, add to the day's total but cannot efficiently replace dairy foods.

For women the need for calcium is particularly great. Pregnancy and nursing double the requirement for this nutrient. And during the aging process women tend to lose calcium from the bone. This often results in the bone-demineralizing disease known as osteoporosis. For women, especially those past menopause, it's a good idea to take daily calcium supplements. Medical authorities recommend a daily total intake of 1000 milligrams or more. The best source of calcium in supplement form is calcium carbonate, since it provides the greatest percentage of actual calcium to the body.

Iron combines with protein to make hemoglobin, the red substance in red blood cells, which facilitates oxygen transport to all parts of the body. There is a continuous turnover of iron in the body, resulting in a regular need for this nutrient. This is particularly true for menstruating women, who may require supplements of iron to fulfill their requirements. Dietary sources of iron include beef and cereals, especially the fortified types.

Phosphorus combines with calcium to form bone tissue and assists in a number of regulatory functions. Sources include milk and other dairy foods, meat, fish, poultry, eggs, whole-grain cereals, and legumes. Soft drinks and other processed foods also provide a great deal of phosphorus in the diet. Some authorities have proposed that we consume too much phosphorus, causing an imbalance between calcium and phosphorus. They recommend cutting back on soft drinks and processed foods.

Iodine helps to regulate the rate at which the body uses energy and prevents the formation of goiter. Dietary sources include seafoods of all sorts and iodized salt. There is absolutely no problem with iodine deficiency, even for those who have totally eliminated the use of table salt. In addition to the normal sources of iodine, there is a considerable amount of the nutrient in all forms of milk, owing to current farming techniques.

Magnesium aids in metabolism and assists in the functioning of nerve and muscle fibers. Sources include legumes, whole-grain cereals, milk, meat, seafood, nuts, eggs, and green vegetables.

Zinc becomes part of several enzymes and insulin. It is found in meat, eggs, oysters and other seafoods, and whole-grain cereals.

Copper is involved with iron storage and plays a role in the formation of red blood cells. This nutrient has no designated RDA but is found in a wide variety of foods, including seafood, meat, eggs, legumes, whole-grain cereals, nuts, and raisins.

FAT

While it's certainly true that the vast majority of Americans and others eating a Western-style diet consume far too much fat, a certain amount is essential for life and health. Fat supplies indispensable essential fatty acids, carries the fat-soluble vitamins, and is an integral aspect of the metabolism of all food. In the body it is a component of cell walls, cushions vital organs, and provides insulation.

Fats are found in both animal and vegetable foods as well as in all varieties of cereals. Based on the molecular structure of the fat, it is classified as saturated, monounsaturated, or polyunsaturated.

Saturated fats include those from animal sources as well as coconut oil, palm oil, and hydrogenated oils. Saturated fats are solid or semi-solid at room temperature. Olive oil, canola oil, and peanut oil, cashews, and avocados contain sizable amounts of monounsaturated fats. Polyunsaturated oils include corn oil, safflower oil, and other vegetable oils. No food has one type of fat exclusively, but rather contains predominantly one type or another.

Most authorities recommend that the average American consumption of fat be reduced from the typical level of 40 or even 50 percent of calories to a maximum of 30 percent of calories. This means a reduction in total fat— fats of all kinds. Typical recommendations call for 10 percent of calories as saturated fat, 10 percent as monounsaturated, and 10 percent as polyunsaturated. For a normally active 150-pound adult male this translates to about 65 to 75 grams of fat daily, 20 to 25 grams of each of the three types. Those wishing to modify their diets further, say to 20 percent of total calories as fat, would consume only 50 grams of fat, one-third from each of the three types.

Interestingly enough, while such reduction may at first seem dramatic, the most obvious modifications do a large part of the job. Fried foods, whether at home or away, provide a large amount of the fat we consume. Baked goods contain as much as 50 percent of calories as fat. Fats added to foods, including butter, margarine, oils, and mayonnaise, contribute a great deal. When such foods are reduced, there is less need to be concerned about the more hidden forms of fats.

Cholesterol is found only in animals fats. There is no cholesterol at all in any foods of plant origin. Even if all cholesterol were eliminated from the diet by means of a strict vegetarian program, the body would produce enough to meet its needs. For many individuals, in fact, the body produces too much and even dietary cholesterol restrictions are insufficient to completely normalize levels in the blood. Fat must also be reduced, since the body produces cholesterol from fat sources. And for certain individuals additional measures must be considered, such as the inclusion of oat bran and higher-than-RDA doses of niacin.

CARBOHYDRATES

Sugars and starches are the two main types of carbohydrates in the diet. These are chemically related and are principally classified by molecular complexity. Hence the term "complex carbohydrates," which are the preferred form of carbohydrates in the diet.

While it's true that most of us consume far too many "simple sugars" we also have to remember that the body does not distinguish between sugar taken in as sucrose and that eaten, say, as fruit juices. All sugars provide the same number of calories and are ultimately converted by the body to glucose, the sugar found in the blood. Complex carbohydrates, the starches, are metabolized by the body more slowly than simple sugars, thus keeping a more stable, constant blood-sugar level. Those simple sugars are also more likely to elevate triglyceride levels. Finally, simple sugars contain no fiber.

Fiber is a form of carbohydrate we've heard a great deal about. There are two main types of fiber, soluble and insoluble. The insoluble types, such as wheat fiber, have a beneficial effect in the intestines by speeding along the process of fecal elimination. Many authorities believe that fiber has a protective effect against colon cancer. Such insoluble fibers are termed non-nutritive, since they are not absorbed by the body. Soluble fibers, on the other hand, do provide a valuable amount of nutrition.

WATER

If asked to name the nutrients essential for health and life, few persons would include water. Yet this nutrient accounts for one-half to three-fourths of the body's entire weight.

Water is used in the production of tissue, acts as a solvent, and regulates body temperature. It carries nutrients to cells and carries wastes away in the urine. Water is the principal component of blood. It aids in digestion and is required for a wide spectrum of chemical reactions.

We lose water every day in a number of ways. Of course a great deal is used to produce urine to flush out the body's wastes. Water loss also occurs through sweat, both perceptible and imperceptible. The feces contain a large quantity of water. All this fluid must be replaced.

Remember the old advice to drink eight eight-ounce glasses of water each day? Well, the wisdom of that advice holds true today. This is particularly true for those consuming oat bran and other fiber foods; the water needs increase in order to form the feces and prevent constipation.

Bear in mind that oat bran absorbs water readily. It takes a great deal of fluid to keep this fiber in a soft state as it passes through the digestive tract.

Water is the ideal thirst quencher, with no calories or added chemicals. Whether it's straight from the tap or out of an imported bottle, water hits the spot. But other fluids can be counted in the day's intake. Diet sodas, decaffeinated coffee and tea, juices, and milk all contribute to the total.

Nutrition Supplements

Traditional nutritionists and dietitians state rather unequivocally that diet alone provides all the nutrients we need. They say supplementation simply results in expensive urine. On the other side of the argument are those who say supplementation is more important than the foods we eat. The truth probably lies somewhere in between.

As we have seen, large doses of the vitamin niacin can be very effective in controlling fats in the blood. The evidence is overwhelming. But does evidence exist for supplementing other nutrients as well?

Calcium supplements can supply the bone-building mineral missing in so many diets. Reaching the one or one-and-a-half gram level recommended by many authorities to prevent osteoporosis may be difficult if not impossible with diet alone, though diet is the place to start. And calcium has also been shown to slow down the proliferation of epithelial cells in the colon, thereby protecting against cancer.

Survey after survey shows most women's

diets are too low in iron. Again, diet alone cannot bring the level of this mineral up to the amounts needed for women during the years between puberty and menopause. Supplementation certainly would help.

Next, women taking oral contraceptives are very likely to be deficient in folic acid. The same applies to those who smoke cigarettes. Again, diet alone is unlikely to supply sufficient folic acid.

The controversy regarding vitamin C is unlikely to be resolved in the near future. Nutrition surveys show diets of many men and women to be low in this vitamin. Many dentists recommend vitamin C for patients with gingivitis (tender and bleeding gums). And, of course, Dr. Linus Pauling and others maintain that large doses of vitamin C can both prevent and lessen the severity of the common cold. It's no surprise that many persons routinely take additional vitamin C.

What about vitamin E? Few people actually believe that supplementation with this vitamin can improve sexual performance unless an actual deficiency state exists. That was a claim frequently encountered a few years ago. But today there may be other reasons to consider adding vitamin E to the diet in amounts beyond those found in grains and other foods. Vitamin E is an antioxidant, and as such it may protect against the effects of pollution in the air and the rancidity of fats and oils in our foods. Most researchers now agree that vitamin E protects against heart disease by preventing the oxidation of LDL cholesterol.

The same kind of logic applies to supplementation of trace nutrients, those found in only minute amounts in our foods. Do you know for certain the amount of copper, zinc, and other minerals in the foods you eat daily? Probably not. On the other hand, no harmful effects have ever been shown in terms of supplementation short of massive amounts.

There is, however, some potential harm in large doses of vitamin A. This is one of the fat-soluble vitamins; it is stored in the tissues of the body rather than being excreted in the urine. Long-term damage has been reported when individuals supplement their diets with megadoses.

Especially for those reducing the amount of red meats in the diet, there may be concern about vitamin B_{12}. This is particularly a consideration for vegetarians. Adding a small amount of vitamin B_{12} to the diet seems logical.

Similarly, other B-complex vitamins may come up short in the diets of those under stress either mentally or physically. Moreover, it may be wise to balance the B vitamins for those of us who take large doses of niacin.

Table 17. Recommended Daily Dietary Allowances (RDA) for Major Nutrients

	AGE (YEARS)	WEIGHT (KG)	WEIGHT (LBS)	HEIGHT (CM)	HEIGHT (IN)	ENERGY (KCAL)	PROTEIN (G)	VITAMIN A ACTIVITY (RE)	VITAMIN A ACTIVITY (IU)	VITAMIN D (IU)	VITAMIN E ACTIVITY (IU)
									FAT SOLUBLE VITAMINS		
Infants	0.0–0.5	6	14	60	24	kg × 117	kg × 2.2	420	1,400	400	4
	0.5–1.0	9	20	71	28	kg × 108	kg × 2.0	400	2,000	400	5
Children	1–3	13	28	86	34	1300	23	400	2,000	400	7
	4–6	20	44	110	44	1800	30	500	2,500	400	9
	7–10	30	66	135	54	2400	36	700	3,300	400	10
Males	11–14	44	97	158	63	2800	44	1,000	5,000	400	12
	15–18	61	134	172	69	3000	54	1,000	5,000	400	15
	19–22	67	147	172	69	3000	54	1,000	5,000	400	15
	23–50	70	154	172	69	2700	56	1,000	5,000		15
	51+	70	154	172	69	2400	56	1,000	5,000		15
Females	11–14	44	97	155	62	2400	44	800	4,000	400	12
	15–18	54	119	162	65	2100	48	800	4,000	400	12
	19–22	58	128	162	65	2100	46	800	4,000	400	12
	23–50	58	128	162	65	2000	46	800	4,000		12
	51+	58	128	162	65	1800	46	800	4,000		12
Pregnant						+300	+30	1,000	5,000	400	15
Lactating						+500	+20	1,200	6,000	400	15

SOURCE: Food and Nutrition Board, National Academy of Sciences/National Research Council

		WATER SOLUBLE VITAMINS							MINERALS					
	AGE (YEARS)	ASCORBIC ACID (MG)	FOLACIN (MCG)	NIACIN	RIBOFLAVIN (B₂) (MG)	THIAMIN (B₁) (MG)	VITAMIN B₆ (MG)	VITAMIN B₁₂ (MCG)	CALCIUM (MG)	PHOSPHORUS (MG)	IODINE (MCG)	IRON (MG)	MAGNESIUM (MG)	ZINC (MG)
Infants	0.0–0.5	35	50	5	0.4	0.3	0.3	0.3	360	240	35	10	60	3
	0.5–1.0	35	50	8	0.6	0.5	0.4	0.3	540	400	45	15	70	5
Children	1–3	40	100	9	0.8	0.7	0.6	1.0	800	800	60	15	150	10
	4–6	40	200	12	1.1	0.9	0.9	1.5	800	800	80	10	200	10
	7–10	40	300	16	1.2	1.2	1.2	2.0	800	800	110	10	250	10
Males	11–14	45	400	18	1.5	1.4	1.6	3.0	1200	1200	130	18	350	15
	15–18	45	400	20	1.8	1.5	2.0	3.0	1200	1200	150	18	400	15
	19–22	45	400	20	1.8	1.5	2.0	3.0	800	800	140	10	350	15
	23–50	45	400	18	1.6	1.4	2.0	3.0	800	800	130	10	350	15
	51+	45	400	16	1.5	1.2	2.0	3.0	800	800	110	10	350	15
Females	11–14	45	400	16	1.3	1.2	1.6	3.0	1200	1200	115	18	300	15
	15–18	45	400	14	1.4	1.1	2.0	3.0	1200	1200	115	18	300	15
	19–22	45	400	14	1.4	1.1	2.0	3.0	800	800	100	18	300	15
	23–50	45	400	13	1.2	1.0	2.0	3.0	800	800	100	18	300	15
	51+	45	400	12	1.1	1.0	2.0	3.0	800	800	80	10	300	15
Pregnant		60	800	+2	+0.3	+0.3	2.5	4.0	1200	1200	125	18+	450	20
Lactating		80	600	+4	+0.5	+0.3	2.5	4.0	1200	1200	150	18	450	25

Faced with all these considerations, I have made a personal decision to supplement my own diet. While I do not necessarily recommend following my own regimen for others, I do not hesitate to say what I take. In addition to niacin, I take a full-spectrum vitamin-mineral supplement which includes all the trace nutrients. I take a balanced B-complex tablet, a 500-milligram vitamin C tablet, and a 400-IU vitamin E capsule as well. I feel confident that this provides the safeguard or insurance I want.

When I began writing about health and medicine twenty years ago, nutrition supplementation was considered in the realm of faddism. Solid scientific research has shown the benefits of many aspects of supplementation. And I believe we will see additional proof of such benefits as research continues.

FOOD SELECTION

It certainly would be inconvenient to go to the supermarket or restaurant with a list of the nutrients needed for the day. Most of us don't think in terms of milligrams of this or grams of that. So there must be a better way to select the day's foods.

As it turns out, one of the best ways is not

new. The Daily Food Guide was first developed by the U.S. Department of Agriculture back in the forties. It was and is a system by which nutrition scientists determined average nutrient intake achieved by eating a number of servings of various kinds of foods, often called the "four food groups."

Diabetic patients use a variation on this theme in the form of "exchange groups." Whatever form or name given, this approach specifies the number of servings of foods from the four basic food groups, which will provide the required nutrients to prevent deficiencies. Those four groups are the meat group, milk group, fruit-vegetable group, and bread-cereal or grain group. Today nutritionists and dietitians also refer to the "extras" group or the "others" group to talk about foods that offer insignificant nutrients but that contribute flavors and calories. Condiments, oils, butter, sugar, and alcohol are included in such "others."

While it is certainly true that many different foods offer a particular nutrient, the four groups are based on certain foods that are especially rich in particular nutrients.

The so-called "meat" group should probably be termed the "protein" group since that's the nutrient the foods in this classification contribute most. In addition to meats, this group includes fish, poultry, eggs, nuts, and dry beans, such as lentils or pinto beans.

Obviously some of the foods in this protein group also contain a great deal of fat and should be limited. Although nuts, for example, contain no cholesterol, they are very high in fat. Does this mean one should eliminate them? Not at all. Simply limit the total amount eaten. Moderation is the key word. The same applies to meats. Certainly they are much higher in fat content than fish, but when properly trimmed and broiled rather than fried, meats have a place in a fat-and-cholesterol-controlled diet. Even eggs make a wonderful contribution. But, for those of us watching cholesterol intake, the yolks go down the drain or into the dog's food dish. Egg whites are an excellent source of protein, have no cholesterol, and are very low in calories.

The ideal way to approach the selection of foods from the protein or meat group is to go for a wide variety. One day have fish, another day turkey, the next day a vegetarian bean-and-rice dish, then a veal entrée, and so on. By seeking such variety, one may eat a bit more fat and cholesterol on one day and make up for it by eating less on another. That way the fat and cholesterol intake over the long term remains reduced.

How much is enough? That question reflects the major problem with typical eating habits. For many men, a 24-ounce porterhouse steak is a "serving" of meat. To a dietitian or nutritionist, however, a serving of meat is 3½ ounces or so. Two daily servings of meat, fish, or other foods from this group will satisfy one's protein requirements and provide a variety of other nutrients as well.

When choosing which of the great variety of foods to eat, spend a few moments with Table 11 included in Chapter 4, "Winning by the Numbers." You'll see that the fat content of these foods varies tremendously. As a result, in our household turkey has replaced beef as the dominant meat. We still enjoy beef and veal, but only as an occasional treat rather than the practically daily routine of old.

Besides, when trying to vary the diet as widely as possible, there really isn't "room" to have any one type of food too frequently. And, when we do have beef, we try to enjoy it in smaller quantities than in the past. An excellent example is skewered beef with vegetables (see recipe p. 588). We use marinated chunks of filet mignon (four ounces raw per person) along with mushrooms, tomatoes, green peppers, and onions. Broiled over the charcoal, this is a sumptuous treat that looks as good as it tastes. Yet the meal has a very reasonable amount of fat and cholesterol. Served with a baked potato or rice and a fine bottle of red wine, it's a fabulous example of how delicious a low-cholesterol diet can be.

At first it may appear difficult to consider the serving size so carefully. But here's a very simple way of dealing with this: when you buy a pound of beef, simply divide it into four equal portions for storage. That way when it's time to cook you'll have a proper four-ounce serving for each person. The same applies to fish, poultry, or any other meat.

It's just as easy to determine your needs from the milk group. This group contributes calcium as its predominant nutrient. Included are milk, yogurt, and cheese. Adults need two or more servings each day. That means two eight-ounce glasses of milk, two cups of yogurt, two one-and-a-half-ounce servings of cheese, or any combination of these dairy foods. Needless to say, the best are the low-fat or nonfat varieties. Read the label to see just how much fat you're getting per serving. Some of the new yogurts, for example, are being advertised as "premium." This means they're made with whole milk or even cream rather than low-fat milk, and the fat, calorie, and cholesterol levels soar as a result.

The next group gives us no such problems with cholesterol. The fruit-vegetable group provides our vitamins A and C along with a substantial amount of fiber. Some authorities feel there should be separate fruit and vegetable groups, rather than combining them in one group. Each day an adult needs two servings of fruit and two servings of vegetables at a minimum. Here's the place to satisfy your appetite without guilt. Pile on that corn, squash, spinach, and salad! Enjoy all the seasonal fruits as well as splurging on imported delicacies.

The same also applies to the bread-cereal or grain group. This includes all the breads, cereals, and grains, especially the whole grains. Here's the source of abundant fiber, thiamine (B_1), iron, niacin, and good complex carbohydrates. For many societies around the world, foods from this group comprise the staple diet: Rice in the Orient. Pasta in the Mediterranean. Hearty breads in Europe. Instead of thinking "meatballs and spaghetti" think in terms of "spaghetti with a little meat." As an additional benefit, you'll be able to enjoy more food on your plate for fewer calories. Adults need a minimum of four servings daily from this group. This is where to balance off your caloric needs for the day. Eat all the grains, breads, and pastas you like without gaining weight.

Most of us were taught to believe that starchy foods are fattening and should, therefore, be limited by those watching their weight. Actually, it's the butter and sauces that add the calories. Breads, pasta, and a wide variety of whole-grain foods supply a lot of nutrition for the calories. Remember, too, that you'll be replacing fat calories with carbohydrate calories. Each gram of fat contains nine calories, while a gram of carbohydrate provides only four. You'll find that eating more carbohydrate-rich foods will give you a tremendous feeling of satisfaction. In fact, you'll be amazed at how much you'll eat while either maintaining or actually losing weight.

The only warning or caution flag that goes up here is in the bakery. Many or most of the commercially prepared baked goods have a high content of fat and cholesterol. Choose sourdough and rye bread and commercially baked breads that do not contain eggs and shortenings on the ingredients label. Unfortunately, this excludes virtually every cookie, pie, and cake in the bakery. Angel-food cake is an exception, made only with egg whites. Your best bet for such baked goods is to prepare them at home from scratch, using low-fat milk and egg substitutes.

Read Chapter 13, "Let's Go Shopping," for tips and hints about selecting the best foods for a cholesterol-controlled diet. You'll find that with a little thought you can enjoy practically all the dishes on your list of favorites. It simply takes a modification here and an adjustment there.

This book does not include any suggested menus for the day. In my opinion, based on a number of years of experience, no one pays any attention to such menus, or takes the time and effort to follow them faithfully. I do, however, show some examples of typical days' food intake to demonstrate how a wide variety of foods can be chosen while remaining within reasonable limits of fat and cholesterol. See page 394.

Your best approach is to modify your existing eating habits, using your favorite recipes and favorite restaurants. It's ridiculous to expect that anyone is going to change a lifetime of eating patterns overnight—or ever. But it's not at all out of the question to make a few adjustments. If a recipe calls for heavy cream, use evaporated skim milk. If baking, replace butter with tub-type margarine—in half the quantity. Use two eggs whites instead of one whole egg. Fry with just a spray of Pam.

Such recommendations apply to the entire population rather than only those with a particular need to reduce the cholesterol risk factor. A diet high in fiber and complex carbohydrates and low in fats and cholesterol has been generally regarded as best for all

Americans, male and female, young and old alike. The same principles, with particular emphasis on simple sugars, apply directly to those trying to control diabetes. Such a diet is widely believed to offer protection against a number of cancers, especially colon and breast cancers. The low-fat diet is inherently lower in calories, benefiting those many Americans who are overweight. All necessary nutrients are provided in abundant quantities, ensuring proper growth and maintenance even for children. On the other hand, there are absolutely no contraindications for following this type of diet for the entirety of one's life. The nutrition plan described in this book assures one of a balanced diet, complete with sufficient protein, vitamins, and minerals.

Moreover, this approach to nutrition puts a high value on the pure enjoyment of food. Our abundance of food should be relished and cherished. The variety most authorities encourage allows one to savor all the many flavors and textures in our cornucopia of foods.

Bear in mind that those rich French sauces were originally developed to mask spoiled and rotten meats in the days prior to refrigeration. Remember that those fast-food nuggets of chicken are up to half chopped skin and gristle. Hot dogs contain ingredients that virtually no man or woman would eat if they were not disguised. Read the ingredients on some snack-food labels and ask yourself if you really miss nibbling at a chemical factory. Remember the times you overindulged and suffered with gastric upset and indigestion.

Instead of those "delights" plunge into the wealth of natural, delicious flavors of foods as they were meant to be. Enjoy! That's all the nutrition you need to know for a healthful diet!

13

Let's Go Shopping

The place to start improving your eating habits and those of your entire family is the supermarket. A bit of planning can make a huge difference in the way you eat, and in the success of lowering your cholesterol levels. And, in the process, you'll save time and money and you'll come to a whole new enjoyment of food.

For years home economists have urged cost-conscious homemakers to use a shopping list. Now that may not sound like an earth-shaking idea, but the fact is that many or even most shoppers go into the market without much idea of what they'll buy. Purchases are based on impulse, and the bill at the checkout counter often is more than expected. Making a list and sticking with it helps to save dollars.

At the same time, calorie-conscious shoppers are warned not to venture into the aisles of the market while hungry. We've all done that, and the result is always the same. We buy more food than we really want or need—and the wrong kinds of food. And again, the foods are based on impulse decision making.

You've probably heard this advice before.

But now it's time to put these suggestions into practice in order to purchase foods in a more logical manner for more healthful eating. And let me add one more suggestion, especially for your first few trips: Go to the market when you have plenty of time. Don't rush. Make shopping a learning experience.

Now let's get down to some details. First we'll consider a new approach to making the shopping list. Remember that the best way to select nutritious foods is on the basis of the four food groups. Each day we want to eat foods from the meat, milk, fruit-vegetable, and bread-cereal groups. By doing so, as we discussed in the chapter on nutrition, we'll get all the nutrients we need, without a lot of calories, and without a lot of fat and cholesterol.

THE MEAT-GROUP SHOPPING LIST

The meat-group category includes a wide variety of protein-rich foods. Some are better choices than others. Too often when we think of meat, the mental image is that of a rare cut of beef. But the word "meat" includes veal, fish, chicken, turkey, and, in terms of protein contributions, eggs and dried beans.

Let's start with beef. There's no reason to completely eliminate red meat from the diet, especially if you really enjoy it. Select those cuts that are lowest in fat content, as shown in the charts in Chapter 4, "Winning by the Numbers." Notice also that those figures refer to a three-ounce cooked serving that has been well trimmed of visible fat. So when shopping count on four ounces per person.

But, if you haven't already started to do so, broaden your selections of meats. Veal, for example, is a delicious alternative that's considerably lower in fat content. Ground veal contains only about 10 percent fat, while the leanest ground beef has about 15 percent. It's also a good value when compared with lower-fat-content ground beef, and gives you a greater cooked yield. Try it for hamburgers, chili, sloppy joes, or in any other recipe calling for ground beef.

Today there's a wonderful way to enjoy all your favorite cuts of juicy beef without fat. Ozark Belgian Blue Beef sells specially bred cattle called Belgian Blue. Naturally raised and processed, without antibiotics or hormones, this beef has all the flavor and tenderness you love. Imagine New York strips, ribeyes, sirloin, roasts—even ribs—that average a mere 3 grams of fat per serving. At that rate you can dig into a 10-ounce slab of rare beef and still be heart healthy. And you can have it delivered to your door at a very reasonable price. You'll want to keep a freezer-full for every time nothing but beef will do. Write for more information to Ozark Belgian Blue Beef, LCC, Route 4, Box 2220, Stockton, MO, 65785. Or call (877) 425-8363.

You can also get very lean ground beef in any supermarket by selecting a piece of top round or a London broil and asking the butcher to trim off all the visible fat before grinding. That will give you about 5 percent fat, as compared with the 15 percent found in the leanest pre-ground beef. Some supermarkets now offer very-low-fat ground beef, labeled as low as 5 percent fat. Then you can use the ground beef in all your recipes calling for hamburger.

But for the lowest fat content of all, shop for poultry. Turkey breast has a mere trace of fat, less than 4 percent. Note that I'm referring to turkey breast, not skin or dark meat. Skin contains more than 39 percent fat. Dark meat has more than 8 percent. These figures are on the average, with young birds having less fat, and mature birds having more.

When shopping, read the label on prepackaged ground turkey or turkey sausage and you'll see that these products are made from the entire turkey, skin and all. This results in a fat content of about 15 percent, no better than lean ground beef.

For something different and delicious, try replacing beef with ostrich meat. This delicious red meat—not white like chicken—has all the flavor of beef with just a gram or two of fat per serving. Call Cal-Pride Ostrich at (800) 495-7743.

Chicken is another excellent source of protein without a lot of fat and cholesterol. But again note that dark meat contains higher amounts of fat. Chicken breasts are best, and there are hundreds of ways to prepare them.

Other poultry is not as good a choice. Both duck and goose contain high levels of fat, and should be kept for special occasions if you really like those birds.

Wild game, even if raised on commercial farms, offers low-fat meat in a tasty variety. New Zealand now exports delicious venison, so tender you won't have to marinate it. If there's a hunter in your family, wish him or her luck.

Next on your shopping list should be lots of fish. If you're not already an avid fish eater, there are a number of ways to start appreciating and enjoying this meat alternative. Most fish haters still like tuna fish in salads or sandwiches. Try using canned salmon in some recipes that call for tuna. This is even easier now that Hormel has started to can salmon without the skin and bones. You can use it straight out of the can, just like tuna.

Shellfish lovers learned in Chapter 7 that previous figures for cholesterol content were greatly exaggerated because of faulty testing methods. Shrimp contains a fair amount of cholesterol. But all shellfish have only traces of fat. And, for the most part, we tend to eat smaller amounts of shellfish at a time than meat, so having a few shrimp really won't hurt at all. The winner of the low-fat, low-cholesterol contest, though, goes to the popular and versatile scallop.

For those of us who also have to watch the price tags of the foods we buy, *surimi*, or imitation crabmeat, is getting better and better.

If you prefer your fish in the convenient frozen and breaded form you can still enjoy it, but start to read the labels carefully. Some of the batters are made with egg yolks and a lot of fat. Others, including the very delicious Lite Cod and Lite Sole entrées from Morton, contain no egg yolks and have a low fat content, considering that they are fried foods. Even so, limit fried foods of any kind.

When selecting fresh fish, let your taste buds be your guide. As more and more Americans have learned to enjoy fish, the variety and selection have grown all over the country.

You don't have to live near an ocean to get the freshest fillets.

Moving down the aisle of the meat section, we come to luncheon meats—the downfall of many of us. The unhappy fact is that such meats, even when made from turkey or chicken, contain an unhealthful amount of fat. Just one slice of salami has 9 to 12 grams of fat. And I've never known anyone who eats just one slice. One slice of Canadian bacon, on the other hand, has only two grams. Other good choices are sliced turkey breast and ham. Surprised that ham is on the list? Read the labels on these foods and you'll see that some ham products contain as little as 2 percent fat.

The all-American hot dog, unfortunately, is another source of excessive fat in the diet. All-beef Oscar Mayer frankfurters have 13.5 grams of fat each. Even the Tyson chicken frankfurter gives you 8.5 grams. Today you can find virtually any hot dog or sausage you want in a low-fat version. Oscar Mayer, Hormel, Ball Park, Healthy Choice, and many others offer 97% fat-free varieties.

Bacon and sausage have far too much fat and contain a walloping amount of sodium as well. A good alternative is turkey breakfast sausage. This has 15 percent fat, but you can reduce the amount by parboiling before you brown the patties. Try your homemade variety using ground turkey breast and the recipes found at the end of this book. You can make your own salami, bologna, pepperoni, jerky, and breakfast sausage by mixing ground turkey or another lean meat with a product called Spice 'n' Slice. Each box contains separate packs of spices and salt, so you can limit the amount of sodium to your own needs. You can place an order by phone, using your charge card, by calling (800) 310-4094.

Eggs—an excellent source of protein—have one of the highest contributions of cholesterol. Depending on the size of the egg and the method of measurement, a large egg contains from 200 to 250 milligrams of cholesterol. For 10 years I did not eat a single egg yoke. Then I made a wonderful discovery that now allows me—and you—to enjoy all the eggs I want, as well as other cholesterol-rich foods.

Just as all animal tissues contain cholesterol, an animal sterol, all plant tissues have phytosterol, a plant sterol, not to be confused with steroids. It turns out that the molecular structures of cholesterol and phytosterol are virtually identical. So similar, in fact, that the human body cannot tell the difference.

Phytosterols are now available in concentrated tablet form. Taken 30 minutes or so before a meal, they dissolve in the stomach and enter the digestive tract where cholesterol is normally absorbed, blocking the cholesterol receptor sites. So when cholesterol in the food you eat comes along, there's no room at those sites, and it gets passed out.

There's plenty of scientific evidence to back this up, and because phytosterols are of plant origin, there are no possible side effects or adverse reactions for anyone. So all of us can enjoy all the eggs, shrimp, and other cholesterol-rich foods we want.

To order phytosterol tablets, call (800) 483-2532. They will also send you a complete report answering all your questions about this revolutionary breakthrough. See also page 442.

Because the meat group is comprised of those foods that offer a significant amount of protein, dried beans and peanut butter are also included. Dried beans include lentils, navy beans, pinto beans, garbanzos, kidney beans, and other; you can also buy them canned to avoid the process of cooking. Dried beans have also been shown to significantly reduce cholesterol levels. Try them in salads, soups, and a number of dishes such as dips.

Peanut butter poses somewhat of a problem. While it contains no cholesterol, it does have a large amount of fat. One tablespoon contains more than 7 grams. A sandwich typically will have two or even three tablespoon-fuls. Keep this to a once-in-a-while treat.

The same applies to nuts of all sorts. One tablespoon of chopped walnuts contains 4.8 grams of fat. Peanuts have 7 grams. One ounce of almonds provides more than 16 grams in the roasted and salted variety.

But there's good news about nuts. Research has shown that, as part of a healthy diet, nuts do not raise cholesterol levels. In fact, those who enjoy nuts regularly actually have a lower risk of heart disease, perhaps owing to the amino acid arginine richly present in all nuts. Just don't forget the calories, and keep your enjoyment in moderation.

THE MILK-GROUP SHOPPING LIST

Dairy foods, as we've all learned from school days, provide the majority of calcium in the diet. While it's certainly true that we never outgrow our need for calcium, we don't need the fat and cholesterol. So selections from this group should be made accordingly.

Choose nonfat or low-fat milk rather than whole milk. The differences are enormous. Whole milk contains 9 grams of fat per eight-ounce serving. Low-fat milk has 5 grams. And nonfat milk has only a trace remaining. The cholesterol disappears right along with the fat. After a while, you'll actually prefer the lighter, fresher taste. Start weaning yourself away from whole milk. Go first to the low-fat and then on to nonfat types.

The same applies to cheese. Start reading those nutrition labels. One ounce of American cheese has a whopping 8.4 grams of fat. But Borden's Lite Line has only 2.0. One cup creamed cottage cheese contains 9.5 grams, but the 2-percent type reduces that down to 4.4. And you can go all the way down to 1.6 grams with 1-percent cottage cheese. Regular mozzarella cheese contains 6.1 grams of fat per ounce. The low-moisture, part-skim variety brings it down to 4.8.

One nice way to get the flavor of cheese in your foods without all the fat is to use grated Parmesan cheese. One tablespoon has only 1.5 grams of fat. But a one-ounce portion of hard Parmesan bounces the total up to 7.3 grams.

Bear in mind that cholesterol levels drop right along with the fat content. So there is, of course, a lot less cholesterol in the low-fat varieties than in the regular types.

Keep reading those labels when you come to the yogurt section. You'll find a big difference from one container to another. The most commonly found and eaten kind of yogurt is low-fat, which has about 3.4 grams of fat per cup. Nonfat brands have a mere 0.4 grams. Whole-milk types, on the other hand, have 7.7 grams per eight-ounce container. And the newly introduced "premium" yogurts made with cream in addition to whole milk have even more. Those "premium" yogurts are an example of how a delicious, nutritious food can be turned into a fat- and cholesterol-laden disaster—a junk food. Calorie content varies widely in various kinds of yogurt, depending upon the amount of fat and sugar. Read the labels.

What about some other dairy products? Sour cream can easily be replaced with nonfat brands for a big saving in fat and cholesterol. Eggnog has 19 grams of fat and lots of cholesterol in every eight-ounce glass. But you can make a delicious version with Egg Beaters and evaporated skim milk (see recipe p. 525).

Cream contains a lot of fat and cholesterol. Nondairy creamers cut out the cholesterol, but the fat content is just as high—and the fat they use is saturated. The perfect alternative is canned evaporated skim milk. Use it any time a dish calls for cream, whipping cream, or whole milk. It has a lot of "body" owing to the addition of nonfat milk solids. In fact, it can even be whipped. Try this with a touch of egg white, a dash of sugar, and a trace of vanilla extract. For best results, chill the mixture and your beaters in advance. Pet and Carnation make evaporated skim milk. You may have to search around in order to find it near you. Or have your supermarket manager order a case.

You probably think you shouldn't even be looking at the whipped-cream products in the dairy case, so I'll point you in that direction to look for Reddi Whip or other fat-free aerosol whipped cream.

THE FRUIT AND VEGETABLE SHOPPING LIST

Spend some time in the produce section of your store. Go to some of the specialty shops. Stop at roadside stands. Try all the different kinds of fruits and vegetables from all over the nation and around the world. Talk to the manager to find out how to prepare and cook some of the more exotic varieties.

Now that you're saving money by cutting down on the amounts of meat and cheese you're eating, you can spend some on fruits and vegetables you may have avoided before.

There's only one fruit that you should limit during your trips to the supermarket. Avocados have 16.4 grams of monounsaturated fat per 3½-ounce serving. Of course there's no cholesterol, since that's limited to animal foods. Though monounsaturated fat is better than saturated, that's still a lot of fat to consume. If you enjoy the special flavor and delicate texture of avocados, keep the servings small. I like to use a nice, ripe avocado to spread on bread instead of mayonnaise when making turkey sandwiches.

With that one exception, you can enjoy all the fruits and vegetables in the marketplace. Canned and frozen vegetables contain all the nutrients in fresh varieties, at typically lower cost. But, if using the canned types, read the labels for sodium content or choose the salt-free brands. Canned refried beans may contain lard. Select those labeled "vegetarian."

Canned fruits can also be a welcome treat for dessert or as a snack. It's best to choose the types canned in plain water or the fruit's own juices rather than heavy syrup, which adds a lot of sugar.

THE BREAD-CEREAL SHOPPING LIST

This group includes all the foods made from grain. They're an important part of the diet, providing fiber, carbohydrates, and many of the B vitamins. But, again, read the labels to see exactly what you're eating.

Commercially baked goods frequently are made with egg yolks, fat, or both. Soft white bread, for example, has one gram of fat per slice. That adds up quickly. The same applies to many of the whole-wheat breads. Again, read the ingredient labels carefully to spot those "partially hydrogenated fats."

Most oyster crackers, the kind sprinkled in soups and stews, are made with lard. I prefer to buy the Sunshine brand, which is made with only vegetable oil. Buy bagels made with water rather than the egg types.

How about pasta and noodles? Most spaghetti and other pastas are made with only flour and water. But egg noodles contain, of course, eggs. This adds 50 milligrams of cholesterol per cooked cup of noodles. But you can find noodles made without eggs. They're marketed as "lite" noodles. Or substitute fettuccine. No Yolks was the first cholesterol-free brand of noodles on the market. Today there are many others. Or you can simply take a phytosterol tablet to block the cholesterol and enjoy any cholesterol-rich food you wish! See page 371.

Another source of hidden cholesterol includes all the packaged cake and pancake mixes, which are made with egg yolks. Your best bet is to make your own pancake or cake mixes, using the recipes found at the end of this book, and keep them stored in the freezer.

When it comes to breakfast cereals, fat and cholesterol are not a problem, but sugar is. The old-fashioned cereals, free of added sugar, are still the best. And, of course, you'll want to increase your consumption of oat bran both in cereals and made into muffins. You can purchase oat bran in one-pound packages found in the hot cereal section. Some stores now carry oat bran in bulk, bringing the price down considerably. You might consider approaching the store manager to discuss a discount for large purchases.

One last comment about the foods in the bread-cereal group. Advertisers have convinced the buying public that granola bars are a healthful, nutritious, "natural" snack. A closer look shows them to be no more than candy bars in disguise. The Nature Valley coconut bar, for example, has a whopping 6.1 grams of fat. Plus lots of sugars. The Carnation cinnamon breakfast bar contains 11 grams of fat. And, again, the rest of the calories come mainly from sugar. You'd be better off with a candy bar. A Snickers bar has "only" 6.2 grams of fat.

OTHER FOODS SHOPPING LIST

In addition to the basic foods we've discussed, most shopping lists include a wide variety of foods best listed as "others." In this category one can group the oils and fats, sugars, spices and herbs, and many condiments. These offer more enjoyment than nutrition, and selection should be carefully made.

When it comes to fats and oils, there are some items it's simply best to avoid completely. These are butter, lard, and hard margarine. Coconut, palm, and palm kernel oil come packed with more saturated fat than even butter and lard. Avoid products made with these tropical oils as much as possible. As a result of pressure from consumers, Keebler has removed all tropical oils from its products. Continental Baking Company has taken out both animal shortening and tropical oils from its Wonder Bread products. General Foods continues to use tropical oils only in cereals and desserts. Keep reading the labels to see which products use these oils and which do not.

The advertising on TV seems to make selection of vegetable oil difficult, but the facts make the choice a lot simpler. Regardless of what advertisers say about their particular products, the fact is that *no* vegetable oil contains cholesterol. As far as cholesterol is concerned, then, one oil is as good as another.

The next point in those advertisements regards how much polyunsaturated fat the oil contains. Yes, safflower oil has more than corn oil. But the difference is made up by monounsaturated fat, which is just as desirable. In fact, monounsaturated fats have more capability of maintaining the protective HDL levels than do polyunsaturated fats.

For a general-purpose cooking oil I prefer Puritan or other brands of canola oil. This offers the same monounsaturated fats as olive oil, without the overbearing flavor you want to avoid in certain recipes.

But you may wish to buy two oils in addition to your routine vegetable oil. As discussed in Chapter 7, olive oil and peanut oil are primarily monounsaturated fats; their use in certain world populations has been correlated with reduced cholesterol levels with no reduction in protective HDLs. Both add their own flavors to certain kinds of cooking. We use all three—vegetable oil, olive oil, and peanut oil—in our house.

Regardless of the type of oil, though, it's best to limit the total amount you use. One very nice way to do that is by cooking with Pam or one of the other vegetable-oil sprays on the market; they provide a fine, uniform coating on the pan. It's remarkable how little oil one really needs to sauté a piece of fish or chicken.

I've also found another interesting and delicious use for such sprays. I've always enjoyed garlic bread, but had virtually eliminated it from my diet to get rid of the butter. Then I came up with this recipe: spray a piece of sourdough bread with butter-flavor Pam, sprinkle on garlic powder to taste, and bake for five minutes in a hot oven. It's delicious, without much fat at all.

Another way to cut down on total fats is to use a marvelous product called Butter Buds. They've been able to capture the flavor of butter in these packets of powder, with no fat or cholesterol. We use them in a number of ways. They're terrific when sprinkled over hot vegetables. They add butter's flavor to baked goods. And they're a wonderful ingredient in cooking. We even sprinkle them on popcorn. Every time you use Butter Buds, that's another time you're not consuming fat—and that's the whole idea. Two other products, Molly McButter and O'Butter, have entered the market. These are similar to Butter Buds, but come in shaker containers.

Moving down the cooking-oils aisle we come to the salad-dressing section. Again, your best bet is to start reading labels. See how many grams of fat are to be found in each tablespoonful. This doesn't necessarily mean buying only those that have the lowest amount, regardless of personal taste. Rather, it may be a matter of using a bit less of one particular type. It's a trade-off.

You may be surprised to see that the traditional bottled oil-and-vinegar dressings contain more fat per serving than a similar amount of Thousand Island or Ranch dressing. Make your shopping trips a learning experience by standing in the aisle and reading those labels before you buy the foods. Many products are available with no oil at all. As time goes on, you'll know the brands and types to select.

Tartar sauce, for example, varies enormously from product to product. Read the label. If the product's ingredient list includes egg yolks, move on to the next one. The same applies to salad dressings.

Many people already buy packets of salad dressing seasonings to mix together at home. The directions often call for mayonnaise. One suggestion would be to use low-fat mayonnaise. Another is to substitute nonfat yogurt. If directions call for oil, simply use half the amount listed and increase other liquids.

But what about mayonnaise? Again, read the labels. There are a number of reduced-fat brands on the market. I'm particularly fond of Hellman's/Best Foods Low Fat. And, while mayonnaise is made with egg yolks, the actual amount of cholesterol is so small in a single serving that it's almost insignificant. On the other hand, you may prefer the taste of salad dressing, which contains no cholesterol at all. Pick the reduced-fat brands.

The next big source of calories in the supermarket and in the diet is sugar. Brown sugar, granulated sugar, "natural" turbinado sugar—they're all the same in terms of calories and the way your body digests them. Sucrose is sucrose, no matter where it comes from. And *all* sugars, including honey and fructose, eventually get broken down by the body into blood sugar, called glucose.

Your choice of the type and amount of sugar you want in your diet, then, depends only on personal taste and your waistline. While sugar does not directly elevate cholesterol levels, it may lead to overweight or raised triglycerides.

That brings us to the next category in the "others" group. Desserts pose somewhat of a problem for those of us trying to limit fat and cholesterol. The same applies to snacks. Ice cream, pies, cakes, cookies, and other treats are loaded with fat and cholesterol. And the richer and better tasting they are, the higher the levels of those offenders. In many cases it's a matter of complete avoidance.

Instead of ice cream, choose sherbet. Try some of the newly introduced sorbets. Read the labels and you'll see that the principal ingredient is fruit purée. They are truly delicious, long a special treat in Europe.

Another alternative is frozen yogurt and various frozen-yogurt dessert confections. Johnson's frozen yogurts are available in chocolate, peach, and other flavors, all with very little fat.

Also consider new products as they come on the market. One example is gelatin pops, which contain only 35 calories per bar. And instead of having an ice-cream bar for a snack opt for the popsicle.

When it comes to cakes and cookies, there are few acceptable types other than angel-food cake, which is made with only egg whites, no yolks. If you are a true cake and cookie lover, it may be worth the effort to return to baking homemade goods from scratch so that you can use egg substitutes and vegetable oils instead of fat- and cholesterol-laden ingredients.

But let's face it: now and then there's just no substitute for a rich, gooey cake. Birthdays, parties, anniversaries, and the like call for sweet confections. For these special times, you can choose from a myriad of cakes by Entenmann's. While fat-free, don't forget that the baked goods have just as many calories as the original, since sugar is used to replace the fat. If weight loss is important in your case, enjoy these very moderately and stick with a true serving size rather than half the cake.

While you're shopping you'll also want to pick up some packages of raisins and dried fruits. Arrange them attractively in bowls so they are available whenever you get the urge to munch. For a special treat, why not buy a gift platter of fancy fruits for yourself? You deserve it.

Finally we come to the category of beverages to wash down all those foods. There are few limitations here. America has really caught on to the idea of drinking bottled water, both bubbling and still, both imported and domestic. You can even find reduced-sodium waters. And today there are a spectrum of calorie-free soft drinks, sweetened with NutraSweet, which leave no bitter aftertaste.

Here's a bit of personal preference and practice: I've cut out the sugar in soft drinks, and use it in my cooking and baking. Again, a nice trade-off. I can't tell much of a difference in a cola drink, but I appreciate the touch of sugar sweetness in my oat-bran muffins and in my home-baked cookies.

The goal of your shopping list, then, is to

select foods that will add up to your daily target of fat, cholesterol, and sugar without going over that target. And, of course, you'll also want to count the milligrams of sodium in tallying your lists.

There are two things that make the dietary-modification part of this program work. First, knowing just how many grams of fat should be included throughout the day. Second, reading the labels on prepared foods and the charts listing fats and cholesterol in this book.

If, like me, you limit your fat to 50 grams per day, it's fairly easy to keep track of your intake. The three muffins I eat in the morning provide a total of 10.5 grams of fat. Using the oil-free recipe cuts out even this fat almost completely. Milk, coffee, juice, and other beverages have little or no fat. At lunch I may have a tuna-salad sandwich. The tuna has only 0.8 grams of fat for a 3½-ounce serving; that's half a can of water-packed tuna. I also use a tablespoon of Weight Watchers' reduced-fat mayonnaise, which adds 4 grams of fat. My beverage, again, adds no fat. Nor does the fruit I nibble on throughout the afternoon as snacks.

So far I'm up to a total of 15 grams of fat. I've got 35 grams to go. For dinner I can have veal cutlets (9.0 grams per 3½ ounces), mixed green salad with blue-cheese dressing

(7.3 grams per tablespoon), spaghetti with commercial sauce (1 gram for 3 tablespoons), a tablespoon of grated Parmesan cheese (1.5 grams), and tapioca pudding for dessert (3.1 grams per 3½-ounce serving). That comes to about 22 grams for dinner, still short of my allotted total. I remember that, and the next day I might be at a restaurant where I won't feel guilty about ordering the French-fried potatoes.

Try it for yourself. Think of a day's food. Make up some menus for yourself and start tallying up the grams of fat contained in each of the foods. You'll be absolutely amazed at how much food, and how many different kinds of food, you can eat and enjoy each and every day.

The only times you'll run into problems are when you want to eat foods you already know should be avoided. Like greasy fast-food meals. Or hollandaise sauce. Or a hot fudge sundae topped with whipped cream and chopped nuts.

After a while, you'll almost instinctively know when you're within your own permissible fat-intake level. You won't have to specifically count each food's fat content because you'll be selecting foods you know are within your set limits.

But be prepared for one frustration in the

supermarkets. Not every food has a nicely spelled-out nutrition label listing the content of fat, cholesterol, and sodium. The laws are not strict along these lines. As time goes on, more and more foods will be labeled. In the meantime, the food industry is making every effort to keep such information off food packages. They don't want you to know how much fat there is in an ounce of cheese, or a handful of peanuts, or a half-dozen crackers, or in any of a number of other foods.

If you feel that manufacturers should list the amounts of fat, cholesterol, and sodium to make it easier for you to keep track of your healthy diet, write to your representatives in Congress and let them know. You'd be amazed at how much they pay attention to such letters. Constituents ultimately count more than lobbyists if they stand up to be counted. But, until all foods are labeled, rely on the charts in this book.

While making that shopping list, think also in terms of the meals you'll prepare. One nice and practical approach is to plan the meals for the entire week. That way you'll know what foods to purchase from each of the groups, and you'll see at a glance when you're choosing the widest variety of foods. Next comes the matter of cooking those foods.

To make them taste their best, you'll want

to experiment with all kinds of herbs and spices. Every kitchen should be supplied with a broad assortment of dried herbs and spices. As you read through recipes, you may see some that you'll want to pick up. And, while you're at it, try some of the fresh herbs that are available in your produce section. There's nothing like fresh basil, for example, to put a zing into a tomato sauce. Or fresh garlic.

You'll also find that when you use herbs and spices there'll be less need for salt. A dash of this or a splash of that can replace the sodium very nicely.

The Equipment You'll Need

A lifetime of food enjoyment deserves a bit of financial investment. Some of the items that make low-fat and low-cholesterol cooking easier cost quite a few dollars. But they're worth it in the long run. Add to your kitchen as you're able.

A set of fine, sharp knives are a joy in the kitchen. There's nothing more frustrating than to try to chop and slice foods with a dull blade. A good set of cutlery is a lifelong investment. Add a cutting board and you'll be all set.

Two appliances that also greatly help are

the blender and the food processor. Both have come down in price considerably over the years, and are frequently on sale. Owning a food processor facilitates cooking so much that you'll be able to enjoy foods and dishes you'd otherwise pass by.

While you're slicing, dicing, and otherwise preparing your foods, you'll want to know exactly how much you'll be serving. That's why a food scale is an essential piece of equipment. As you use the scale, you'll start to develop an eye for measurements.

Then it's time to cook those foods. To do so, you'll want at least one nonstick pan for sautéing. This cuts considerably into the amount of oil needed. A good steamer, the kind placed in a pot with a cover, lets you prepare crisp, delicious vegetables. And a wok gives you access to the whole world of stir-fry Oriental cooking.

Whether a recipe is simple or complicated, it still takes some time to prepare. Why not double the recipe? Store the extra portions in the freezer for times when you simply don't have the time to cook.

It's often the hurried meal that's packed with the most fat and cholesterol. Think about it. It's been a long day at work, you're tired, it's late in the evening, and you don't feel like cooking. So you pick up a double cheeseburger on the way home—complete with French fries and a milkshake. Take a look at the numbers for such a meal in the charts to see just how much fat and cholesterol you're eating just because you don't have the time or energy to cook.

Instead, think how nice it would be to remember all the pre-prepared meals waiting for you in the freezer. Chili made with ground turkey breast. A few Chinese entrées. Or perhaps one of the new lite entrées along with a salad.

As you put your shopping list together, plan on having some "emergency meals" in your freezer. Plan the snacks you'll have when that midnight hunger strikes. Be ready for all the times when the choice comes down to healthful versus harmful food selections.

Each time you go shopping, read those labels. Try to find something different in the produce section. Soon your new eating patterns will become second nature, and you'll wonder why you didn't start doing this years ago.

MENU PLANNING

Everyone's tastes and preferences are different, and trying to follow a specific, day-by-day diet is almost bound to fail, since those preferences are not taken into consideration. But, strictly for the sake of illustration, let's look at three "typical" days' meals made from the foods we talked about buying in the market. All the recipes are listed in the book, and the listings of fat and cholesterol for each dish are based on the assumption that you'll be cooking with egg whites rather than yolks, and following the other ideas for reducing fat and cholesterol in your foods.

I've compiled these meal plans to fit my own needs as a 150-pound male, limiting fat intake to 50 grams and cholesterol to less than 250 milligrams. In order to calculate the values, I had to look up the numbers in the chart right here in the book. Why not try to add up some of your own favorites? If you near the end of the hypothetical day, and you've gone over your own limit, remember to cut back the next day. If you've got a few grams and milligrams to spare, that might be the day for a treat of some sort.

Certainly no one will calculate the exact figures for fat and cholesterol each and every day. That's just asking too much, even for the most dedicated person. But after a while, just a short while, you'll start mentally coming up with an average total and you'll be right on target.

Day One

	FAT (GRAMS)	CHOLESTEROL (MILLIGRAMS)
Breakfast		
3 oat-bran pancakes with maple syrup	4.5	0
1 three-oz. turkey-sausage patty	4.2	66
1 four-oz. glass of orange juice	—	—
Decaffeinated coffee or tea	—	—
Lunch		
1 tunafish sandwich made with 3½ oz. tuna and 1 tbsp. low-fat mayo on sourdough bread	4.8	63
1 oat-bran muffin made with bananas and dates	4.5	—
1 eight-oz. glass skim milk	0.4	5
Snack		
1 medium apple	—	—
Dinner		
Mixed green salad with 2 tbsp. Green Goddess or similar creamy dressing	5.0	—
5 oz. roast chicken or turkey, white meat only, without skin	7.0	110
Mashed potatoes made with Butter Buds and evaporated skim milk	—	—
Vegetable with 1 tsp. margarine	4.0	—
Dinner roll (whole-wheat) with 1 tsp. margarine	4.0	—
½ cup sherbet	4.0	—
Day's total:	**42.4**	**244**

NOTE: Vary total calories for personal needs by adding or subtracting amounts of nonfat foods such as potatoes.

Day Two

	FAT	CHOLESTEROL
	(GRAMS)	(MILLIGRAMS)

Breakfast

²/₃ cup (uncooked) oat-bran cereal with raisins	4.0	—
¹/₂ cup skim milk for cereal	0.2	5.0
¹/₂ cup tomato juice	—	—
Decaffeinated coffee or tea	—	—

Lunch

Ham sandwich made with 3¹/₂ oz. ham on sourdough or whole-wheat bread with lettuce and tomatoes	5.0	50.0
1 tangerine	—	—
1 eight-oz. glass skim milk	0.4	5.0

Dinner

Green salad with creamy dressing	5.0	—
7 oz. broiled salmon with lemon squeeze	14.8	94.0
Rice with 1 tsp. margarine	4.0	—
Vegetable with 1 tsp. margarine	4.0	—
Dinner roll with 1 tsp. margarine	4.0	—
¹/₂ cup vanilla custard	0.3	3.0

Evening Snack

Air-popped popcorn seasoned with Butter Buds	—	—

Day's total:	**41.7**	**157.0**

NOTE: If you can do without the margarine during dinner, you may prefer to "spend" the fat grams on your popcorn.

Day Three

	FAT (GRAMS)	CHOLESTEROL (MILLIGRAMS)
Breakfast		
3 oat-bran muffins made with blueberries	10.5	—
½ cup grapefruit juice	—	—
1 eight-oz. glass skim milk	0.4	5
Decaffeinated coffee or tea		
Lunch		
1 peanut-butter sandwich made with 2 tbsp. peanut butter and jam or jelly, on sourdough or whole-wheat bread	14.4	—
1 eight-oz. glass skim milk	0.4	5
Grapes	—	—
Dinner		
Mixed green salad with creamy dressing	5.0	—
4-oz. lean filet mignon, broiled	12.0	144
Baked potato with Butter Buds	—	—
Vegetable	—	—
3½ oz. tapioca pudding	3.1	53
Snack		
Raisins	—	—
Day's total:	**45.8**	**207**

NOTE: Here's an example of two fairly high-fat menu items, peanut butter and beef, both in the same day—possible when you watch the other foods eaten.

14

The Proof of the Pudding

I'll never forget the day I heard about my own positive results with the diet-oat-bran-niacin program. I was working out at the Santa Monica Medical Center Cardiac Rehabilitation Center. Specifically, I was sweating on the rowing machine when my blood-test data came through. When the nurse read those wonderful numbers, tears actually came to my eyes.

Remember that just a few months earlier I had had a total cholesterol level of 284 mg/dl. A highly restricted diet of absolutely no red meat, no eggs, and nonfat milk got it down only to a disappointing 271.

Then, after just eight weeks of eating my oat-bran muffins and taking my niacin tablets, I received the good news. My total cholesterol level had plummeted to 169. And my ratio of total cholesterol to HDL was a nice, healthy 3.4—far below risk.

A year later, subsequent blood testing came up with the same kinds of numbers time and time again. For me, I knew I had found the answer. And, being a writer, I wanted to share the news with others.

The fact of the matter is I probably had enough of a story to tell so that I could have published the book simply on the basis of my own spectacular results. But I also have scientific training and an ingrained scientific curiosity. Would the approach work for others as well?

Moreover, as a medical writer I've often been critical of books that make claims without very much documentation. I became determined that not only would I back up every statement in the scientific chapters with references from the most trustworthy scientific literature, but also I would tell how the program can and has worked for many others.

We have the results now, and for many they are simply spectacular. Total cholesterol levels drop by 100 points and more. Reductions total 30, 40, even 50 percent. The protective HDL levels often double. Triglycerides are cut in half. And these cases are documented.

I began by approaching Dr. Albert Kattus, then Director of the Cardiac Rehabilitation Center and a renowned cardiologist. We had developed a nice rapport during the time of my own treatment pre- and post-surgery. And I have enormous respect for his opinions. Dr. Kattus is now deceased.

Dr. Kattus shared my enthusiasm and arranged for a meeting with the hospital's

Medical Research Committee. After explaining our research proposal and pointing to its promise of success with little if any expectation of side effects, we received permission to go ahead with the study.

The idea was to recruit a number of people with elevated cholesterol levels. Potential subjects were told about the program through a brief memo and signed an informed consent form. The program lasted eight weeks, with weekly meetings every Monday evening. Those meetings gave participants an opportunity to talk about all the aspects of cholesterol now covered in this book, to ask questions, and to share experiences.

After a series of lectures, with handout materials and personal conferences, a total of twenty participating men and women were asked to follow a moderately restricted diet as discussed in Chapter 4, "Winning by the Numbers," to consume fifty grams of oat bran daily either as cereal or muffins, and to gradually work up to three grams of niacin as described in Chapter 6, "The Amazing Story of Niacin."

In addition, three individuals, unable to take niacin owing to contraindications including diabetes and gout, came to the meetings, followed the diet, and took oat bran. Therefore we had a total of twenty-three persons coming to our Monday get-togethers. There were also two persons who followed the program outside the hospital setting.

Of the twenty people beginning the full program at the hospital, five failed to follow the modified diet, did not eat the suggested amounts of oat bran, forgot to take the niacin, or combinations of all three. Their results were predictably poor. But for the fifteen faithfully staying with the program, the results were more than merely encouraging.

The average fall in total cholesterol was 22 percent. Remember that authorities strongly believe that for every 1 percent drop in cholesterol, the risk of coronary heart disease falls by 2 percent. That means the subjects in our study had their risk of heart disease slashed by nearly half.

In addition, the two individuals who went on the program outside the hospital setting were particularly motivated. One cut her total cholesterol from 260 to 168 in eight weeks. The other slashed his level from 251 to 145. In just eight weeks!

But that's just the beginning. For the participants at the hospital, the levels of the protective HDL (high-density lipoprotein) *rose* by an average of more than 22 percent. Sometimes the numbers doubled or even tripled. That meant that the ratio of total cholesterol to HDL, a very important predictor of heart-disease risk, went to normal in every single individual who complied!

Simply stated, those results have never been seen in medical science before without the use of potent prescription drugs. Every single person who followed this program eliminated totally the risk of heart disease from cholesterol. There is no reason to believe that others following the program should have anything but success.

Two of the men on the program during our study were physicians themselves. Both remained on the program after the formal research came to an end, and both have demonstrated even greater improvements. Needless to say, they are now actively prescribing the program for their own patients. Everyone who has an elevated cholesterol level learns about miracle muffins and niacin.

The results for each of the participants in the study at Santa Monica Hospital Medical Center are listed in the tables beginning on page 416. I've also commented on their compliance. And the three persons listed at the end of the tables took only the oat bran, without the niacin.

Oat bran, when combined with a modified diet as discussed in Chapter 5, "Getting the Scoop on Oat Bran," can lower LDL cholesterol. HDL levels are not affected. Of the three persons taking oat bran without the niacin, cholesterol levels fell by 15, 10, and 5 percent. Compliance with the dietary modifications probably determined their levels of success.

How can we tell about compliance? Niacin compliance is the easiest to detect. Those subjects taking niacin experienced a considerable decline in levels of triglycerides, often by 50 percent or more. The average drop was 44 percent. Typically triglycerides will come down when one takes niacin whether one follows other aspects of the program or not.

Compliance with oat bran was a matter of simply asking the participants. Practically everyone enjoyed this part and compliance was good.

Dietary compliance was more difficult. We asked all the participants to keep a dietary diary for two weeks during the program. They listed all the foods and beverages taken during each day. This served two purposes. First, we had a better idea of what people were actually eating. Second, the exercise was very educational. Often we don't realize what we're eating unless we actually list all those foods, step back, and take a look. After doing so, many were able to see where they were consuming fats and cholesterol they easily could reduce or replace.

Some individuals, however, were simply unable or unwilling to modify their diets even moderately. While this is the most practical and effective program for reducing cholesterol and improving ratios described anywhere, it will not work if one continues disastrous eating habits. Most people in the study found that suggested modifications made reducing their fat and cholesterol levels of intake relatively easy.

Easy, yes, but totally effortless, no. As one of the men said in response to a complaint about missing fatty cuts of beef and cheese, "You have to bite the bullet." It's kind of like quitting the cigarette habit. The first few weeks are particularly difficult, and it gets easier as time goes on. After a while, the craving is gone completely. Sure it's tough, but it's more than worth it.

While every one of the compliant individuals left the study with completely normalized cholesterol ratios, some did better than others in terms of total cholesterol levels. Some who were content to make very few alterations in their diets achieved lowering of 10, 12, 15 percent or so. Others who made a greater effort brought their levels down by 30, 35, and even 55 percent.

In my own case, I limit my daily intake of animal meat of all types to six ounces. I rather carefully look at food labels, avoiding or at least limiting the amount of saturated fats. I enjoy cheese only rarely. And butter and eggs are completely out. But that still means I can enjoy a hamburger, an occasional steak, desserts, and a cornucopia of other foods. Many years later and I'm still compliant, with few if any real cravings. The result? My cholesterol level remains in the 160s every time I have it tested. From my original level of 284 mg/dl, that represents a 40 percent reduction. Yet most people I have dinner or lunch with for business or pleasure never know I'm modifying my diet in the least.

It also appears that the three aspects of the program have to come together. One man who dropped his level under the 200 mark later stopped taking niacin. His cholesterol level rose quickly.

Unfortunately, it also is true that not all people can tolerate the niacin. Most are willing to put up with the flushing sensation that occurs at the start of therapy but which diminishes once the three-gram level is achieved. A certain number of individuals, however, develop a rash that forces them to stop taking the tablets. One of our participants developed such a rash.

Bear in mind that *any* substance, even foods, can cause reactions in some people. Many are allergic to strawberries. Others are intolerant of dairy products. And a large number experience gastric upset from plain old aspirin. Some get an upset stomach from a single multiple vitamin-mineral supplement. There's no way to predict who might have an adverse reaction. But even if one does occur, cessation of the vitamin reverses the condition within just a few days. There are no long-term ill effects.

As indicated earlier, niacin appears to be safe even in long-term use. The vast majority of people will experience no difficulties whatever. In our study, we excluded from niacin those persons with either diabetes or gout or pre-existing liver malfunctions. Those with ulcers should also see their physicians before starting on niacin.

Out of both personal and professional curiosity, I decided to have a complete panel of blood studies done on myself a year after starting niacin. Every indicator came back completely normal after that year.

Upon completion of the study, I conducted a survey of everyone who had participated. Most agreed that the program was easy to follow and that they intended to stay with it. The results appear in Table 19 on pages 416–17.

MEET THE PARTICIPANTS

B.R. was the first person I met. She was early for the first weekly meeting and we chatted as I set up my slides and other presentation materials. B.R. made it clear that she really didn't think the program would work, since she had tried to lower her cholesterol levels many times in the past. But she figured she'd give it a try. B.R. gave it her best effort, followed the dietary modifications, ate the oat bran regularly, and took the niacin without any problems. Skeptical to the point of cynicism throughout the study, she was happy to learn that after just eight weeks her cholesterol level had dropped by 27 percent and her ratio had gone from 12.3 to 3.1. A real success story, B.R. is now telling everyone about the program.

C.O. had tried desperately to lower her dangerously high levels. Even drugs had been ineffective. But on this program her total cholesterol level dropped by 159 points, for a 35 percent reduction, and brought her ratio down to 3.4.

B.H. is retired and she and her husband travel extensively. Even for a vacation in Europe, B.H. took along a supply of oat bran and her bottle of niacin tablets. She was well rewarded with a 19 percent dip in cholesterol and a safe ratio of only 2.3.

A.J. attended every meeting without fail. He was bound and determined to make the program work for him. His perseverance paid off: his cholesterol fell from 243 to 163 in just eight weeks, with a doubling of HDL levels, resulting in a very healthy ratio of 2.6.

Similarly, the two physicians, R.G. and

C.K., took the program very seriously and followed it faithfully. Both achieved results they knew were important but were unable to reach with what medicine had to offer before R.G. went from 289 to 204. C.K. watched his level fall from 257 to 186.

Even those who complied poorly achieved notable success. L.S. had a difficult time with diet, admitting that he didn't try as hard as he should have. Yet he saw his cholesterol level fall by 14 percent and his ratio improve from 6.6 to 5.2. J.C. also was unable to control his diet, but with a 45 percent rise in HDL, his ratio fell to a normal 4.1. The same applied to E.P., whose protective HDL level rose by 20 percent.

There is still a great deal medical science must learn about cholesterol and how the body deals with it. In the meantime, however, we do know that total cholesterol should be under 200. The ratio of total cholesterol to HDL should be no higher than 4.4 for females and 5.2 for males. Achieving those numbers virtually eliminates this important risk factor of coronary heart disease.

"Do-It-Yourself Programs"

The participants in our hospital study had the distinct advantage of those eight Monday-night meetings. They learned just about everything there is to know about cholesterol, how oat bran and niacin work, and how to improve their diets painlessly. Plus they had the reinforcement of meeting every seven days to ask questions, get support from the group, and perhaps to get back on the wagon after falling off for a while. An advantage, yes. But not a requirement for success.

A medical colleague of Dr. Kattus referred to me a 28-year-old nurse who had just learned her cholesterol was a disturbingly high 260. Trained in the value of preventive medicine, she knew that if her level wasn't changed, she would be certain to develop coronary heart disease.

When I met her in Dr. Kattus's office, S.B. told me she was very health conscious. She ran twenty to thirty miles weekly, and her diet could best be described as "California healthy." S.B. ate meat only occasionally, and preferred fish and poultry. Her diet was loaded with fresh fruits and vegetables. Only the cheese had to be reduced in her otherwise perfect diet. (And, of course, those rich desserts she had always tried to limit because of the calories anyway.)

S.B. had no problem in getting to the therapeutic three-gram level of niacin. She enjoyed the oat bran. And in just eight weeks her blood chemistry was totally turned around.

From 260, S.B.'s cholesterol level dropped to 168. Her HDL rose from 41 to 98. The destructive LDL levels dropped from 205 to 63. The result was a change in ratio from 6.34 to 1.7. At the same time, her triglycerides went down from 67 to 33. To say that she was happy with the results is an understatement.

The same goes for my printer. R.R. runs the local Kwik Kopy Printing Shop, and has done all my printing for many years. One day, coincidentally, he asked me if I knew anything about cholesterol. R.R. didn't know about the book or the research study at that time, but he was aware that I wrote about medicine.

This is a guy who holds a black belt in karate, works out five days a week, and frequently runs in IOK races. In general, he's highly fitness conscious, also eating a "California healthy" diet. That's why he was so surprised—and appalled—when his doctor told him his cholesterol level was at 251. For this 37-year-old man, coronary heart disease was ready to knock on the door if he didn't do something about that dangerous level.

Here's a good example of someone for whom a healthful diet wasn't enough. R.R.'s diet was already fine-tuned. He needed more.

I felt that R.R. would be splendid proof of the program. The only modifications his diet required were cutting back on butter and cheese. The butter was used moderately, but cheese was a frequent part of the diet. He still eats it, but far less often.

R.R. enjoys three oat-bran muffins each day. He finds they fit perfectly into his busy life, and he brings them to the shop for breakfast and snacks.

At the beginning, I'd come into the shop and ask how the program was going. R.R. said all was well but that the flushing from the niacin was uncomfortable. Later, the flushing persisted and kept him from going any higher than two grams daily.

One afternoon I came in with some printing to be done and noticed that R.R.'s face was a bright red. I asked whether he'd been out in the sun that weekend, surprised since he wasn't a typical California sun worshiper. R.R. said that was his usual niacin flush.

I suggested that he switch to Nicobid, a time-release niacin formulation, to ease the flushing. At that time Endur-acin was unavailable. Nicobid worked well for R.R., but it doesn't eliminate the flush as well as Endur-acin does for most people. Fortunately R.R. did not experience the gastric upset Nicobid can cause.

At the end of R.R.'s "test" period of eight weeks, I asked him what numbers he'd be happy with—how much of a cholesterol reduction he was expecting. He didn't know that I had just come back from the hospital laboratory with his test results. R.R. said he'd be pleased with anything under 200, the danger point for cholesterol levels. He was ecstatic when he learned that he had achieved a drop to 145!

R.R.'s complete "lipid profile" was a joy to behold: from 251 to 145, a more than 100-milligram drop in total cholesterol. His level of destructive LDL had gone down to just 77. His protective HDL was up to 66. Triglycerides fell to 42. And the predictive ratio had improved to a very, very healthy 2.2—less than half the normal risk level.

"No Excuses Acceptable"

Even with R.R.'s flushing, he continued to take the niacin. Fortunately, the Nicobid was able to solve his problem completely. But the important thing was that R.R. stuck with it. He could have quit early on, and we'd never have known how well he could succeed.

When S.B. started the program, she knew that she'd have to watch her diet, especially when out on dates. But she knew the importance of getting that cholesterol level down to normal. She stuck with it then, and stays with it now.

B.H. can afford all the finest foods at expensive restaurants throughout Europe as she travels with her husband. And it's also quite a problem to stay with the oat bran during their many lengthy trips. Yet she has decided that her health is more important than a fancy sauce Béarnaise. So B.H. selects broiled chicken and fish whenever she can. And her suitcase is never packed without a supply of oat bran to take along.

On the other hand, one of the study participants, who will remain not only unnamed but without even initials, gave in to excuses easily. A bachelor, he got his girlfriend to make muffins for him at the beginning. After an argument she stopped baking and he stopped eating the oat bran. It was too difficult to prepare them himself, so he simply stopped.

Can a bachelor or anyone else living alone be expected to bake muffins? Why not? The recipes are easy to follow and require just a bit of time each week. After my surgery, I prepared my own muffins just two weeks after the doctors had repaired my clogged arteries. Even though my energy reserves were low, I put a high priority on baking those muffins. There's no excuse for not doing it yourself.

Some have asked whether muffins will become boring after a while. Remember the French who eat their daily croissant for their entire lives. Actually the muffins are less tiresome, since they can be prepared in an almost infinite variety. Moreover, one day one can enjoy muffins and another day hot cereal.

There's also no excuse for forgetting even one dose of niacin. Many individuals, myself included, find that the best bet is to have a supply wherever they go. I keep a bottle in my bathroom for the morning and evening, one in the kitchen for lunch, another in the glove compartment of the car for when I'm out on the road, still another in my office, and a final container in my travel kit. No excuse to miss.

For most individuals, the diet is the toughest part, yet it remains crucial for the total success. Yes, you can improve significantly without much change in diet, just by including oat bran and niacin. Yet for best results, the fat and the cholesterol intake must be modified. Sticking with the diet sometimes can be difficult.

I'm reminded of the business outing I was on some time back. In an unfamiliar neighborhood, the only restaurant I could find was a Straw Hat Pizza place. There was no time to find an alternative, and I was starving. So in I went and ordered a pizza with green peppers, mushrooms, onions, sliced tomatoes, and, please, hold the cheese. It was delicious! And the person taking my order wasn't even surprised—it turns out that many strict vegetarians do the same thing. Now I can go into such pizza restaurants with family or friends, enjoy the environment, and relish the crispy crust and the fresh ingredients without concern or guilt. At home I frequently make pizzas with preformed crusts, pizza sauce, fresh vegetables, and a sprinkling of low-cholesterol low-fat cheese. Even my kids think they're great.

There are lots of other suggestions for enjoying restaurants while complying with cholesterol modifications in Chapter 11, "Dining Out: To Your Health!" In many ways it's even easier to follow the diet when eating out than when preparing foods in one's own home. Even airlines provide a low-fat low-cholesterol menu for travelers. You just have to ask for it in advance.

What are some other excuses? How about "My family shouldn't have to 'suffer' because of my special diet." First of all, the word "suffer" doesn't apply. The foods best for this program are best for everyone. Second, with a few simple modifications, practically every favorite family recipe can still be enjoyed.

There simply are no good excuses, no valid excuses, for not following the program and reducing one's cholesterol to healthy levels. Any more than there are good excuses to continue smoking cigarettes. In both cases, the choice is completely yours and the rewards so totally

Table 18. Average Results with the 8-Week Cholesterol Cure Program

	TOTAL CHOLESTEROL REDUCTIONS (%)	TRIGYCERIDE DECREASE (%)	LDL DECREASE (%)	HDL INCREASE (%)
Participants with good compliance	31.67	42.08	47.45	60.58
All participants	22.05	41.10	32.61	43.85

outweigh the efforts that the decision should be immediate and final.

The program has been clinically proven to be safe and effective (see Table 18). Followed properly, it can dramatically reduce cholesterol levels to completely healthy in just eight weeks. The risk of coronary heart disease will be greatly diminished. The chances of living a longer, healthier life are tremendously improved.

Personal Notes

Charles E. Keenan, M.D.
General Practice
Santa Monica, California

I appreciated being a part of the study just completed. It was quite revealing. I had a

Table 19. Lipid Profile Records of Study Participants: Baseline and After Two Months

SUBJECT NUMBER	TOTAL CHOLESTEROL	IMPROVEMENT (%)	TRIGLYCERIDES	IMPROVEMENT (%)	HDL	IMPROVEMENT (%)	LDL	IMPROVEMENT (%)	RATIO	SEX	COMMENTS
1	251	43	81	50	40	65	177	60	6.3	M	Good compliance outside hospital
	145		42		66		71		2.2		
2	260	36	67	50	41	114	205	70	6.3	F	Good compliance outside hospital
	168		33		98		63		1.7		
3	257	27	—	—	74	0	—	—	—	M	Good compliance
	186		95		65		102		2.9		
4	243	33	360	88	31	100	140	35	7.8	M	Good compliance
	163		47		62		92		2.6		
5	289	29	211	40	47	0	200	33	6.2	M	Good compliance
	204		115		47		134		4.3		
6	234	25	65	0	54	33	167	52	4.3	M	Good compliance
	175		64		72		90		2.4		
7	321	27	232	76	26	200	249	40	12.3	F	Good compliance
	244		81		78		150		3.1		
8	458	35	103	34	73	20	364	46	6.3	F	Good compliance
	299		68		87		198		3.4		
9	269	19	194	69	53	81	177	39	5.1	F	Good compliance
	217		62		96		109		2.3		
10	220	55	72	05	35	0	171	65	6.3	F	Good compliance
	98		69		24		60		4.1		
11	303	30	228	40	42	24	215	39	7.2	F	Good compliance
	212		136		52		133		4.1		

#										Sex	
12	248	10	194	53	67	90	142	43	3.7	F	Good compliance
	224		91		127		81		1.8		
13	326	15	102	30	90	36	216	30	3.6	F	Fair compliance
	289		72		123		152		2.3		
14	233	16	121	28	53	0	155	19	4.4	M	Fair compliance
	196		88		52		126		3.8		
15	289	14	165	30	44	09	212	16	6.6	M	Poor dietary compliance
	250		115		48		179		5.2		
16	256	0	377	64	36	80	147	0	7.2	M	Poor dietary compliance
	266		138		65		173		4.1		
17	265	0	147	24	57	25	179	0	4.6	M	Poor dietary compliance
	275		142		71		182		3.9		
18	252	12	132	55	100	0	—	—	3.4	F	Poor dietary compliance
	222		60		97		113		2.3		
19	249	06	215	30	42	0	164	0	5.9	M	Poor dietary compliance
	234		155		40		163		5.9		
20	237	06	164	50	—	—	—	—	—	M	Poor dietary compliance
	222		83		31		174		7.2		
21	225	07	270	47	37	0	134	0	6.1	M	Total noncompliance
	209		144		28		152		7.5		
22	308	15	209	0	46	0	220	20	6.7	F	Oat bran only niacin contraindicated
	262		203		43		178		6.1		
23	245	10	102	0	34	0	191	17	7.2	M	Oat bran only niacin contraindicated
	222		179		26		160		8.5		
24	224	05	48	13	77	09	137	12	2.9	F	Oat bran only
	213		42		84		121		2.5		

— = Data not available.

good deal of personal interest as my cholesterol has been slightly elevated throughout the
years. I'd used the things available to me,
other than drugs, but to no avail.

I must confess to a bit of initial skepticism
and pessimism regarding the results of such a
simple change of dietary habits. Many large
drug firms are spending millions of dollars trying to find a medicine to counteract the cholesterol disease. Medically, it has been very
frustrating to prescribe medications and have a
limited amount of success, occasionally with
significant side effects. Patients on these medications are on them for life. This makes one
very hesitant to prescribe medications that
have any significant side effects. Another concern is that medications either have to be
given too frequently or cause significant diarrhea and so forth, making it difficult to keep
patients on them. They are also, in my experience, quite expensive.

I had tried and recommended yogurt, garlic,
exercise, and a few other environmental
changes, again with rather questionable results.

I decided to try this approach to see how
difficult it would be for my own compliance.
It seemed too good to be true, just a mild dietary change and additional vitamin pills. I
must admit to have been buoyed up by testing
my cholesterol very early in the program. I was

astounded to find it down by 33 percent. This made my enthusiasm and excitement for the experiment much greater.

Some of the interesting things that were byproducts of my becoming a part of it were uncovering the talent for being a cook (baking bran muffins), enjoying the weekly lectures, and having a unique approach to tell my earlier hypercholesterol patients who had failed on other regimes. I was so encouraged that I told other patients to contact the program for possible admittance to the study. I've subsequently been encouraging all my patients to make this dietary adjustment as it seems to be a painless change with dramatic results.

My results, I think, were as exciting and as successful as one could hope for. My initial cholesterol was 246 and the subsequent level was 186. It really makes me an apostle for the program and I hope I can spread this simple, inexpensive, and drugless approach to health and longevity.

Exercise certainly is a valuable tool, but I doubt if it has anywhere near the effectiveness of this. I was amazed at the relatively little change in my lifestyle and the significant results I had with just the oat bran and niacin. If a person tries this approach and it is successful, there is no need to go on costly medications with significant side effects.

If my initial enthusiasm proves accurate, this could be the greatest boon to longevity since penicillin. As with any other form of therapy, this may not be the panacea for everyone, but for many this will be a very significant factor in their future health.

I can recommend this wholeheartedly to everyone for their initial use and have them individually check their pre- and postcholesterol levels. This could well be their passport to longevity.

In closing, I might raise my glass and toast saying "long live oat bran and its users."

Dr. R.G.
Santa Monica, California

Having discovered my serum cholesterol and serum triglycerides to be at the upper limit of normal (289 mg/dl and 211 mg/dl, respectively) several years ago, I was interested in a method of lowering these values.

Approximately three years ago I modified my diet by eliminating all eggs and significantly decreasing the amount of red meat, cheese, and other dairy products. This dietary change did not alter the serum cholesterol or serum triglycerides to any significant degree.

In January of 1985, I learned of the niacin-oat-bran study at Santa Monica Hospital and became a participant in that study. The study required the daily intake of niacin (three grams) and one-half cup of oat bran. Some initial flushing symptoms from the niacin (which can be almost completely ameliorated with one aspirin tablet) are no longer present. Since I had already modified my diet three years ago, there was no additional alteration in my diet during the course of this study.

I was pleasantly surprised to find that my serum cholesterol levels decreased by approximately 30 percent (below 200) and my serum triglycerides decreased by 50 percent over a three-month period of time. In addition, the ratio of total cholesterol to HDL changed from 6.15 to 3.4 over a similar period of time.

Because of this success and the paucity of side effects, I fully intend to maintain this program indefinitely.

Sigrid Broderson, R.N.
Private Duty Nurse
Los Angeles, California

Since I was young, I've always been very physically active. I've enjoyed sports, and have spent a lot of time snow skiing, even to the point of teaching others. I also enjoy windsurfing, tennis, racquetball, swimming, you name it. Last year I took up running and have done a few 10K races, and in 1986 I'm planning to do my first marathon. The point of all this is that I'm in good physical condition, and I'm interested in maintaining good health in general.

My health interests, of course, are both personal and professional. As a registered nurse, since 1979 I've been involved with intensive care.

My own health, I've thought, has always been good. My heart rate has been in the forties, and my blood pressure has always been in the low-normal range. I've watched my diet carefully.

In April, after I had an accident, I decided to have my cholesterol checked. I'd been working closely with a patient who had a cholesterol problem, and I'd been giving nutrition counseling and helping him with his diet. So I became curious as to what my own cholesterol level was. To my surprise, the cholesterol was extremely elevated. I found this hard to believe. In fact, I had the test repeated the next week, this time a complete lipid panel to see not only my total cholesterol but also the levels of the protective HDL and the harmful LDL. Again the results were disappointing, with a high total cholesterol of 260 and high LDL of 205, along with a fairly low HDL of only 41.

I couldn't believe that one of the major aspects of health was so threatening since I'd been taking such good care of myself in terms of exercise and diet. It was particularly alarming to me since I'd spent so much time with coronary patients, those who had had heart attacks and open-heart surgery. I was very much aware of the risk factors of heart disease, and I knew that I was at risk. I had inherited the condition from my mother, whose cholesterol level was also high and who had developed heart disease.

I returned to my cardiologist, and he referred me to Mr. Kowalski and his research study. After our first meeting I was more than eager to begin the new program.

Taking the niacin, for me, was not much of a problem. I only remember a couple of days, as I was increasing my intake, that I experienced any flushing. It was mild, went away quickly, and wasn't really a problem. If I'm a bit a late with my niacin dosage now, I occasionally get a little tingly feeling, but that only reminds me that I'm on the road to good health.

Another positive aspect of taking the niacin is that it gives me a schedule, a routine, that reminds me to take my other vitamins. It also reminds me regularly to watch my diet, since I take my niacin near mealtimes.

At first I started with oat bran as hot cereal, but after a month I tired of that and switched to the muffins from the recipes Mr. Kowalski developed. Now I find myself often eating more than the three muffins a day, since I think they're so delicious. I actually have to limit myself, only because of my total calories.

Dietary changes weren't difficult at all, since my diet was pretty good to begin with. I've always enjoyed fruits and vegetables, and never had much fat in my diet. I did eliminate egg yolks and cut back a bit on red meats. But I still enjoy eating out, and now I don't really think of this as a "restricted" diet since there are so many foods to choose from.

It was all so easy during the first two months that I was actually scared when it was time to take my blood test again. Surely the results couldn't be very good when the program was so painless. To my surprise, the results came out extremely well. What a terrific motivation to keep it up. My total cholesterol dropped from 260 to 168. My harmful LDL level went from 205 to 63. My protective HDL rose from 41 to 98. And the important ratio of total cholesterol to HDL dropped from 6.34 to 1.7.

Now I know I'm doing everything I possibly can to reduce the risk of heart disease. My health is my own responsibility, and it's up to me to protect my life.

On a professional level, this program has motivated me to a new commitment to health counseling on a preventive basis. And I'm proud that I practice what I preach.

MORE PROOF

Since Dr. Keenan succeeded in lowering his own cholesterol levels with the 8-week cholesterol cure, he's prescribed the program for hundreds of his patients in Santa Monica. Thanks to the introduction of Endur-acin, which makes it possible for the vast majority of patients to take niacin without the original problems of flushing and gastric upset, he finds the program even more successful today.

Moreover, hundreds of other physicians across the country now advocate the program for their patients as well. More often than not, men and women learn about the 8-week cholesterol cure from their doctors, who tell them to read the book, follow the program, and return in eight weeks when they have their cholesterol levels and liver function tested.

The data collected by Dr. Joseph Keenan at the University of Minnesota provided the final, definitive proof that the 8-week cholesterol cure offers the ultimate protection in lowering cholesterol levels after just eight weeks—and for a lifetime.

15

Drugs, the Final Resort

For the vast majority of people, dietary measures alone can bring cholesterol levels under control. This is especially true now that we know how effective the foods containing soluble fiber can be in getting those numbers down. And for those of us with particularly high concentrations of cholesterol in our blood owing to the body's overproduction, for whom dietary action isn't enough, the addition of niacin, particularly the sustained-release niacin preparation Enduracin, can be dramatically effective. But certain individuals may have to resort to prescription drugs in order to eliminate the deadly risk factor of elevated cholesterol levels.

First, there are some people for whom niacin in any form is contraindicated. As mentioned in Chapter 6 those contraindications include liver dysfunction of any kind, past history of hepatitis or cirrhosis, heavy alcohol use, gout, cardiac arrhythmias, diabetes, and pregnancy. Such individuals will learn from their physicians that niacin is not for them.

Second, a very few people will find that, despite the absence of contraindications, their livers are unable to tolerate niacin in dosages needed to be effective. That may be shown in the liver study I strongly recommend after two to three months of niacin therapy and again at one-year intervals thereafter. Again, the number of such men and women is quite small, but when one considers the fact that literally millions of men and women have very high cholesterol levels that don't respond to diet alone and for whom niacin would be medically recommended, those numbers become significant. That's especially true if *you* happen to be one of those people!

In the years that I've been involved with cholesterol control I've spoken with and received letters from some readers of my book who are dismayed that niacin is not for them. Some have developed a persistent skin rash that wouldn't go away until they ceased taking niacin. Others found that while their liver functions were perfectly normal at first examination, elevated liver enzymes later detected by their physicians forced them to stop taking niacin. Often they admitted that they had been heavy alcohol drinkers for years, and that their livers had been compromised in the process.

"What do we do now?" they all want to know.

As you know from reading my book thus

far, I personally prefer to avoid prescription drugs. But the most important consideration is to lower cholesterol levels to normal. If my program of diet, oat bran, and niacin had not worked for me way back in 1984 after my second bypass, by all means I would have given those prescription drugs another look. One must do whatever it takes to lower cholesterol levels into the safe range.

Today virtually every expert in the field agrees that for those who have had heart attacks, bypass surgery, or angioplasty—in other words anyone who has a serious development of heart disease—aggressive measures to lower cholesterol levels are vital to stop the progress of that disease. If that means taking drugs, so be it.

Moreover, there have been significant developments in drug therapy since I began writing my book, and these developments certainly warrant a closer look. In the following pages I listed the drugs your doctor may prescribe, depending on your particular condition and needs. In each case I include information on the benefits of the drug, how it should be taken, and potential side effects. Remember that even aspirin has the capability of producing adverse reactions in some individuals, and that the actual incidence of side effects is relatively low for any given drug. Moreover, if one drug isn't just right for you, your physician can then try another one. As a final thought regarding side effects or adverse reactions, remember that the lists include every possible reaction, regardless of how seldom such a reaction might occur. Again using the example of aspirin, one of the potential adverse reactions listed in the medical textbooks is death; but of course the actual incidence of death is infinitesimal. With all this in mind, let's look at the currently available drugs that affect cholesterol and lipid levels. Collectively these are called hypocholesterolemic agents.

Bile Sequestering Agents. Currently there are two drugs in this category, which are also referred to as the resin drugs. They have been on the market since the mid-1960s and are considered to be a first-line consideration for physicians prescribing drugs to lower cholesterol levels. The two drugs are colestipol (*Colestid— The Upjohn Company*) and cholestyramine (*Questran—Mead Johnson Laboratories*). Both are believed to work in the same way.

These substances are not absorbed by the body, and pass directly through the digestive tract. Along the way they bind onto the bile acids in the intestine, which are manufactured by the body from cholesterol in the liver and are used in the digestive process. The bound bile acids are then eliminated as part of the bowel movement. As the bile acids are voided, the body must make more. To do so, additional cholesterol must be used, thus gradually decreasing the amount circulating in the blood.

Since the resin drugs are not absorbed, there are no systemic adverse reactions, that is, reactions taking place outside the digestive tract. Whatever side effects may occur are usually limited to the gastrointestinal tract.

Both drugs must be mixed with water, juice, or carbonated beverages. Neither dissolves entirely, and must be swallowed quickly after mixing lest the drugs settle out or thicken in the mixture. It's best to refill the glass with additional fluid and drink it in order to get whatever resin may be clinging to the glass.

Ultimately your physician will prescribe the dosage he or she feels is best to start with. That dosage may be raised or lowered, depending on your response in terms of lowered cholesterol. In terms of cholesterol lowering, five grams of colestipol is the equivalent of four grams of cholestyramine. These agents work best in divided doses, rather than taken at one time. The bedtime or evening dose has been shown to be most effective.

I've noted elsewhere in this book that I'm a

terrible medicine taker and that I find these drugs to be rather unpleasant. On the other hand, one physician I know very well takes cholestyramine regularly and has no difficulty with it at all. And the same can be said for millions of men and women who have taken these drugs successfully for many years. Some people prefer the unflavored colestipol, while others opt for the flavored cholestyramine. Moreover, cholestyramine can be taken as a newly developed tablet or in the form of a "candy" bar. Since we're talking about very long-term use, do a bit of experimentation to find out which might be most acceptable to you. One of the major drawbacks of these drugs is that patient compliance is less than 100 percent.

Cholestyramine, in a dose of 8 to 12 grams twice daily, or colestipol, with a dosage of 10 to 15 grams twice daily, typically decreases cholesterol levels from 10 to 20 percent. Most of that reduction comes from the LDL subfraction, with little or no effect on the HDL levels.

Side effects in the upper gastrointestinal tract include burping, heartburn, and a bloated feeling or at least a feeling of fullness. To reduce those side effects, you might try swallowing the mixture more slowly and using less fluid in which you mix the drugs, and by not taking the drugs right along with a heavy meal.

Adverse reactions in the lower gastrointestinal tract include constipation, increased quantity of stool, or diarrhea. Frequently such side effects diminish with time. And you can ease the problem of constipation by increasing the fiber in your diet, especially the insoluble fiber in whole-grain cereals such as wheat and bulky vegetables.

While both colestipol and cholestyramine may interfere with absorption, and thus effectiveness, of other drugs your physician may prescribe, colestipol is less likely to pose this problem. Cholestyramine is more likely to affect absorption of drugs, including thiazide diuretics, used to control high blood pressure; warfarin, used to prevent clotting of blood; and certain other agents. Ask your physician or pharmacist about such drug interactions.

The bile sequestering agents are the only drugs that have been used with children, since they are not absorbed through the digestive tract. They have been used, though infrequently, with children with exceptionally high cholesterol levels.

Both colestipol and cholestyramine are extremely expensive drugs. Buying in bulk rather than individual packets can save some money. And by all means you should shop for the best price in town, since you'll be using the drugs regularly.

All the other cholesterol and lipid-lowering drugs available today come as tablets or capsules, which are, of course, much easier to take. But, since they are absorbed into the bloodstream, they have the potential for side effects outside the digestive tract. (Although cholestyramine may be taken as a tablet, no such concerns exist since the drug does not get absorbed.)

Probucol (Lorelco—Merrell Dow) is chemically unrelated to any other cholesterol-lowering drug. While its mode of action isn't absolutely certain, it appears to cause the metabolic breakdown of LDL cholesterol. Unfortunately, while LDL levels fall, this drug also results in a decrease in HDL levels. In some patients this fall in HDL could be significant. Some patients have been given niacin along with probucol in order to counteract this adverse effect. There is little if any effect on triglyceride levels.

Probucol typically is prescribed in dosages of 0.5 gram twice daily. At that dosage level, moderate cholesterol reductions of 10 to 15 percent can be expected.

Serious toxicity has been reported with probucol when tested in laboratory animals.

Some individuals may be hypersensitive. Women should not become pregnant within six months of taking probucol, nor should they take the drug when pregnant or breast feeding.

Gastrointestinal side effects include diarrhea or loose stools, flatulence, abdominal pain, nausea and vomiting, indigestion, and gastrointestinal bleeding. Some effect may be seen in electrocardiograms, with changes in heart rhythms. On very rare occasions adverse reactions have included rash, impotency, anorexia, and other significant side effects. One interesting but unpleasant reaction may be a particularly fetid, stinky perspiration.

Owing to probucol's tendency to lower the protective levels of HDL, its use by physicians has lessened considerably.

Clofibrate (Atromid-S—Ayerst) has largely fallen into disuse. While it may lower LDL levels by way of reducing the very-low-density-lipoprotein (VLDL) precursors, it may on occasion actually elevate those levels. This has been shown when clofibrate was used with patients with type IIb hypercholesterolemia, in which both the cholesterol and triglycerides are significantly above normal. Moreover, even when successful, only modest reductions of LDL cholesterol have been seen.

In 1978 a study was published in the *British*

Heart Journal that ended clofibrate's widespread use. The World Health Organization Clofibrate Trial results published in that journal indicated that significant increases in death rate were associated with the drug's use.

Gemfibrozil (Lopid—Parke-Davis) is chemically related to clofibrate, but happily does not have the same poor record. It works by lowering VLDLs and thus causing a decrease in LDLs. Gemfibrozil also results in a modest but significant elevation in the protective HDLs. Typically gemfibrozil is taken as two 300-mg capsules twice daily, for a total of four capsules each day. It decreases triglycerides significantly.

Contraindications for this drug include liver or kidney impairment and pre-existing gall-bladder disease. The reason for the latter is that gemfibrozil increases levels of cholesterol in the liver, though levels drop in the blood. This increase of cholesterol in the liver can lead to the development of gallstones, potentially necessitating gall-bladder removal by surgery.

On the whole, however, reports of side effects and adverse reactions are relatively low. Most such reactions involve the gastrointestinal tract, including abdominal pain, diarrhea, nausea and vomiting, and flatulence. However, adverse reactions including rash, headache, dizziness, blurred vision, anemia, muscular pain, insomnia, and ringing in the ears have been reported rarely.

Gemfibrozil was used in research referred to as the Helsinki Study, which was reported during the American Heart Association meeting in November 1987. Those taking the drug over a long period of time had a significantly lower rate of heart attack and death than those receiving a placebo. Many believe this may be owing to gemfibrozil's ability to raise levels of HDL.

Lovastatin (Mevacor—Merck Sharp & Dohme) was approved by the Food and Drug Administration in September 1987. Since then it has become widely prescribed by physicians all over the country. This is the first drug in a totally new class of cholesterol-lowering agents, working at the site of the liver to interfere with the normal production of cholesterol. Technically, it is a potent inhibitor of HMG co-A reductase (hydroxymethylglutaryl coenzyme-A reductase), an enzyme necessary for cholesterol production. This drug is capable of very significant reductions in LDL and total cholesterol. HDL levels either remain unaffected or may rise modestly.

Researchers at the West Virginia University

School of Medicine reported a fall in total cholesterol of 24 percent, with a drop of 32 percent in LDL, on a dosage of 20 mg of lovastatin daily, taken in the evening. HDL levels increased by 5 percent.

A number of studies have been published demonstrating the effectiveness and apparent safety of lovastatin, and many in the medical community are excited about its potential. The principal concern at this time is lovastatin's lack of a track record. Since it has been used for only a very short period of time, we don't know about long-term safety.

Depending on the individual response to the drug, dosage of lovastatin may be limited to one tablet daily (20 mg) or up to 80 mg per day. Since this drug acts at the site of the liver, higher dosages are associated with more frequent liver-function abnormalities as seen by way of liver-enzyme tests.

Contraindications to lovastatin include liver disease or unexplained elevations in liver enzymes. Patients should be tested for liver function prior to beginning the drug and every four to six weeks for the first year and a half of lovastatin usage. Pregnant and lactating women should not take lovastatin, and because the drug's effects on future children have not been established, lovastatin should not be taken by any woman of childbearing age unless she is certain not to have another baby. During initial testing with the drug, some changes in the eye were noted in laboratory dogs. As a result, physicians were encouraged to check their patients' eyes when prescribing lovastatin. However, Dr. Donald Hunninghake, a leading authority in drug therapy, later reported that no problems involving lens opacity or cataracts had been noted in humans, and that concern in this area could be relaxed.

In 23 centers 744 patients have been participating in a long-term study of of lovastatin. The average age of the patients when they began taking the drug was fifty, and 68 percent of patients are male. As of May 1988, the total number was down to 670 after two and a half years. Of those no longer in the study, some were lost to follow-up and others were discontinued. Sixteen dropped out because of drug-attributable adverse reactions. The group will be continued for study into the future, but the conclusions of the interim report presented at the First National Cholesterol Conference in Washington, D.C., in November 1988, were that the drug appeared to be on its way to a safe record during prolonged use.

It is very important to note that all drugs, including lovastatin, should be used as part of total therapy, including a prudent, low-fat, low-cholesterol diet. At no time should drugs be viewed as an alternative to diet. In fact, without substantial change in the diet, the drugs are not nearly as effective.

The principal concern about lovastatin is that it will be overprescribed by physicians. It may be tempting to reach for the prescription pad, rather than first attempt to work with the patient to lower cholesterol levels by diet. In fact, some patients receive lovastatin prescriptions from their doctors without even knowing the LDL/HDL breakdown of the total cholesterol. As a result, a large number of women are taking the drug; while their total cholesterol levels may be on the high side, their levels of HDL may be high enough to offer sufficient protection from heart disease.

Lovastatin is a potent drug with great potential for significantly reducing cholesterol. Efforts should be made to keep dosage as low as possible in order to minimize any adverse reactions. This can be done by maximizing the impact of a low-fat, low-cholesterol diet. It should be realized that lovastatin, like any other therapy for cholesterol control, could potentially be taken for the rest of one's life.

For most people, the cost of lovastatin is a significant consideration. This is an extremely expensive drug that could cost thousands of dollars annually.

Since this book was first written, a number

of chemically similar drugs have been introduced. All are in the category referred to as the "statin." While Mevacor (lovastatin) is still routinely prescribed by physicians, other statins including pravastatin (Pravacol), simvastatin (Zocor), fluvastatin (Lescol), and atorvastatin (Lipitor) appear to be more potent. Of all of them, Lipitor is probably best since it actively reduces cholesterol, has some lowering effect on triglycerides, and mildly elevates HDL counts. Research has also shown that the statin drugs can be successfully combined with niacin to provide the benefits of both while also reducing the dosage of each.

Of course, your physician is the right source to decide whether you should use drugs.

OTHER METHODS OF CHOLESTEROL CONTROL

Patients with extremely high cholesterol levels owing to a hereditary condition known as familial hypercholesterolemia often do not respond to normal dietary and drug therapy. Some of these patients have been treated with a procedure that actually cleans the cholesterol out of their blood. The process, known as LDL-pheresis, is similar to dialysis therapy used for kidney patients.

In this procedure patients are hooked up to

a machine in the laboratory. Blood is taken through a needle in the arm and is pumped into a centrifuge, which separates the liquid plasma from the white and red cells of the blood, along with platelets and other blood components. The plasma then goes through a glass chamber, where it is exposed to antibodies or a chemical called dextran sulfate to remove microscopic particles of LDL cholesterol. After the LDL has been filtered out, the patient's blood is reconstituted and returned through a needle in the other arm.

Very few patients have been treated in this way, and the process is extremely expensive. However, after undergoing treatment periodically for an average of twenty months, patients' cholesterol levels dropped from an average of 372 mg/dl to 138, and their HDL levels rose. For those patients with this genetically rare condition, LDL-pheresis can literally be a lifesaver. One center using the procedure is the Rogosin Institute, which is affiliated with the Cornell University Medical College and New York Hospital in New York City.

A much less dramatic approach to cholesterol control is based on the idea that plant sterols, closely related to cholesterol in chemical structure but unable to cause blockage in the arteries, the sterol that comes from animal sources. These plant sterols, the phytosterols, have been around for a long time, and many tout their effectiveness. One pharmaceutical company, Eli Lilly, actually introduced a product in the early 1960s that contained one of the plant sterols, beta sitosterol. At that time, there was less emphasis on cholesterol control, and the product never caught on, so the company discounted its manufacture. And since phytosterols are naturally-occurring plant substances, no one can have an exclusive patent on their manufacture and sale. Thus other companies have not rushed into the arena to do additional research or to launch other products.

One of the newest weapons in the anti-cholesterol war is, at the same time, one of the oldest. When this book first came out, I wrote that phytosterols were probably of little if any value. These are plant sterols with molecular structures virtually identical to cholesterol, the animal sterol.

The problem with phytosterols in the '80s was a matter of inadequate dosages and poor quality in terms of bioavailability. In other words, to get a good effect from phytosterols, one needs to take a large enough dose, and the tablets need to properly dissolve before reaching the part of the digestive tract—the first third of the intestine—where cholesterol is absorbed. Products on the market at that time simply didn't pass muster.

That was, of course, frustrating, since research dating all the way back to the '50s showed a very positive benefit of taking phytosterols. Moreover, the safety record was spectacular. Since phytosterols are simply plant substances, there are no side effects or adverse reactions possible. No down side whatsoever.

Nutritionalists had long bemoaned the fact that one of nature's most perfect foods—eggs—were being avoided owing to the concern over cholesterol. Especially for older persons and those living alone, eggs represent an inexpensive, tasty, easy-to-prepare source of the highest quality protein. Using phytosterols prior to a meal of eggs—or, for that matter, any animal foods such as meat or cheese or sea foods—could totally block the absorption of cholesterol.

But phytosterols provide cholesterol-reducing benefits beyond merely blocking dietary cholesterol. Taking a sufficient dosage, as demonstrated by the most recent research in Finland in 1996, on a regular basis can result in a cholesterol reduction in the blood of 10 and 13 percent. That's a major improvement! The Finns did that by adding phytosterols to margarine which was then used by subjects in place of their regular spread. In fact, following their spectacularly successful research, the Finns marketed the phytosterols-laced margarine as Benecol. Food stores there can't keep it on the shelves.

Fortunately, we Americans can get our phytosterols in a far less expensive, easier and more convenient form. The Endurance Products company now produces a high-quality, high-dosage phytosterol tablet. Just take one or two 400-mg phytosterol tablets prior to animal-food-containing meals, and watch other foods once again. While other products are also on the market in drug and health food stores, I can't vouch for their quality. To order the Endurance Products phytosterols, call (800) 483–2532.

CHOLESTEROL QUACKERY

Prefer a tasty chewable phytosterol tablet that you can munch at the beginning of meals? This has a big advantage over phytosterol-laced margarines. You can carry a supply in pocket or purse wherever you go, and add no fat or calories to the meal. Order the chewable phytosterols, called Kholesterol Blocker, from Nutrition For Life International at (888) 688–6354. Use the identification number 152097 to receive a 10 percent discount for readers of this book. There will be no shipping charges.

If you were to believe every claim for every potion, pill, and nostrum you read about here and there, and every advertisement in health-food stores, you'd think you could lower your cholesterol level by 150 percent. You'd have no cholesterol left in your body!

I've been approached a number of times about one or another miracle potion, with those touting them hoping I'd write about them in my books and newsletters. When I receive such a request, I make a very simple request in return: Send me clinical evidence of effectiveness. So far no one has done so, because no such evidence exists.

I'm certain I'll receive a lot of hate mail for saying so but it's what I believe to be the truth. Does vitamin E raise HDL levels? No. Does evening primrose drop total cholesterol levels? No. Does lecithin make cholesterol melt away? No. Sorry, those things may look good on paper, but they just don't work. They won't do you any good, but they won't do you any harm either, except to your wallet.

But there's one kind of quackery that can do you harm, and that does no good whatever: chelation therapy. I'll get a lot of nasty mail about saying that, too. Chelation therapy is viewed as quackery by the American Heart

Association, the American Medical Association, and the American Council on Health Fraud.

After years of poor diet, smoking, stress, lack of exercise, and general neglect, not to speak of genetic predisposition to heart disease, many people would like an easy way to erase the damage done. Enter the quacks who advocate what's called chelation (kee-lay-shun) therapy to dissolve away the cholesterol-laden plaques in arteries.

The theory sounds good: the chemical EDTA has been shown to cling (chelate) to minerals in the blood. It's been used successfully, for example, to treat patients with lead poisoning, removing the mineral from the blood. Advocates take the next step on faith by then saying that therefore the EDTA can remove the calcium in the plaques, thus softening them so that they can dissolve away, eliminating the risk of heart attack. But the theory just doesn't hold up in practice. The EDTA, injected into the bloodstream, binds to calcium in the blood but has no effect on the calcium in the plaques.

Practitioners charge very high fees for regular EDTA injections in their offices. People who know they have significant blockage often turn to chelation as an alternative to bypass surgery or angioplasty. While I can certainly understand the desire to grasp at straws, the sad fact remains that chelation therapy is a fraud and that people who put their faith in such treatment may be at risk by rejecting the advice of their physicians who can offer life-saving procedures. By all means seek second opinions, and even third opinions, from other qualified sources. But don't turn to quacks.

I've been accused by practitioners of chelation therapy of having a closed mind on the subject. They point to a pile of articles, which, upon closer examination, turn out to be nothing more than testimonials, without scientific validation. How can some people swear by chelation while others, including myself, swear at it?

Let's take a look at the value of testimonials in this regard. The subjective judgment of an individual that he "feels better" or that he can now walk without angina is without merit. One cannot feel elevated cholesterol levels in the blood or clogged arteries, so one cannot feel the difference chelation claims to make. As far as angina goes, that can be affected by a number of simultaneous lifestyle changes, including diet and exercise. When a patient feels better after chelation, the practitioner takes all the credit. But when the treatment fails to produce satisfactory results, the practitioner sadly proclaims that the person didn't come to him soon enough.

Will I ever change my mind about all this? Only if a valid study involving angiographic investigation of the arteries is done, proving that some difference can be actually measured. If chelation therapy can cause the regression of arterial plaque, then one can measure the blockage in an angiogram done before the procedure and then compare it with the occlusion after therapy. Angiographic studies determined the effectiveness of my program on the progression of my own disease by way of my lowered cholesterol levels. I showed that, at least in my own case, I was able to stop the disease dead in its tracks. The only reason advocates of chelation refuse to do such studies is that they're afraid of poor results.

Chelation advocates claim a lack of funding for such studies. Yet they charge thousands for their unproven therapy. Those advocates also claim that the medical "establishment" is trying to block their "alternative" approach because it poses competition. The fact is that anyone can buy a bottle of EDTA and begin to use it in medical practice. If there was any validity to the procedure, the medical community would jump at the opportunity to add the therapy to their armamentarium, just as they readily accepted the angioplasty.

Ultimately your own physician is the best source of treatment for heart disease and other ailments. If you're confident of his or her judgment, follow the advice given. If you have doubts, seek a second or even third opinion. And if the consensus is that a surgical procedure such as angioplasty or bypass is needed, don't be afraid to have it done.

Similarly, if your physician has determined that the best way to lower your cholesterol level includes the use of drugs, by all means don't reject that advice. Certainly I personally prefer my diet-oat-bran-niacin regime over the use of prescription drugs. But if, for any reason, you cannot follow that program, and normal dietary restrictions fail to lower your cholesterol level sufficiently, by all means listen to your doctor's advice.

If you do resort to drug therapy, don't think that removes all responsibility for improved diet from your shoulders. In order for any therapy—and that includes my own oat-bran-niacin approach—to be effective, a good diet must remain the foundation for success.

16

Yes, You Can Reverse Heart Disease!

Coronary artery disease has traditionally been considered an incurable, progressive disease. The outcome of heart disease too often has been death, making it the killer of nearly half of all Americans. Thus, when my readers and those attending my presentations asked the often-repeated question, "Can heart disease be reversed?" my reply was always cautious and conservative. But today we can be a lot more positive: Yes, heart disease *can* be reversed. And at the least we can stop the disease process dead in its tracks.

When my battle with heart disease began at the tender age of thirty-five in 1978, I merely hoped to buy some time. After my second bypass surgery in 1984, my hopes grew stronger and more ambitious. By lowering cholesterol levels significantly, I prayed, I might be able to stop the insidious progress of the disease. Granted, that was wishful thinking, because no proof existed that we could do much more than slow the process down a bit.

Then, piece by piece, the evidence started to build. Today the data we have in hand shows without doubt that we can certainly stop the progress of heart disease and in some cases actually reverse the process.

The concept of reversal of atherosclerosis goes back at least fifty years. First there was circumstantial evidence in various populations that when fatty substances were limited in the diet, very striking decreases in the incidence of heart disease and heart attacks occurred. But that did not tell us whether anything was happening to the lesions known as atherosclerotic plaque.

For example, during the Second World War the availability of cream, butter, and fatty meats was greatly limited, especially in the civilian population. Ironically, America and her allies tried to supply as much of such foods as possible to our fighting men. "A nation fights on its stomach," the saying went. After the war ended, fatty foods regained their place in shopping carts and in homes across America and Europe. Much later, medical scientists looking at historical data noticed that during the war years heart disease appeared to lessen, and following the war it returned in full strength.

Using such data as proof, a number of physicians and scientists began urging their own professional organizations and institutions to recognize the link between diet and heart disease. Unfortunately, their efforts were to little avail, and heart disease continued to grow as a major killer.

Then a wonderful study project, now considered a medical historic landmark, began in the little town of Framingham, Massachusetts, more than thirty years ago. Dr. William Castelli and his colleagues offered men in that town a free medical examination, with follow-up every two years. They measured height, weight, blood pressure, various chemicals in the blood, including the little-understood lipid known as cholesterol. They also kept track of heart attacks and death due to heart disease.

On men who died of heart attacks, autopsies were performed. Universally their arteries supplying blood to the muscle of the heart were clogged with a concretion of dead cells, calcium, clotting factors from the blood, and, very notably, cholesterol. It was noted that during their lives those men typically had high levels of cholesterol in their blood.

Whether dietary cholesterol was related to blood cholesterol, and, most importantly, whether reducing cholesterol levels would help to prevent heart attacks were questions that raged for years. We knew that men with lower levels of cholesterol had fewer heart attacks. But we didn't know whether an aggressive effort to keep cholesterol levels down could play an influence on the incidence of heart disease.

Today, of course, we have that evidence. The data, discussed in Chapter 1, were available to me when I began to write the first edition of this book in 1985. It was with that information that I began my personal war on cholesterol in an effort to save my own life. But was I simply putting off the inevitable?

There had been a number of hints as to the possibility of reversing heart disease. In work done at the University of Chicago under the leadership of Dr. Robert Wissler, rhesus monkeys developed the clogged arteries of heart disease when fed a fatty, cholesterol-rich diet. When the fat and cholesterol were removed from the diet, the atherosclerotic lesions began to disappear.

In 1970, researchers at the University of Iowa, also working with rhesus monkeys, found that one could reverse the lesions even when rather advanced. Those results were repeated again and again in twelve separate studies at the University of Chicago.

Those findings have been corroborated by Dr. Thomas Clarkson at Bowman-Gray Medical School, at Louisiana State University, and in a total of about twenty studies in primate models that show consistently that lesions can be reversed. Lesions become smaller and smaller; injury to the inner lining of the arteries known as the *intima* gradually heals; and cell proliferation, a major marker of atherosclerosis, lessens.

The question remained, however, whether these findings could be applied to humans. Until 1987, we had to make do with less-than-convincing anecdotal, testimonial data.

For example, Nathan Pritikin's arteries were studied in autopsy after his death. The results of that autopsy were flaunted in a letter published in the *New England Journal of Medicine*. It was said that Mr. Pritikin's arteries were completely clear. But that statement was questioned by many. First, there was no absolute evidence that Pritikin had heart disease in the first place. Second, he had never had an angiogram to determine that his coronary arteries were initially clogged. Third, he never submitted to an angiogram when he was living to show that his arteries were clear. And fourth, he had fought a long battle with leukemia, a disease that is well known to significantly reduce cholesterol levels in the blood and that could have leached the cholesterol out of the arteries if, indeed, they had been occluded. Thus there was no proof that Pritikin's efforts to keep cholesterol levels down by way of his dietary program were actually responsible for his clean arteries at death.

Then the first carefully controlled study to determine the effectiveness of cholesterol reduction to stop or reverse the atherosclerotic process was done. The landmark study, conducted by researchers at the University of Southern California in Los Angeles, was reported in the June 19, 1987, issue of the *Journal of the American Medical Association*. For two years 162 coronary bypass patients were studied. Each of the men was given an angiogram at the start of the study, and blockage in the arteries was carefully measured. Then the group was divided into two. The first group were given a fat-modified diet in which fat comprised about 20 percent of total calories, the bile acid-binding drug colestipol, and niacin. The second group, the control group, were placed on a modified diet, about the same as American Heart Association recommendations, and given a placebo in place of the colestipol and niacin.

At the end of the two-year period, the first group showed a 26 percent reduction in total plasma cholesterol, a 43 percent drop in LDLs, and a 37 percent rise in HDLs. Looking at angiograms done at the end of the study and comparing them with those done two years earlier, the researchers found that not only was the progress of the disease stopped in those on the diet-colestipol-niacin program, but also there was reversal of the atherosclerotic plaque buildup in more than 16 percent of patients.

Dr. David Blankenhorn, director of the project, known as the Cholesterol Lowering Atherosclerosis Study (CLAS), has presented his data at numerous medical meetings since that time. He believes unequivocally that heart disease is, indeed, reversible. But even more important is his adamant advice that everyone having a bypass operation should receive aggressive therapy to reduce cholesterol in order to prevent the need for a second surgery. In fact, the impact of the CLAS work has led to a strong commitment to "secondary prevention" in those treating patients with a history of heart disease. Unfortunately, however, only about 20 percent of bypass patients currently receive this kind of advice and treatment.

Dr. Blankenhorn joined the University of Chicago's Dr. Wissler at the annual November meeting of the American Heart Association in Washington, D.C., in 1988, and the two stated unequivocally that lowering cholesterol levels significantly was essential for everyone with advanced heart disease. To achieve reversal of heart disease, or even to halt its progress, one must not settle for the 200 mg/dl suggested for the general population, but rather one must shoot for levels below 160.

Serving on a panel along with Drs. Blankenhorn and Wissler at the November AHA meeting was a man who had demonstrated that such cholesterol reduction could be achieved without drugs of any kind. And his patients demonstrated the benefits of his program by reversing their advanced cases of coronary heart disease.

Dr. Dean Ornish, of the University of California at San Francisco and Director of the Preventive Medicine Research Institute of San Francisco, randomly assigned fifty-five patients with coronary artery disease to one of two groups. The comprehensive-change group went on an ultra-low-fat vegetarian diet, did an hour of meditation daily to help control stress, and engaged in regular physical exercise. The moderate-change group ate a prudent low-fat diet as typically advocated by the AHA, did some exercise, and quit smoking. Twenty-nine patients in total submitted to an angiogram at the beginning of the study and one year later.

The results were dramatic. Ten of twelve patients in the total-lifestyle-change program complied with the program and achieved an overall regression of artery blockage. The average blockage went down from 44.1 percent to 40.8 percent during the year. Conversely, those in the ordinary-care group had an overall progression of heart disease, with blockage going from 44.1 percent to 46.2 percent. Dr. Ornish's study will continue, and patients will receive another angiogram in four years, in 1992, to determine, we all hope, how much additional regression was achieved. Dr. Ornish stated that his preliminary findings strongly suggest that lifestyle changes can have a beneficial impact both on cholesterol levels and atherosclerosis.

All the authorities on the AHA panel agreed that cholesterol must fall significantly lower than the 200 mg/dl level in order to begin to reverse heart disease. Recognizing that other risk factors such as high blood pressure and cigarette smoking must also be included in the equation, they recommended that optimum cholesterol levels drop to 150 mg/dl with levels of the artery-clogging LDL falling to under 100 mg/dl. So we seem to have a consensus that a range of 150 to no more than 200 is the goal, with those demonstrating current heart disease needing to get closer to the lower figure.

Dr. William Castelli, director and founder of the Framingham study, has pointed out that in all his years of experience, working with thousands of patients, he has never seen a heart attack in anyone whose cholesterol level was under 150 mg/dl. In Dr. Ornish's reversal program, total cholesterol fell from an average of 227 to 136. In the control group there was no significant change in cholesterol levels and, as noted, the disease worsened.

Dr. Ornish admits that his program probably couldn't be followed by everyone. It takes a tremendous commitment. One man in the project actually quit his job so he could devote more time to his meditation, exercise, and food preparation. And even with all the time in the world not many individuals could continue on a diet that goes even beyond Pritikin, eliminating all meat, poultry, and fish, and avoiding any added oils or fats. But the value of his study is recognition that the achievement of lowered cholesterol can, indeed, lead to regression. However, we don't know from his work just what role was played by either the meditation or exercise. No effort was made to separate out those factors in terms of success.

Another study, however, focused entirely on cholesterol. Dr. Stanley Dudrick of the University of Texas Health Science Center in Houston gave patients by intravenous needle a specially formulated total parenteral nutrition (TPN) solution designed to lower cholesterol and reduce atherosclerotic plaque buildup in the arteries. A standard TPN solution, given, for example, to burn patients and others unable to eat solid food, contain 20 to 25 percent fat. This lowers cholesterol by 20 to 40 percent. To get more lowering effect, Dr. Dudrick removed all fat.

After one week of continuous intravenous infusion with two to three liters of the solution, during which time they did not eat normal foods, 35 patients showed a 40 to 60 percent cholesterol reduction. The patients all showed plaque reduction after three months on the mixture and water.

Plaque reduction was measured by magnetic resonance imaging, not angiograms. And measurements were done on the aorta, and on the carotid arteries in the neck and the iliac arteries in the abdomen. Coronary vessels were not measured, as accurate diagnosis cannot be achieved without angiographic study.

These are extremely preliminary findings, and many have voiced skepticism over them. Much additional research will be needed, including controlled, double-blind trials, to determine whether this approach is truly useful. Even then, the procedure will be limited to those with extremely high levels of cholesterol, owing to hereditary disorders, who are likely to be willing to comply with such drastic measures.

But what about those of us following a more reasonable approach to cholesterol reduction? What happens when total cholesterol falls significantly by following the 8-week cholesterol cure? Since I realized that my own mortality depended on getting my own cholesterol under control, I've not only been following the findings of research studies described here, but I've been following just what was happening, very specifically, to Bob Kowalski.

Remember that six years after my first bypass surgery I needed a second operation. I had changed my diet a bit, but my cholesterol levels remained elevated. Four and a half years after the second bypass and after I'd gone on my oat-bran-niacin regime I began to wonder very seriously what shape my own vessels were in at the time.

As I've been traveling around the country, physicians have often inquired about my health. I told them my cholesterol levels and the very good results of my treadmill stress tests. But I hadn't had an angiogram, which is the only way one can tell conclusively about the condition of the arteries, since just prior to the second bypass.

As you may know, an angiogram is the invasive procedure in which a physician inserts a catheter through an incision in an artery in the arm or groin and threads it carefully into the heart vessels. Fluoroscopic cameras then show the actual anatomy of those vessels. No non-invasive procedure can provide absolute diagnosis at this time, although research and development efforts are leading in that direction. Today, however, the angiogram remains the gold standard.

I was feeling absolutely terrific. My cholesterol remained controlled, at a level research had shown to stop if not reverse heart disease. My blood pressure was perfect. I worked out very actively in the gym five days a week, each and every morning, and my resting heart rate was a nice low 48 to 52. Moreover, my 1988 treadmill stress-test result was as good as the previous year's, if not better.

During that year, however, my cardiologist, Dr. Albert Kattus, had retired. His colleague, Dr. Carter Newton, performed the stress test for me in Santa Monica. As we discussed the results, he said, "I know Al Kattus would give you an all-clear on the test, Bob, but to be absolutely on the safe side, have you thought about having an angiogram? I think you should."

Just about that time, the singer-songwriter Roy Orbison died of a massive heart attack. He had had bypass surgery ten years earlier. Unfortunately, he continued to smoke heavily after his surgery and probably his diet wasn't the best. As a fan of his, with many Orbison records in my collection, I was sorry he hadn't had a thorough examination to reveal that he needed further treatment.

Coincidentally, I'd been working with Dr. Jack Sternlieb, director of the Heart Institute of the Desert in Rancho Mirage, just outside Palm Springs. Dr. Sternlieb had performed bypass surgery on Betty Ford, and had been written up as having one of the best records in bypass surgery in the country, if not the best. He had invited me to the Heart Institute to do a couple of presentations. I was extremely impressed by his facilities, his record, and his dedication to prevention. Very few cardiac surgeons have his devotion to stopping heart disease before it continues on to another heart attack or another operation. I knew that if I ever needed to return to the operating room I'd want to place myself in Dr. Sternlieb's able hands.

That's one of the reasons I elected to have my angiogram done right there at the Heart Institute. I guess I don't have to tell you that I was nervous, not so much about the angiogram itself, but about the results.

I felt I really couldn't lose, one way or the other. On the one hand, if there was something that just didn't show up by way of the treadmill test, I wanted to know about it so something could be done to remedy the situation. On the other hand, if the results were good I'd know with even more certainty that both my readers and I were on the right track in following the 8-week cholesterol cure.

Well, the results were so good that I'm still celebrating! Dr. Sternlieb put it this way: "Your vessels look like they were put in last week!" In other words, no clogging of any kind occurred in the grafted veins used in the bypass four and a half years earlier. He felt the results were remarkable.

Dr. Surender Vuthoori, the cardiologist who actually performed the procedure, agreed the vessels showed no signs of any progress of the disease. He pointed out that four to five years after bypass, one would expect the beginnings of reocclusion, the clogging that ultimately leads to either another operation or worse. It's a wonderful thing to watch the angiogram screen and see the bypassed vessels fully open and bringing life-giving blood to the pumping heart, and the native arteries open and flowing.

Both men said they believed all their patients should be on my program. In fact, my books are for sale in the Heart Institute lobby. And niacin—specifically Endur-acin—is prescribed for all high-cholesterol patients who have no contraindications. They want all their patients to have the success I enjoyed.

I had a subsequent angiogram at the Heart Institute in 1993, and the results were just as good. Since then, I've had a thallium treadmill test every other year, and each time the report has been excellent. At the time of this edition of my book, it has been 14 years since my second bypass, and I'm feeling terrific!

Should everyone have an angiogram? Definitely not. First, there is some risk attached to the procedure. There is a very slight chance of having a heart attack as a result of the catheter's entering the heart and vessels; there's even a small risk of death. Next, the cost of an angiogram is significant. And at the very least the procedure isn't exactly pleasant. For the vast majority of patients, noninvasive procedures are more than adequate to determine the state of their health. Listen to your physician's advice as to what's best for you.

But here I offer another word of strong caution. It takes many, many years for the atherosclerotic process to clog our arteries. Yes, we certainly can stop that process from going any further. In most instances, that's enough, since the heart already receives an adequate flow of oxygen-carrying blood. In the case of bypass patients we can be quite confident that one operation will be all it ever takes to ensure a long life. In some instances, we can even expect to see reversal. Yet we have to remember that since the atherosclerotic process of clogging took place over many years we can expect that it will take many more years for significant regression to occur.

In the meantime, the disease state may already be life-threatening. At the least it can be debilitating, owing to the pain of angina. The immediate answer may be angioplasty with a balloon catheter to clear a blockage or two, bypass surgery to bring blood to deprived areas of the heart, or perhaps medical therapy to keep vessels as open and flowing as possible.

Please do not consider any cholesterol-reducing program, including my own, to be a replacement for potentially life-saving surgery if that's what's needed in your case. Don't think you can start eating oat-bran muffins and taking niacin and doing exercise in order to circumvent your physician's advice to take more serious steps.

If your cardiologist recommends surgery and you feel you'd like another opinion, terrific. You should feel confident in this major decision, which has a huge impact on your life. But don't play ostrich to hide from the unavoidable truth.

When I first sat down to the typewriter to write this book in 1985, I was elated that my recent second bypass had been successful and that I'd developed a program that could keep my cholesterol under control. I felt that I had gotten out from under the Sword of Damocles that had hung over my head for the past six years, and that I'd have many more years to look forward to enjoying.

But there was always a nagging feeling that maybe someday the bubble would pop. Yes, my cholesterol was way down there, but, owing to my genetic background of heart disease, would my bypass vessels eventually begin to clog? Yes, I'd learned to control stress levels to a great degree, but was I overdoing it by working as much as I do and traveling all over the world to do presentations and media interviews? Yes, my exercise regime had resulted in tremendous stamina, but could I exceed my limits on a ski trip or an arduous mountain hike? I was far, far from a "cardiac cripple" but I still thought of myself as a heart patient.

No more. I've seen the insides of my own heart, arteries, and bypass vessels. Heart disease, for me, is a thing of the past. And I intend to spend the rest of my hopefully long and healthy life telling the rest of the world how they, too, can know the joy and health I now enjoy. Thank you, God, for the wonderful gift of life!

17

To Tomorrow and Tomorrow and Tomorrow

Call it an instinct for survival. Call it a love of life. There is a desire, a burning need to survive, to live for tomorrow and tomorrow and tomorrow.

I have my own reasons. Their names are Ross and Jenny. You have your reasons. All of them are worthwhile and defy description on the printed page.

I'll never forget that day I came back from the surgeon's office when he told me of the mortality risk of the surgery. All I could think of was leaving my little children behind, with them not understanding why.

Think of it: By taking some vitamins, eating some muffins, and following a sensible, delicious diet, you and I can cut our risk of heart disease in half. We don't have to undergo "heroic" measures. We'll never be written about in *Time* magazine, but we'll be pioneers nonetheless, proving that heart disease *can* be defeated.

No, I don't deny that I often envy those who dig into a gooey piece of chocolate cake, apple pie with crust made from lard, prime ribs of beef, and even the burgers and fries from the fast-food stands here in Southern California. There's a place here that serves, as I recall, the most scrumptious double cheeseburger in Los Angeles. The memories of those burgers are tempting and strong, but they don't stand a chance when I look at the faces of my two kids.

Ross and Jenny are my fortification. Each time I might be tempted to bite into one of those burgers, or a thick slab of prime rib, or a cheese-laden pizza I think that I might miss a day with them. Maybe I'd miss the graduation. Or the special award ceremony. Or the wedding. Maybe even the grandchildren!

You have to find your own reasons. It takes more than just a momentary decision to carry on a lifetime of commitment.

Think of those deeply committed to religious beliefs. The decision to attend those Sunday services on a day the sun is shining is based on deep commitment. It goes beyond a logical, scientific decision.

We all have our disappointments, and times when we think it may not be worth it. Those are the times when the temptations to forget the oat-bran muffins, the daily doses of niacin, the low-fat diet are the strongest. It's so easy to feel sorry for oneself, to give oneself a "consolation prize" in the form of a dozen doughnuts or a 24-ounce sirloin steak.

I had the opportunity to consult for a

weight-loss group for two years. Many of the clients failed to achieve their intended "goal" weight or to stay with it once they reached that goal. Why? Often because they didn't have a good enough reason to become slender or to stay slender. Their excuses could fill a book. But those made it who came to realize that their own satisfaction was the ultimate reason for success.

If you skimmed over or skipped Chapter 8, on weight loss, go back and read it. I discuss a lot of the motivational drive needed to succeed. Those motivations are the same for *anyone* who sincerely wants to make a change in his or her life.

Face it: the changes you need to make could be the difference between living and not living. The next time you think that the flush you get from the niacin is uncomfortable and not worth it, think again. The next time you feel that a doughnut or a croissant would be better than another oat-bran muffin, think again. The next time you'd rather select the tournedos with béarnaise sauce over the broiled swordfish, think again.

Think about whether those choices are worth a year, a month, a week, or even a day. I think about that time with my kids. You think about the time with whomever or whatever.

Wake up tomorrow morning and look at the

sky. Even if it's raining or gloomy, it's beautiful because you're there to experience it. Like the words in the song, stop to smell the roses. As the bumper stickers advise, hug your kids today.

Every man and woman in the world is lucky in one way or another. You have to define your own luck. You have to count your own blessings. If you can honestly say there is nothing you enjoy anymore, no one you care to hug today or tomorrow, then by all means, don't make another batch of muffins. Throw your niacin tablets away. Forget the diet and gorge on butter and eggs. Maybe you'll even want to start smoking, or smoke more, to speed the process.

No thanks, not for me. Jenny's smile makes the gloomiest day bright. Ross's every success and milestone is important to me. You never saw two more terrific kids. Or maybe you have. Maybe they're yours. Maybe they're your grandchildren. Or the children you haven't had yet. Maybe your children are your work, your hobbies, your church, your friends. All of these are important. All of them are the *most* important.

What's your reason for tomorrow? And tomorrow? And tomorrow?

Make your commitment today to a heart-healthy lifestyle. And keep up-to-date on all that's happening through my quarterly newsletter. See page xviii for details.

18

Miracle Muffins and Breads

Since discovering the vital role oat bran can play in living a healthful life, I've worked on a number of ways to incorporate oat bran into my own diet. Personally, I don't care much for hot cereal, which is the principal way oat bran is normally served. For me, the best way has been using oat bran in baking muffins.

Before you start saying to yourself that you don't have time to do any baking, consider the fact that in just 10 minutes of preparation time and 17 minutes of baking time you can have a week's supply. And you'll more than save that time when it comes to eating. Muffins are the ideal fast food for someone on the run all the time as I am. Just gobble down two or three muffins along with a glass of skim milk or a fruit milkshake and you're set for hours.

I try to get one-half cup of oat bran into my diet each and every day. Three muffins supply that whole amount. And with the variety of muffins and other baked goods I've suggested here, plus others you may come up with on your own, you'll never get tired of them—any more than people get tired of bread.

To get started, you'll need one or two metal

muffin pans and a supply of paper baking cups to line the cups with. All the ingredients you'll need are listed in the Shopping List chapter, except for any fresh fruit you may wish to add for variety.

A Few Words About Muffin Making

While all the muffin recipes you're about to read have been extensively tested, a few words of explanation are in order. First of all, let me say that all these ideas were developed in my own kitchen, based upon the original recipe on the oat-bran box. But I've made changes and additions.

For example, I have omitted salt entirely. I find that this makes no perceptible difference in flavor, and I'd rather not have the sodium in my food. The two tablespoons of cooking oil provide only one-half teaspoon of oil per muffin. You'll find that most muffin and biscuit recipes call for much more oil. You can also substitute corn syrup (Karo) for oil.

Next, I have experimented with sugar content. I tried eliminating sugar entirely, relying instead on all-fruit sweetening. Both the flavor and texture of the product suffered. So now I routinely use one-quarter cup of brown sugar for a 12-muffin recipe. Again, note that this is just four tablespoons per batch, or one tea-spoonful per muffin.

Don't forget that these oat-bran muffins have become a staple part of my daily diet, and hopefully they will be part of yours also. With this in mind, the amount of oil and sugar in the muffins, as part of your total diet, is really quite small.

If you prefer, however, you certainly may experiment on your own, trying less sugar or replacing some of it with additional fruit. But just for your interest and information, don't forget that the body metabolizes all sugars in the same way. Whether it's sucrose in brown sugar, glucose in honey, or fructose in fruit and juices, the chemical formula is similar and the effects the same. That doesn't mean you should go hog-wild and double the recipe's sugar content. Just keep the word "modera-tion" in mind.

As I mentioned earlier, I did the first muffins in my own kitchen. I used a standard electric oven, and recommend an oven ther-mometer to be sure of the temperature: 425 degrees.

To have these muffins come out as perfect as possible, time is critical. For all recipes, use a timer and note that you set the time at *ex-actly* 17 minutes. When the timer rings, use a toothpick to test doneness. The toothpick should come out of the muffin just slightly tacky to the touch, not wet or dry.

If you overbake by even a minute or two, you'll have dry muffins. Other recipes are not as critical since they have more sugar and oil to retain moisture. It's better to return the muffins to the oven for an additional minute than to regret the extra minute if they are already overbaked. Depending on the particular recipe or the amount of fruit you're using, the batter will take more or less time. The pineapple muffin recipe, for example, is quite moist and probably will require an extra two minutes.

By all means, experiment. Each time you try a recipe or a variation, jot down the temperature of the oven and the exact amount of time it took to bake the muffins. Also make a note as to just how juicy the fruit was that you used. These things all make a big difference.

A word of caution so you don't make the same mistake I did at the beginning of my own muffin experience. These muffins do *not* get browned easily. At first you may think they don't look done. Use that toothpick. If you bake them until they're as brown as a typical flourbased cake would be, the muffins will be dry.

Unlike commercially prepared baked goods, these muffins do not contain any preservatives. If you don't expect to eat them within two or three days, by all means keep the muffins in the freezer or refrigerator. A large plastic storage bag is best to retain moisture. If you have a microwave oven, pop cold or frozen muffins in for a moment to warm them beautifully. Standard ovens have a tendency to dry out the muffins, if you leave them in too long.

Don't be discouraged if all this seems like a lot of trouble. Baking with oat bran is simply different from baking with wheat flour and butter- and sugar-laden recipes. You'll be comfortable with the procedures after just two or three batches, even if you've never baked before in your life. And the rewards you'll reap are simply spectacular!

IF YOU OWN A FOOD PROCESSOR . . .

After trying a few of the muffin recipes, you'll find that they come out a bit on the crumbly side, rather like cornbread. Some people really like that texture. And I enjoy it, too. But there's a way I discovered to give your muffins, breads, and brownies a more cake-like structure.

Take the whole box of oat bran and just empty it right into your food processor with the large blade set to grind. Let the machine run during the full time it takes to get all your other ingredients out and measured. When it's time to add the oat bran and mix the batter, you'll find that you've milled the oat bran down to a flourlike, powdery consistency. It makes a *huge* difference in the way your muffins turn out.

● ●

Basic Muffins

2 ¼ cups oat-bran cereal
¼ cup chopped nuts (walnuts, pecans, or
    even peanuts)
¼ cup raisins (or dates, currants, or
    whatever)
1 tablespoon baking powder (not baking
    soda)
¼ cup brown sugar
        or
¼ cup honey or molasses
1 ¼ cups skim milk or evaporated skim milk
2 egg whites or egg substitute for two eggs
2 tablespoons vegetable oil

This is basically the recipe listed on the side of the Quaker Oat Bran box. But I've substituted a few items and increased the amount of milk to get better, lighter muffins. Start off with this one. Later you may wish to cut down on the amount of sweetenings added. Some of the other recipes for muffins offer excellent alternative sweeteners, such as frozen apple-juice concentrate.

Preheat the oven to 425°F. In a large bowl combine the oat-bran cereal, nuts, raisins and baking powder. Stir in the brown sugar *or* liquid sweetening. Mix the milk, egg whites, and oil together and blend in with the oat-bran mixture. Line muffin pans with paper baking cups, and fill with batter. Bake 15 to 17 minutes. Test for doneness with a toothpick; it should come out moist but not wet. *Makes 12 muffins.*

Store in a plastic bag to retain moisture. Keep the muffins in the refrigerator if they will not be consumed within 3 days, as they contain no preservatives.

Nutrition Information per Serving

Serving: 1 muffin
Cholesterol: 0.42 milligrams
Protein: 2.53 grams
Carbohydrates: 17.8 grams
Fat: 5.2 grams
   Saturated: 0.41 grams
   Polyunsaturated: 2.32 grams
   Monounsaturated: 0.89 grams
Fiber: 3.98 grams
Sodium: 109 milligrams
Calories: 137

Oil-Free Muffins

2¼ cups oat-bran cereal
1 tablespoon baking powder
¼ cup brown sugar
½ cup dry fruits (raisins, dates, prunes)
1¼ cups skim milk or evaporated skim milk
2 egg whites
2 tablespoons corn syrup

One can also make muffins without any oil at all by substituting corn syrup for the oil. You can also make this substitution in any of the other muffin recipes in this section. Try substituting corn syrup for oil in ther baking recipes as well.

Preheat the oven to 425°F. Mix the dry ingredients in a large bowl. Mix the milk, egg whites, and corn syrup together and blend with dry ingredients. Line muffin pans with paper baking cups, and fill with batter divided equally. Bake 13 to 15 minutes. Test for doneness with a toothpick. *Makes 12 muffins.*

NOTE This oil-free recipe requires a bit less baking time than the recipe for basic muffins.

Nutritional Information per Serving
Serving: 1 muffin
Cholesterol: 0.42 milligrams
Protein: 1.99 grams
Carbohydrates: 22.4 grams

Fat: 1.48 grams
  Saturated: 0.04 grams
  Polyunsaturated: 0.01 grams
  Monounsaturated: 0.01 grams
Fiber: 4.01 grams
Sodium: 111 milligrams
Calories: 120

Apple Cinnamon Muffins

  2¼ cups oat-bran cereal
  ¼ cup brown sugar
  1¼ teaspoons cinnamon
  1 tablespoon baking powder
  ¼ cup chopped walnuts
  ¼ cup raisins
  ¼ cup skim milk or evaporated skim milk
  ¾ cup frozen apple-juice concentrate
  2 egg whites
  2 tablespoons vegetable oil
  1 medium apple, cored and chopped

Mix the dry ingredients in a large bowl. Mix the milk, apple-juice concentrate, egg whites, and oil in a bowl or blender. Add to the dry ingredients and mix. Add the chopped apple. Line the muffin pans with paper baking cups and fill with batter. Bake in a 425°F. oven for 17 minutes. *Makes 12 muffins.*

After cooling, store in a large plastic bag to retain moisture and softness.

TIP Serve with applesauce or spread with apple butter.

Nutritional Information per Serving
Serving: 1 muffin
Cholesterol: 0.17 milligrams
Protein: 2.1 grams
Carbohydrates: 22.3 grams
Fat: 4.13 grams
  Saturated: 0.27 grams
  Polyunsaturated: 1.67 grams
  Monounsaturated: 0.62 grams
Fiber: 4.28 grams
Sodium: 103 milligrams
Calories: 142

• •

Banana Nut Muffins

2¼ cups oat-bran cereal
1 tablespoon baking powder
¼ cup brown sugar
¼ cup chopped walnuts or pecans
1¼ cups skim milk
2 very ripe bananas (the riper the
    better), mashed
2 egg whites
2 tablespoons vegetable oil

Preheat the oven to 425°F. Mix the dry ingredients in a large bowl. Mix the milk, bananas, egg whites, and oil in a bowl or blender. Add to the dry ingredients and mix. Line the muffin pan with paper baking cups and fill them with batter. Bake for 17 minutes. *Makes 12 muffins.*

TIP Serve with a banana milkshake.

Nutritional Information per Serving

Serving: 1 muffin
Cholesterol: 0.42 milligrams
Protein: 2.64 grams
Carbohydrates: 20.1 grams
Fat: 5.29 grams
  Saturated: 0.45 grams
  Polyunsaturated: 2.33 grams
  Monounsaturated: 0.9 grams
Fiber: 4.2 grams
Sodium: 108 milligrams
Calories: 146

Canned-Fruit Muffins

2¼ cups oat-bran cereal
1 tablespoon baking powder
¼ cup raisins
2 tablespoons vegetable oil
1 cup evaporated skim milk
2 egg whites
1 16-oz. can pears (drained)

Preheat the oven to 425°F. Mix the dry ingredients in a bowl. Mix together all other ingredients except the pears. Add the liquid mixture to the dry ingredients and mix. Chop the canned pears fine and add to the batter. If the batter seems dry, add a bit of the fluid drained from the pears. Line the muffin pan with paper baking cups and fill with batter. Bake for 17 minutes or until a toothpick comes out dry.

NOTE Always look for canned pears without any added sugar. Not only are they lower in calories, but they also taste better. And don't stop with pears. Look for all the other canned fruits you can store and use when you don't have any fresh fruit and it's time to make muffins. Peaches are good. Or, for something really colorful and delicious, try fruit cocktail. Save the cherries to put on top. Even the kids will love these.

Nutritional Information per Serving
Serving: 1 muffin
Cholesterol: 0.33 milligrams
Protein: 1.63 grams
Carbohydrates: 12 grams
Fat: 3.1 grams
   Saturated: 0.32 grams
   Polyunsaturated: 1.34 grams
   Monounsaturated: 0.56 grams
Fiber: 2.2 grams
Sodium: 106 milligrams
Calories: 86.7

Strawberry Muffins

2¼ cups oat-bran cereal
¼ cup brown sugar
1 tablespoon baking powder
½ cup evaporated skim milk or skim milk
¾ cup canned strawberry nectar or
    strawberry juice
¾ cup fresh or frozen strawberries, cut up
2 egg whites
2 tablespoons vegetable oil

Preheat the oven to 425°F. Mix the dry ingredients in a large bowl. Mix the milk, strawberry nectar, strawberries, egg whites, and oil in a bowl or blender. (Reserve 12 pieces of fresh strawberry to place on top of the muffins.) Combine with the dry ingredients and mix. Line muffin cups with paper baking cups and fill with batter. Place a piece of strawberry on each. Bake for 17 minutes. *Makes 12 muffins.*

TIP Serve as strawberry "shortcake." Place each in a bowl and cover with chilled strawberries. Top with whipped chilled evaporated skim milk.

Nutritional Information per Serving
Serving: 1 muffin
Cholesterol: 0.17 milligrams
Protein: 1.36 grams

Carbohydrates: 17.7 grams
Fat: 3.71 grams
  Saturated: 0.3 grams
  Polyunsaturated: 1.35 grams
  Monounsaturated: 0.56 grams
Fiber: 3.93 grams
Sodium: 101 milligrams
Calories: 119

• •

Pineapple Muffins

2 ¼ cups oat-bran cereal
¼ cup brown sugar
1 tablespoon baking powder
½ cup evaporated skim milk or skim milk
2 8-ounce cans crushed pineapple in its
       own juice (unsweetened)
2 egg whites or 2 ounces egg substitute
2 tablespoons vegetable oil

Preheat the oven to 425°F. Mix the dry ingredients in a large bowl. Mix the milk, 1 can of crushed pineapple with juice, egg whites, and oil in a bowl or blender. Combine the ingredients and mix. Drain the second can of pineapple and add to the mixture. Line the muffin pans with paper baking cups, and fill with batter. Bake for 17 minutes. *Makes 12 muffins.*

TIP Serve with a pineapple milkshake.

Nutritional Information per Serving
Serving: 1 muffin
Cholesterol: 0.17 milligrams
Protein: 1.44 grams
Carbohydrates: 17.5 grams
Fat: 3.73 grams
Saturated: 0.3 grams
Polyunsaturated: 1.35 grams
Monounsaturated: 0.56 grams
Fiber: 3.49 grams
Sodium: 101 milligrams
Calories: 119

• •
Pineapple Upside-Down Muffins

Make these for a special treat.

Prepare the recipe as for pineapple muffins (see previous page). Before filling the muffin cups, place a slice of pineapple and a maraschino cherry in each. Pour in the batter. Bake for 19 minutes.

Another alternative is to use a cake pan instead of the muffin pan. Spray the bottom of the pan with Pam, and line it with pineapple rings with a maraschino cherry in each. Pour the batter over. Bake for 19 minutes. Turn out of the pan and serve as an upside-down cake.

Nutritional Information per Serving
Serving: 1 muffin
Cholesterol: 0.17 milligrams

Protein: 1.64 grams
Carbohydrates: 23.9 grams
Fat: 3.95 grams
  Saturated: 0.31 grams
  Polyunsaturated: 1.42 grams
  Monounsaturated: 0.58 grams
Fiber: 4.28 grams
Sodium: 101 milligrams
Calories: 144

• •
Pear-fection Muffins

  2¼ cups oat-bran cereal
  3 tablespoons brown sugar
  1 tablespoon baking powder
  ½ teaspoon cinnamon
  ¼ teaspoon vanilla
  2 egg whites
  2 tablespoons vegetable oil
  ¾ cup evaporated skim milk
  1 large ripe pear (or 2 small pears),
    peeled and cored

Preheat the oven to 425°F. Mix the dry ingredients in a large bowl. Mix all the other ingredients, including the pear, in a blender at low speed. Combine with the dry ingredients and mix. Line the muffin pan with paper baking cups. Fill the baking cups with batter. Bake 17 minutes or until a toothpick comes out dry.

TIP This is a good example of what to do with fruit that gets a little too ripe. The riper the better for muffins. Following the muffin program, you'll never throw soft fruit away again.

Nutritional Information per Serving
Serving: 1 muffin
Cholesterol: 0.25 milligrams
Protein: 1.5 grams
Carbohydrates: 15.3 grams
Fat: 3.75 grams
  Saturated: 0.31 grams
  Polyunsaturated: 1.35 grams
  Monounsaturated: 0.57 grams
Fiber: 3.82 grams
Sodium: 103 milligrams
Calories: 111

• •

Pumpkin Muffins

2¼ cups oat-bran cereal
3 tablespoons brown sugar
1 tablespoon baking powder
½ teaspoon nutmeg
½ teaspoon cinnamon
¼ cup raisins
½ cup canned pumpkin
½ cup frozen pineapple-juice concentrate
¾ cup evaporated skim milk

2 tablespoons vegetable oil
2 egg whites

Preheat the oven to 425°F. Mix the dry ingredients in a large bowl. Mix all other ingredients in a blender. Combine with the dry ingredients and stir just to mix. Line the muffin pans with paper baking cups. Fill the cups with batter and bake for 17 minutes or until a wooden toothpick comes out dry. *Makes 12 muffins.*

TIP The pumpkin in these muffins is a fine source of both vitamin A and vitamin C. Serve them with turkey and cranberry sauce.

Nutritional Information per Serving

Serving: 1 muffin
Cholesterol: 0.25 milligrams
Protein: 2.23 grams
Carbohydrates: 18.1 grams
Fat: 3.14 grams
    Saturated: 0.33 grams
    Polyunsaturated: 1.34 grams
    Monounsaturated: 0.57 grams
Fiber: 2.25 grams
Sodium: 112 milligrams
Calories: 113

. . . .

Dinner Muffins

1 ¼ cups oat-bran cereal
1 cup self-rising flour
1 ½ cups evaporated skim milk
2 egg whites
2 tablespoons honey
3 tablespoons vegetable oil

If you'd like to have some of your daily oat bran as dinner muffins, you'll probably prefer this less sweet variation.

Preheat the oven to 425°F. Mix the dry ingredients in a large bowl. Mix the milk and the remaining ingredients in a blender at low speed, then add to the dry ingredients and stir until just mixed. Line a muffin pan with paper baking cups, and fill with batter. Bake 15 minutes or till a toothpick comes out dry.

TIP Experiment a bit with your dinner muffins. Some people prefer to add a few raisins. Or try using other fluids to replace part of the milk.

Nutritional Information per Serving
Serving: 1 muffin
Cholesterol: 0.5 milligrams
Protein: 2.81 grams
Carbohydrates: 18.6 grams
Fat: 4.33 grams
  Saturated: 0.49 grams

Polyunsaturated: 2 grams
Monounsaturated: 0.84 grams
Fiber: 2.23 grams
Sodium: 137 milligrams
Calories: 131

• •

Molasses Muffins

2 ½ cups oat-bran cereal
1 tablespoon baking powder
¼ cup raisins
¼ cup chopped nuts
1 ¼ cups evaporated skim milk
2 tablespoons vegetable oil
2 egg whites
¼ cup molasses

Preheat the oven to 425°F. Mix the dry ingredients in a bowl. Blend all other ingredients in a blender and add to the dry ingredients. Stir just to mix. Line the muffin pan with paper baking cups and fill with the batter. Bake for 16 minutes or until a toothpick comes out dry.

NOTE This is a nice variation from other muffins made with brown sugar. The molasses gives the muffins an entirely different flavor. If you prefer, you can cut down the amount of molasses to reduce calories. And don't forget that you can also substitute the molasses for sugar in any of the other muffin recipes to mix and match flavors.

Nutritional Information per Serving
Serving: 1 muffin
Cholesterol: 0.42 milligrams
Protein: 2.53 grams
Carbohydrates: 13.6 grams
Fat: 5.21 grams
   Saturated: 0.42 grams
   Polyunsaturated: 2.32 grams
   Monounsaturated: 0.89 grams
Fiber: 3.99 grams
Sodium: 108 milligrams
Calories: 121

• •

Dinner Rolls

   ¾ cup oat-bran cereal
   ½ cup self-rising flour
   ¾ cup skim milk
   2 tablespoons honey
   3 tablespoons vegetable oil

Notice that these are not muffins! Yes, you can make rolls and breads with oat bran. This is a very simple recipe that can be made at a moment's notice to have with dinner. It's a variation on a pretty standard recipe.

To get these rolls to come out well, first put

the oat-bran cereal through a food processor or blender. This will further mill the cereal to a more flourlike consistency. Then blend in the self-rising flour. Note that you'll need no baking powder. Blend in the other ingredients and drop the batter onto a cookie sheet sprayed with Pam. Bake them at 375° for 8 to 10 minutes or until just barely browned, and serve them hot from the oven. *This will make about 12 rolls.*

Nutritional Information per Serving

Serving: 1 roll
Cholesterol: 0.25 milligrams
Protein: 1.15 grams
Carbohydrates: 10.5 grams
Fat: 3.94 grams
  Saturated: 0.46 grams
  Polyunsaturated: 2 grams
  Monounsaturated: 0.83 grams
Fiber: 1.31 grams
Sodium: 64.4 milligrams
Calories: 85.3

Cran-Bran Bread

2 cups whole cranberries
1½ cups oat-bran cereal
1 teaspoon grated orange peel
1 cup granulated sugar (reduce amount if you prefer)

⅓ cup brown sugar
2½ cups all-purpose flour
3 teaspoons baking powder
½ teaspoon ground allspice
¼ cup vegetable oil
½ cup skim milk
4 egg whites or egg substitute equal to 2 eggs
½ cup chopped walnuts

My wife found this recipe in our local newspaper and we modified it to suit the program by making a few healthful substitutions. It's really delicious, especially around the holidays. This recipe makes three small loaves; you'll want to wrap them in plastic and store in the refrigerator so they don't dry out.

Preheat the oven to 350°F. Chop the cranberries and add to the oat-bran cereal along with the orange peel and sugars. Next, stir together the flour, baking powder and allspice. Add the oil, milk, egg substitute. Blend in the cranberry mixture and walnuts. Spray three 6-by-3-inch loaf pans with Baker's Joy. Divide the batter between the pans, and bake for 40 to 50 minutes, or until a toothpick comes out dry.

Nutritional Information per Serving
Serving: 1 slice
Cholesterol: 0.07 milligrams
Protein: 2.31 grams

Carbohydrates: 20.5 grams
Fat: 3.48 grams
  Saturated: 3.29 grams
  Polyunsaturated: 1.85 grams
  Monounsaturated: 0.7 grams
Fiber: 1.49 grams
Sodium: 43.9 milligrams
Calories: 123.4

• •

Oatmeal Bread

¾ cup boiling water
½ cup old-fashioned rolled oats
3 tablespoons margarine
¼ cup honey
1 teaspoon salt
1 envelope active dry yeast
¼ cup very warm water
½ teaspoon sugar
½ container egg substitute (equal to 1 egg)
2 cups all-purpose flour
¾ cup oat-bran cereal, milled to flour in blender

Here's another delicious way to get oats into your diet. Even if you've never baked a loaf of bread before, it's a lot of fun and almost goof-proof.

Stir together the boiling water, rolled oats, margarine, honey, and salt in a large bowl until well mixed. Let cool to warm. Sprinkle the packet of yeast over the very warm water in a 1-cup container; add the ½ teaspoon sugar. Stir to dissolve the yeast, and let it stand for about 10 minutes or until the mixture bubbles. Next add the yeast mixture, egg substitute, 1 ½ cups of all-purpose flour, and the oat bran to the oatmeal mixture. Beat with an electric mixer at low speed for 2 minutes while gradually adding the rest of the flour. Put the dough into a 9-by-5-by-3-inch loaf pan sprayed with Baker's Joy. Cover with waxed paper and a towel and put the pan in a warm place away from drafts. (A turned-off oven with a pilot is a good place.) Let the dough double in bulk, about 45 minutes.

Bake in a preheated oven at 375°F. for about 1 hour. The bread is done when it feels and sounds hollow when you tap it. Remove the bread from the pan and let it cool.

Next, beam with pride. Finally, serve and enjoy.

Nutritional Information per Serving

Serving: I slice
Cholesterol: 0
Protein: 3.16 grams
Carbohydrates: 22.9 grams
Fat: 3.45 grams
  Saturated: 1.67 grams
  Polyunsaturated: 0.18 grams
  Monounsaturated: 0.8 grams

Fiber: 1.61 grams
Sodium: 57.1 milligrams
Calories: 139

• •

Bran Brownies

    3 tablespoons cocoa
    1 tablespoon instant coffee
    1 tablespoon water
    2 very ripe bananas
    2 cups sugar (less if you prefer)
    6 egg whites
    1 teaspoon vanilla extract
    1 cup oat-bran cereal
    ¼ teaspoon salt (optional)
    1 cup chopped nuts (or substitute raisins
       to cut fat further)

Here's the way to satisfy that chocolate craving and get some of your day's oat bran at the same time.

Combine the cocoa, coffee, water, bananas, and mix in a blender or a large bowl with a hand mixer. Add the sugar, egg whites, vanilla, and mix well. Sift together the oat-bran cereal and salt, then add to the mixture. Fold in the nuts or raisins. Pour into a 9-inch baking pan sprayed with Baker's Joy (oil and flour mixture) or Pam. Bake at 350°F. for 45 minutes. Cut into individual squares, cool, and serve.

These brownies are fudgy, gooey, and delicious. Your family and friends won't believe they're free of fat and cholesterol! *Makes 19 brownies.*

Nutritional Information per Serving
Serving: 1 brownie
Cholesterol: 0
Protein: 4.69 grams
Carbohydrates: 43.8 grams
Fat: 7.57 grams
  Saturated: 0.98 grams
  Polyunsaturated: 3.93 grams
  Monounsaturated: 1.33 grams
Fiber: 2.99 grams
Sodium: 66.8 milligrams
Calories: 251

19

Taste-Tempting Turkey

Everyone truly interested in eating a more healthful diet owes that great bird the turkey a big thanks. Get rid of the idea that turkey belongs on the table only at Thanksgiving. There are dozens of ways to prepare and enjoy this low-fat, low-cholesterol source of high-quality protein. In fact, just about any dish you'd want to cook that calls for high-fat meat can be done to perfection with turkey.

In addition to the savings in fat and cholesterol, you'll enjoy the savings in your shopping budget. Turkey is a real dollar stretcher. And the food industry helps out by offering not only whole birds but also selected pieces and a variety of ground-turkey and turkey-sausage products. But you must realize that the portion with the least amount of fat and cholesterol is the breast. So here's what I do: go to the market and purchase a large turkey breast and have the butcher skin, bone, and grind it or prepare cutlets. When you get home, you can portion out the meat and store it in the freezer in convenient-sized packages. Figure four ounces per serving.

All the recipes you love that call for hamburger can be made with ground turkey breast.

And those dishes you treasure that include cutlets or chops are delicious made with turkey cutlets. Experiment a bit. Soon you'll be savoring a wide variety of turkey alternatives.

• •

Terrific Turkey Meatloaf

1 pound ground turkey breast
1 egg white
½ cup oat bran
3 tablespoons ketchup
1 tablespoon Worcestershire sauce
½ teaspoon Dijon mustard
½ green pepper, minced
3 slices onion, minced
2 tablespoons chopped green olives
1 large garlic clove, minced (more if preferred)
¼ teaspoon each: sage, black pepper, marjoram, celery salt

When I started to cut back on high-fat foods, I mourned the loss of meatloaf, a favorite since childhood. But, with a few modifications, this recipe turns out extremely well.

Mix all ingredients together and form into a loaf. Bake for 1¼ hours at 350°F. Use a meat thermometer (170°F.) to be sure of doneness. Don't overcook. Serve with mashed potatoes and gravy made the low-fat, low-cholesterol way. *Serves 4.*

TIP Make more of this turkey meatloaf than you'll need, and double the amount of gravy if you prefer. Both freeze beautifully for a fast dinner the next time. And the meatloaf makes a sensational sandwich on sourdough bread with lettuce and tomatoes.

• •
Potatoes

Peel potatoes; cook at a low boil for 20 minutes or till tender to a fork. Mash with evaporated skim milk, white ground pepper, and Butter Buds.

• •
Gravy

¾ cup cold skim milk
¼ cup flour
1 cup hot turkey broth
½ cup egg substitute
½ cup evaporated skim milk
Mushrooms, lightly sautéed or canned
Salt and pepper

Blend the skim milk into the flour until smooth. Blend in the broth. Bring to a boil and cook 1 minute. Set aside. Blend the egg substitute and evaporated skim milk in an electric blender. Dribble hot milk-broth flour mixture slowly into the blender set at low speed. Add the mushrooms, salt and pepper to taste, and your favorite seasonings.

Nutritional Information per Serving
Serving: 2.5 ounces
Cholesterol: 0.27 milligrams
Protein: 1.08 grams
Carbohydrates: 1.37 grams
Fat: 0.18 grams
  Saturated: 0.05 grams
  Polyunsaturated: 0.06 grams
  Monounsaturated: 0.05 grams
Fiber: 0.17 grams
Sodium: 31 milligrams
Calories: 11.3

• •

The All-American (Turkey) Burger

1 pound ground turkey breast
¼ cup oat-bran cereal
1 large minced garlic clove
¼ cup fine-chopped onion
⅛ cup fine-chopped green pepper
1 teaspoon salt or sodium-alternative
    seasoning

It's one thing to cut down on caviar and pâté de fois gras. It's quite another to forget that all-American favorite the hamburger. Just thinking of a patty grilled over the coals, smothered with onions, and nestled in a toasted bun is enough to set anyone's mouth watering. Here's a delicious, satisfying turkey alternative.

Mix all the ingredients and form into 4 patties; grill indoors or out on the barbecue. Serve on the proverbial toasted bun or choose sourdough bread for less fat and cholesterol. Pile high with lettuce, tomato slices, and onion rings grilled on a no-stick pan sprayed with Pam. *Serves 4.*

TIP While you're at it, why not make double the recipe and store the extra patties in the freezer for the next time?

Nutritional Information per Serving

Serving: 1 burger
Cholesterol: 94.5 milligrams
Protein: 34.4 grams
Carbohydrates: 4.16 grams
Fat: 1.34 grams
  Saturated: 0.27 grams
  Polyunsaturated: 0.24 grams
  Monounsaturated: 0.15 grams
Fiber: 1.37 grams
Sodium: 59.6 milligrams
Calories: 179

Oriental Turkeyburgers

1 pound ground turkey breast
¼ cup oat-bran cereal
1 tablespoon low-sodium soy sauce
½ teaspoon powdered ginger (or try
　　freshly grated ginger)
½ teaspoon powdered coriander
¼ cup chopped water chestnuts

Mix all ingredients in a large bowl. Shape into 4 patties. In a nonstick pan sprayed with Pam fry the patties until browned on both sides and cooked to preferred doneness.

Serve with rice and stir-fried vegetables. Don't forget that you can stir-fry the vegetables in a bit of chicken broth rather than oil. Stir in some freshly grated ginger and just a touch of brown sugar for a taste treat. *Serves 4.*

Nutritional Information per Serving

Serving: 1 burger
Cholesterol: 94.5 milligrams
Protein: 34.5 grams
Carbohydrates: 7.08 grams
Fat: 1.37 grams
　Saturated: 0.27 grams
　Polyunsaturated: 0.23 grams
　Monounsaturated: 0.18 grams
Fiber: 1.16 grams
Sodium: 64 milligrams
Calories: 190

• •

Italian Pizzaburgers

1 pound ground turkey breast
¼ cup oat-bran cereal
¼ teaspoon parsley, finely minced
¼ teaspoon oregano
¼ teaspoon marijoram
¼ cup chopped onions
Grated low-cholesterol cheese
4 tablespoons tomato sauce or Pizzaiola
      Sauce (page 516)
2 English muffins, split

Mix turkey, cereal, herbs, and onions and form into 4 patties. On a nonstick pan sprayed with Pam fry until browned. Sprinkle on the cheese. Cover and cook until the cheese is melted.

While the burgers are cooking, spread 1 tablespoon tomato sauce over each English-muffin half. Place the cooked burgers on the muffins. Place in the preheated 350° oven and bake for 3 minutes. *Serves 4.*

TIP Serve these delicious pizzaburgers with a crisp salad of greens, tomatoes, and onions, with an Italian dressing.

Nutritional Information per Serving
Serving: 1 burger
Cholesterol: 99.4 milligrams
Protein: 39.5 grams

Carbohydrates: 18.5 grams
Fat: 4.05 grams
  Saturated: 1.56 grams
  Polyunsaturated: 0.4 grams
  Monounsaturated: 0.75 grams
Fiber: 1.39 grams
Sodium: 35.5 milligrams
Calories: 282

TURKEY MEATBALLS

I have no idea how many dishes in the world include some kind of meatballs. Probably hundreds. There are meatballs and spaghetti, Swedish meatballs, cocktail meatballs, and meatballs eaten all by themselves. Whatever your favorite kind, they can all be made deliciously with ground turkey breast. Just cut down on the amount of fluid normally called for in the recipe, since turkey is more moist than beef. Here are a few recipes to get you going.

• •

Italian Meatballs

  ¼ oat-bran cereal
  ¼ teaspoon oregano
  ¼ teaspoon black pepper
  ¼ teaspoon thyme
  1 tablespoon grated Parmesan cheese

1 large garlic clove, minced fine
¼ cup chopped onion
¼ cup chopped green pepper
1 pound ground turkey breast

Mix the dry ingredients in a large bowl. Add all the remaining ingredients except turkey. Then blend in the ground turkey and form into 12–16 balls. Spray a nonstick pan with Pam. Fry the balls uncovered until browned. Serve with spaghetti and meatless tomato sauce. *Makes 12–16 meatballs.*

Nutritional Information per Serving
Serving: 3–4 meatballs
Cholesterol: 27.4 grams
Protein: 10 grams
Carbohydrates: 12.3 grams
Fat: 0.52 grams
   Saturated: 0.16 grams
   Polyunsaturated: 0.07 grams
   Monounsaturated: 0.82 grams
Fiber: 0.38 grams
Sodium: 25.4 milligrams
Calories: 53.2

• •

Meatballs in Creamy Paprika Sauce

1 pound ground turkey breast
¼ cup oat-bran cereal
1 tablespoon ketchup

¼ teaspoon black pepper
1 garlic clove, minced fine
1 cup chicken bouillon (made from
    bouillon cubes)
1 ½ cups thin-sliced onions
½ cup evaporated skim milk
¼ cup flour
1 tablespoon paprika
2 tablespoons minced parsley

Mix together the turkey, oat bran, ketchup, pepper, and garlic. Shape into small balls. Fry in a nonstick pan sprayed with Pam. Remove the balls when browned.

Add the chicken bouillon to the pan along with the sliced onions. Bring to a boil and simmer till the onions are tender.

In a separate bowl, slowly blend the evaporated skim milk into the ¼ cup of flour until smooth. Then slowly drizzle into the chicken bouillon and onions and blend. Cook over medium heat, stirring, until thick. Add paprika to the finished sauce. Pour over the meatballs. Garnish with sprinkles of parsley.

Serve with mashed potatoes. Use skim milk and Butter Buds for the potatoes. You'd never know you were eating a low-fat dish. *Serves 4.*

Nutritional Information per Serving
Serving: ¼ recipe
Cholesterol: 96 milligrams

Protein: 39.5 grams
Carbohydrates: 19.8 grams
Fat: 2.07 grams
  Saturated: 0.46 grams
  Polyunsaturated: 0.48 grams
  Monounsaturated: 0.33 grams
Fiber: 2.5 grams
Sodium: 284 milligrams
Calories: 266

TURKEY CUTLETS

If you like veal or pork cutlets, try these turkey cutlets. Just tell your butcher to slice the breast meat appropriately. Again, plan on 4 ounces per person. Then, when you see a recipe that calls for medallions or cutlets, just switch to turkey. Of course you'll also want to find substitutes for the high-fat and high-cholesterol ingredients in such recipes. Whenever you see "cream" think evaporated skim milk. Whole eggs convert to egg substitute or egg whites. Butter, of course, is now synonymous with margarine—and then cut the amount in half. Here's an example:

• •

Basic Cutlets

  ¼ cup flour
  ¼ cup oat-bran cereal

**1 pound turkey cutlets (pound on board
    with hand to flatten)
4 ounces Egg Beaters egg substitute
    (1 packet)**

Mix the flour and oat-bran cereal in a large bowl. Dip the turkey cutlets into the egg substitute. Place the cutlets, one at a time, into the flour-bran mixture until well coated. In a nonstick pan sprayed with Pam fry the cutlets until golden brown.

Serve either alone or with any of a variety of sauces.

They are delicious with mashed potatoes and applesauce. Add a crisp salad. *Serves 4.*

Nutritional Information per Serving
Serving: 1/4 recipe
Cholesterol: 94.5 milligrams
Protein: 41.2 grams
Carbohydrates: 27 grams
Fat: 1.37 grams
  Saturated: 0.28 grams
  Polyunsaturated: 0.37 grams
  Monounsaturated: 0.15 grams
Fiber: 1.38 grams
Sodium: 99.2 milligrams
Calories: 215

Turkey Sandwiches

An all-American favorite has always been the turkey sandwich. Think of how you looked forward to having leftover turkey for sandwiches. Instead of just once a year or so, now start enjoying this low-fat, low-calorie, low-cholesterol sandwich throughout the year.

Whether it's a leftover piece of turkey meatloaf, turkey cutlet, or cold turkey breast from a roasted bird, this is a treat.

Select either sourdough bread or wholewheat. Watch labels on bread. You'll want to avoid those with eggs or saturated fats listed. Sourdough bread is baked with no fat or eggs at all.

Next pile on the extras: crisp lettuce, tomatoes, sliced onions, perhaps a bit of avocado, a touch of mustard or ketchup or a dab of mayo. Great!

Sauce for the Turkey

Whether your menu for the evening calls for ground turkey meatballs or turkey cutlets or cold turkey, you can achieve wonderful variety with a number of sauces. Remember that the finest cuisines in the world are based on the sauce, not necessarily what the sauce covers. Here are a few sauces that go particularly well with turkey.

Mustard Sauce

2 tablespoons prepared mustard
¼ teaspoon curry powder (more if you
    prefer)
1–2 dashes Tabasco
¼ cup mayonnaise
¼ cup plain low-fat yogurt

Mix all ingredients together to form a smooth yellow sauce. You may wish to further cut down on fat by reducing the amount of mayo. Serve with cold turkey or seafood.

Nutritional Information per Serving
Serving: 2 tablespoons
Cholesterol: 2.73 milligrams
Protein: 1.43 grams
Carbohydrates: 1.89 grams
Fat: 0.761 grams
  Saturated: 0.238 grams
  Polyunsaturated: 0.127 grams
  Monounsaturated: 0.20 grams
Fiber: 1.72 grams
Sodium: 295 milligrams
Calories: 99

Béchamel Sauce

2 tablespoons margarine
3 tablespoons flour

1 ½ cups evaporated skim milk
½ cup fresh lemon juice
4 ounces Egg Beaters egg substitute
    (1 packet)

Mix the margarine with the flour over low heat. Gradually stir in the milk. Bring to a boil, stirring constantly. Remove from the heat and add the lemon juice. Place the egg substitute in a blender at low speed. Slowly dribble in the cooked mixture and blend until smooth.

This is a basic white sauce. You can also also add a number of seasonings for a variety of tastes. Try some tarragon to make a béarnaise sauce. Or add a tablespoon or so of horserad-ish. Experiment with your favorite herbs.

Nutritional Information per Serving

Serving: ¼ cup
Cholesterol: 1.7 milligrams
Protein: 5.23 grams
Carbohydrates: 8.07 grams
Fat: 2.64 grams
    Saturated: 0.49 grams
    Polyunsaturated: 1.09 grams
    Monounsaturated: 0.925 grams
Fiber: 0.114 grams
Sodium: 101 milligrams
Calories: 74

Cumberland Sauce

2 tablespoons prepared horseradish
½ cup fresh-squeezed orange juice
⅛ cup grated orange rind
2 tablespoons currant jelly
1 teaspoon Grey Poupon mustard
¼ cup red wine

Mix all ingredients and serve with cold or hot turkey.

Nutritional Information per Serving
Serving: ¼ cup
Cholesterol: 0
Protein: 0.46 grams
Carbohydrates: 11 grams
Fat: 0.15 grams
   Saturated: 0.01 grams
   Polyunsaturated: 0.01 grams
   Monounsaturated: 0.01 grams
Fiber: 0.25 grams
Sodium: 103 milligrams
Calories: 64

Dill Sauce

1 cup chicken bouillon
3 tablespoons flour
2½ tablespoons dill weed (or snipped
      fresh dill)
½ cup evaporated skim milk

Stir the cold bouillon into the flour gradually. Bring to a boil, stirring constantly, then reduce to a simmer. Add the dill. Remove from the heat and blend in the milk. Serve over turkey or seafood.

TIP This sauce is also delicious with meatballs and noodles.

Nutritional Information per Serving

Serving: ¼ cup
Cholesterol: 3.44 milligrams
Protein: 3.66 grams
Carbohydrates: 6.61 grams
Fat: 0.95 grams
   Saturated: 0.5 grams
   Polyunsaturated: 0.07 grams
   Monounsaturated: 0.29 grams
Fiber: 0.09 grams
Sodium: 150 milligrams
Calories: 50.3

• •

Onion Sauce

   2 onions, sliced thin and chopped
   ¼ cup chicken bouillon
   2 tablespoons flour
   ¼ cup evaporated skim milk
   ¼ teaspoon sugar

Cook the onions in ¼ cup water until tender, about 10 minutes. Stir the bouillon cube into another ¼ cup water, and slowly blend into the flour until smooth. Dribble into the onions and hot water and stir in the sugar. Add the milk, and heat. Cook on medium heat, stirring, until thick.

Nutritional Information per Serving
Serving: ¼ cup
Cholesterol: 0.56 milligrams
Protein: 1.94 grams
Carbohydrates: 6.55 grams
Fat: 0.21 grams
Saturated: 0.06 grams
Polyunsaturated: 0.05 grams
Monounsaturated: 0.05 grams
Fiber: 0.65 grams
Sodium: 54.2 milligrams
Calories: 35.6

Pizzaiola Sauce

½ cup chopped onion
2 large garlic cloves, minced fine
1 tablespoon vegetable oil
1 can salt-free Italian-style tomatoes, drained and chopped
1 teaspoon dry basil (fresh is even better if you can get it; use 1 tablespoon fine-chopped)
1 teaspoon leaf oregano
4 teaspoons drained capers

This Italian-style sauce is equally good with turkey cutlets or fish fillets. You'll see this listed frequently in Italian restaurants. Enjoy it with a nice little bottle of Chianti and a side dish of fedelini (very thin spaghetti). Buon appetito!

Sauté the onion and garlic in oil until transparent. Stir in the tomatoes, basil, and oregano. Bring to a boil. Lower the heat and simmer uncovered while stirring frequently for 15 minutes, or until the sauce thickens a bit. Add the capers at the last moment before serving.

NOTE This is a very flavorful sauce that you'll come to rely on for frequent meals. Remember that you can make double or triple batches and keep the sauce in the refrigerator or freezer.

Nutritional Information per Serving

Serving: 1/4 cup
Cholesterol: 0
protein: 0.64 grams
Carbohydrates: 3.18 grams
Fat: 1.87 grams
Saturated: 0.24 grams
Polyunsaturated: 1.07 grams
Monounsaturated: 0.43 grams
Fiber: 0.49 grams
Sodium: 6.34 milligrams
Calories: 29.6

See also:

20

You Call This Deprivation?

For most of us, food is an important aspect of life if not one of the major pleasures and rewards. The idea of giving up all those culinary delights would, at least for me, be difficult if not impossible. A few people can remain on diets of steamed vegetables and rice for years without much complaint. But most couldn't comply for very long with a program of such deprivation.

That's why it was important for me to develop reasonable alternatives or modifications for the foods I enjoy so much. Whether in my own home or in a number of restaurants, I frequently point to the foods I'm eating and comment that this is far from deprivation.

Let me tell you a true story that, to me, puts it all into perspective.

One evening my accountant was over for dinner. Needless to say, he was given a meal straight out of this program. On the menu for the evening were turkey cutlets, thin spaghetti with pizzaiola sauce, peas, and garlic bread. Everyone enjoyed it immensely.

The next evening there was some turkey left over, and I decided to repeat the meal for my wife and me. Since there wasn't quite enough to go around, I also prepared a veal cutlet for her. I might point out that the veal was the very finest, brought out fresh from Chicago and selling at a premium price. I didn't tell my wife she was getting the veal instead of the turkey. Her comment? "This doesn't taste as good as it did last night." That's the absolute truth.

Our house is always filled with delicious aromas of baking muffins and simmering sauces. It's an adventure to discover more and more ways of preparing foods that are both delicious and healthful.

This chapter contains just a sampling of the many ways to prepare foods of all sorts without eggs, butter, or excessive amounts of fats and cholesterol. By all means, expand your recipe files with other books and newspapers and magazines.

It may take a period of adjustment, but soon you'll echo my sentiments, "You call this deprivation?"

SCRUMPTIOUS MILKSHAKES: WITHOUT GUILT

Ever since the days when my father owned a drugstore with a soda fountain, milkshakes have been a special favorite. And for a long time

I relied on Instant Breakfast in the mornings to supply some quick nourishment. But the cholesterol and fat in the milkshakes, and the sugar and chemical additives in the Instant Breakfast, made me back off from both. Instead, today I enjoy a variety of special, no-guilt shakes for breakfast or at any other time of day.

Variety is limited only by your own imagination and the types of fruits available at the time. Basically, you throw all the ingredients into a blender, turn it on for a few seconds, and you have a delicious shake. If you want a thicker, richer shake, use evaporated skim milk or low-fat or no-fat yogurt. For a lighter, cooler drink, use fresh skim milk. And, for a summer cooler, add a handful of crushed ice. Here are a few ideas to start with.

Apple-Banana Shake

8 ounces skim milk
1 ripe banana (the riper the better)
2 ounces frozen apple-juice concentrate
1 egg white, uncooked

Nutritional Information per Serving
Serving: 1 recipe
Cholesterol: 4 milligrams
Protein: 13.27 grams

Carbohydrates: 67.81 grams
Fat: 1.26 grams
  Saturated: 0.55 grams
  Polyunsaturated: 0.2 grams
  Monounsaturated: 0.17 grams
Fiber: 2.77 grams
Sodium: 194.2 milligrams
Calories: 322

Strawberry Shake

8 ounces skim milk
1 egg white, uncooked
½ cup fresh or frozen strawberries

Nutritional Information per Serving
Serving: 1 recipe
Cholesterol: 4 milligrams
Protein: 12.38 grams
Carbohydrates: 45.36 grams
Fat: 0.61 grams
  Saturated: 0.3 grams
  Polyunsaturated: 0.1 grams
  Monounsaturated: 0.14 grams
Fiber: 3.57 grams
Sodium: 180 milligrams
Calories: 224.5

Pineapple Shake

   8 ounces skim milk
   1 egg white, uncooked
   2 ounces frozen pineapple-juice
         concentrate
   ¼ cup crushed pineapple (unsweetened)

Nutritional Information per Serving

Serving: I recipe
Cholesterol: 4 milligrams
Protein: 12.96 grams
Carbohydrates: 49.31 grams
Fat: 0.58 grams
   Saturated: 0.3 grams
   Polyunsaturated: 0.06 grams
   Monounsaturated: 0.13 grams
Fiber: 0.3 grams
Sodium: 179.8 milligrams
Calories: 250.8

Fresh Apple Shake

   8 ounces skim milk
   1 apple, cored and chopped into small
         pieces before blending
   2 ounces frozen apple-juice concentrate
   1 egg white, uncooked

Nutritional Information per Serving

Serving: I recipe

Cholesterol: 4 milligrams
Proteins: 12.31 grams
Carbohydrates: 61.01 grams
Fat: 1.18 grams
  Saturated: 0.41 grams
  Polyunsaturated: 0.24 grams
  Monounsaturated: 0.14 grams
Fiber: 3.31 grams
Sodium: 194 milligrams
Calories: 294

Banana-Carob Shake

  8 ounces skim milk
  1 ripe banana
  1 egg white, uncooked
  1 teaspoon carob powder

Use your imagination. Think about your favorite fruits. Combine the fruit with the same flavor of low-fat or no-fat yogurt instead of milk. Or mix different combinations of fruit together.

Nutritional Information per Serving
Serving: 1 recipe
Cholesterol: 4.69 milligrams
Protein: 13.12 grams
Carbohydrates: 40.75 grams
Fat: 1.2 grams
  Saturated: 0.62 grams
  Polyunsaturated: 0.13 grams

Monounsaturated: 0.22 grams
Fiber: 2.77 grams
Sodium: 179.8 milligrams
Calories: 215.5

• •

Low-Calorie Eggnog

1 quart evaporated skim milk
1 cup egg substitute
1 tablespoon rum extract
Sugar substitute equal to ¼ cup sugar
Nutmeg to taste

Blend and serve. *Makes 10 four-ounce servings.*

Nutritional Information per Serving

Serving: 1 recipe
Cholesterol: 4.08 milligrams
Protein: 10.7 grams
Carbohydrates: 12.3 grams
Fat: 0.23 grams
    Saturated: 0.14 grams
    Polyunsaturated: 0.01 grams
    Monounsaturated: 0.07 grams
Fiber: 0
Sodium: 149 milligrams
Calories: 92

Meal in a Mixer

¾ cup skim milk
1 ripe banana
½ cup nonfat strawberry yogurt
¼ cup orange juice

Think about the nutrition packed into this shake: you get calcium from the milk and yogurt, potassium from the banana, and vitamin C from the orange juice. Drink it with a muffin or two and you'll be set for hours. A great way to start the day.

VARIATIONS Keeping the milk and banana the same, vary this recipe by using a variety of flavors of nonfat yogurt and different kinds of juice.

NOTE Whenever possible, do try to use non-fat yogurt. It's available in practically all stores. Why consume even the small amount of cholesterol and fat in the low-fat versions when the flavor is just as good without them?

Nutritional Information per Serving
Serving: 1 recipe
Cholesterol: 4 milligrams
Protein: 10.12 grams
Carbohydrates: 27.99 grams
Fat: 0.6 grams
  Saturated: 0.3 grams
  Polyunsaturated: 0.06 grams
  Monounsaturated: 0.14 grams

Fiber: 1.39 grams
Sodium: 139.5 milligrams
Calories: 154.6

ONE-POT MEALS

Although times have changed, our needs to fix foods that are quick and easy remain the same. Today we stop in at the fast-food stand or buy frozen TV dinners. Yesterday our mothers and grandmothers (men didn't cook much back then) fixed one-pot meals that were really quite simple yet satisfying.

Today we can combine some of our newer food ideas with traditional, tasty one-pot meals that can be prepared in advance and enjoyed with a chunk of sourdough bread. The basic difference will be substituting low-fat and low-cholesterol alternative ingredients. Here are a couple of dishes to start with. Look in your own cookbooks and collections of favorite recipes to find ideas that can easily be altered to fit the more modern healthful way of thinking.

Turkey Chili

1 pound ground turkey breast
1 medium green pepper, chopped

1 medium onion, chopped
1 can kidney beans or chili beans
1 large can tomatoes (28 ounces)
1 package commercial chili mix

Cook the turkey in a large pan sprayed with Pam until broken apart and browned. Add the green pepper and onion, reduce the heat, and cover. Cook over medium heat until the peppers are tender. Add the beans, tomatoes and chili mix. Simmer for 10 minutes and serve.

NOTE Here's a meal that freezes beautifully. Store in individual-serving-sized containers.

Nutritional Information per Serving
Serving: ⅙ recipe
Cholesterol: 6.3 milligrams
Protein: 26.7 grams
Carbohydrates: 16.3 grams
Fat: 1.05 grams
  Saturated: 0.22 grams
  Polyunsaturated: 0.27 grams
  Monounsaturated: 0.13 grams
Fiber: 3.54 grams
Sodium: 390 milligrams
Calories: 179

Turkey-Vegetable Medley

1 pound ground turkey breast
1 can cooked Great Northern beans

1 green pepper, chopped
1 onion, chopped
2 celery stalks, chopped
2 carrots, chopped
1 tomato, peeled and chopped
1 can small peas
1 package Knorr dried vegetable soup
(or other brand)

In a large pan sprayed with Pam cook the turkey until broken apart and browned. Add all other ingredients, including some fluid from the canned vegetables to make a sauce. Cover and simmer just 10 minutes.

NOTE This is the easy way, but not necessarily the best. To do an even better job and have the vegetables come out better, first add the fresh vegetables; then, just a few minutes before serving, add the canned vegetables.

Nutritional Information per Serving

Serving: ⅙ recipe
Cholesterol: 63.3 milligrams
Protein: 28 grams
Carbohydrates: 18.5 grams
Fat: 1.38 grams
   Saturated: 0.31 grams
   Polyunsaturated: 0.32 grams
   Monounsaturated: 0.35 grams
Fiber: 3.86 grams
Sodium: 665 milligrams
Calories: 199

VEGETABLES

Most kids hate vegetables, and too many adults never acquire a taste for them. Maybe that's because they rebel against their parents' telling them that they can't have dessert until they finish every last soggy pea or overdone carrot. The problem for most people is that they never learned how terrific vegetables can taste.

The place to begin is at your supermarket or fresh fruit and vegetable store. Look for roadside stands during the summer and fall. Go to some ethnic neighborhoods and ask about the exotic vegetables you never even knew about before. Make it an adventure in good taste and good nutrition.

The food charts call for at least two servings of vegetables daily. The green ones and the yellow or orange types. But view that as an absolute *minimum*. Shoot for four servings daily. Impossible? Not at all. Vegetables juices, potatoes, salads, finger-sized nibbles with dip—all these add up to lots of vitamins and minerals. And good eating!

Potatoes are a much-maligned vegetable. Unless you smother them with butter and sour cream, they're *not* at all fattening. You can enjoy potatoes several times each week. They're high in fiber and vitamins, tasty, and versatile.

Here are a few recipes to start with. Look through other cookbooks for more.

• •

Gazpacho

1 large (48-ounce) can tomato juice
1 medium onion, chopped fine
1 green pepper, chopped fine
1 jalapeño pepper, chopped fine
    (without seeds)
½ cup chopped fresh cilantro
3 large garlic cloves, minced fine
2 large tomatoes, peeled, seeded, and
    chopped (or canned tomatoes)
⅓ cup fresh lime juice
¼ cup red wine vinegar
½ teaspoon freshly ground pepper

This one's so simple to prepare you won't believe it. Combine all the ingredients in a large bowl or jar, but not an aluminum pot, and store in the refrigerator overnight. Serve cold with sprigs of fresh cilantro.

NOTE This is a favorite California recipe and a frequent noontime meal, especially during the summer. Serve with sourdough bread. What a marvelous way to eat your vegetables!

Serving: 1 cup (8 ounces)
Cholesterol: 0
Protein: 2.2 grams
Carbohydrates: 13.1 grams
Fat: 0.31 grams
   Saturated: 0.37 grams
   Polyunsaturated: 0.13 grams
   Monounsaturated: 0.04 grams
Fiber: 3.29 grams
Sodium: 70.4 milligrams
Calories: 52.1

• •

Oriental Carrots and Green Peppers

6 carrots
4 green peppers
1 tablespoon soft margarine
1 tablespoon vegetable oil
1 tablespoon grated fresh ginger
   (powdered if you must)
1 tablespoon brown sugar
1 teaspoon mild soy sauce

Cut carrots and green peppers into strips about 3 inches long and ½ inch wide. In a medium-size saucepan sauté other ingredients except soy sauce briefly. Next add the carrots and green peppers to the mixture and simmer covered for 10 minutes or until the vegetables are tender. Stir in soy sauce. *Serves four.*

Serve with broiled chicken and some steamed rice.

NOTE Obviously, if you have just enough vegetables for one or two, you'll need less margarine and oil. Use only as much of these fats as necessary.

Nutritional Information per Serving (sauce only)

Serving: about 1 ounce of sauce
Cholesterol: 0
Protein: 0.25 grams
Carbohydrates: 4.39 grams
Fat: 6.34 grams
    Saturated: 0.76 grams
    Polyunsaturated: 3.59 grams
    Monounsaturated: 1.66 grams
Fiber: 0
Sodium: 126 milligrams
Calories: 73.6

Basic Baked Potatoes

You can bake both white and sweet potatoes. Both are delicious. Both use the same techniques equally well. First, if you have a microwave oven you're in luck. It's a snap to wash the potatoes, pierce them with a fork, and bake for 12 to 16 minutes. In the conventional oven or over the coals, first wrap the potatoes with aluminum foil after washing and piercing. This keeps them moist. Bake at 425° for about 45 minutes or until they "give" to the touch.

But what about that butter or sour cream? Here are a few suggestions. Sprinkle on some Butter Buds and white pepper. Try dry vegetable seasonings, such as Mrs. Dash's. How about some salsa or pizzaiola sauce? Or some nonfat yogurt flavored with lemon juice and pepper? Finally, try being really adventurous and taste the potatoes without anything at all to see what they really taste like.

If you still miss sour cream, well, now you can enjoy all you like with either of these mock sour creams. You can also use these "sour creams" as bases for making excellent salad dressings.

Mock Sour Cream 1

- ¾ cup low-fat cottage cheese
- ¼ cup nonfat plain yogurt
- ½ teaspoon lemon juice
- 1 packet Equal artificial sweetener

My personal favorite.

Nutritional Information per Serving
Serving: 2 tablespoons
Cholesterol: 1.91 milligrams

Protein: 3.32 grams
Carbohydrates: 1.47 grams
Fat: 0.42 grams
  Saturated: 0.27 grams
  Polyunsaturated: 0.01 grams
  Monounsaturated: 0.12 grams
Fiber: 0.001 grams
Sodium: 91.5 milligrams
Calories: 23.6

• •

Mock Sour Cream 2

1 cup low-fat cottage cheese
1 tablespoon lemon juice
¼ cup skim milk

With either variation, simply put the ingredients together in a blender and whirl them till smooth. Makes enough to store in the refrigerator for use throughout the week. Enjoy all you want with no guilt at all.

Nutritional Information per Serving
Serving: 2 tablespoons
Cholesterol: 1.67 milligrams
Protein: 2.77 grams
Carbohydrates: 1.04 grams
Fat: 0.37 grams
  Saturated: 0.24 grams
  Polyunsaturated: 0.01 grams
  Monounsaturated: 0.11 grams

Fiber: 0.004 grams
Sodium: 79.1 milligrams
Calories: 19

•••••••••••••••••••••••••••••••••••••

Mashed, Smashed, and Whipped Potatoes

Peel one white potato per person. Bring to a boil in an uncovered pot of water. Reduce the heat to a mild roll and cook for 20 minutes. Drain off the water. Sprinkle the potatoes with Butter Buds and cover for 3 minutes. Mash the potatoes with evaporated skim milk, adding just a few drops at a time until they are whipped perfectly. Season with white pepper.

•••••••••••••••••••••••••••••••••••••

Roasted Potatoes

Boil unpeeled potatoes for about 15 minutes, or until you can pierce them with a fork without too much resistance. Drain them and cut into chunks, still with the peel intact. Sprinkle with Butter Buds and white pepper. Preheat the oven to 375°F. and spray a cookie sheet with Pam. Bake the potatoes for 15 minutes, till they're nice and crisp and browned.

As to salt, follow your own conscience and health needs.

• •
Escarole and New Potatoes

    1 ½ pounds new potatoes (the smaller
        the better)
    ½ cup chopped onion
    2 large garlic cloves, chopped fine
    2 tablespoons vegetable oil
    1 pound escarole leaves
    1 cup chicken broth
    Pepper to taste

Boil the potatoes unpeeled for about 20 minutes, then drain off the water and cover (off the heat). While the potatoes are cooking, in a large skillet sauté the onion and garlic in oil until transparent. Tear the escarole leaves by hand into pieces about 2 inches across. Put the leaves into the pan with the onions, cover, and shake the pan to wilt the leaves and cover them with the onion-garlic oil. Slice the potatoes into chunks and add them to the pan. Stir in the chicken broth, bring to a boil, add pepper, and serve. *Serves 4.*

NOTE The liquid (pot liquor, it's called) is so tasty that you'll want to sop it up with big chunks of sourdough bread. Serve with a piece of broiled chicken or fish. (A nice bottle of white wine wouldn't hurt.)

Nutritional Information per Serving
Serving: $1/4$ recipe
Cholesterol: 0.25 milligrams
Protein: 6.55 grams
Carbohydrates: 39 grams
Fat: 7.64 grams
  Saturated: 1.05 grams
  Polyunsaturated: 4.29 grams
  Monounsaturated: 1.82 grams
Fiber: 3.79 grams
Sodium: 211 milligrams
Calories: 243

French-"Fried" Potatoes

Boil potatoes, either peeled or not, for 10 minutes. Drain them and let cool. Cut them into strips, crinkles, or however you like them best. Preheat the oven to 375°F. and spray a cookie sheet with Pam. Place the potatoes on the sheet so they're not touching. Bake for 30 minutes. Ketchup anyone?

Flavorful Rice Pilaf

4 cups water
1 teaspoon ground coriander (or

1 tablespoon chopped fresh cilantro,
   if available)
1 tablespoon vegetable oil
2 ½ cups uncooked white rice
½ cup dried apples, chopped fine
¼ cup raisins (the golden type are best)
¼ cup apple juice
¼ teaspoon cinnamon (optional)
4 chopped green onions

Put the water into a saucepan with the co-riander or cilantro and bring to a boil. At the same time, heat the oil in a flameproof casse-role. Add the rice to the oil till grains are just coated, then add the water to the casserole. Cover and bake in a preheated 375°F. oven for 25 minutes. By then, the water should all be absorbed into the rice. During the baking, put the apple slices and cinnamon into the apple juice to soak. When the rice is done, drain the apples and blend them into the rice. Add the chopped green onion at the very end.

NOTE Once again, let your imagination go wild. After you've tried this recipe once and you've seen how easy and foolproof it is, you'll want to try a few variations. Instead of apples, next time use apricots and pineapple juice, or prunes with orange juice. Serve with baked chicken or fish.

Nutritional Information per Serving

Serving: 1 cup
Cholesterol: 0
Protein: 5.34 grams
Carbohydrates: 71.8 grams
Fat: 1.29 grams
　Saturated: 0.2 grams
　Polyunsaturated: 0.47 grams
　Monounsaturated: 0.23 grams
Fiber: 1.4 grams
Sodium: 7.93 milligrams
Calories: 323

SALAD DRESSINGS

With the tremendous variety available, everyone should try to eat a salad every day. Whether you prefer it as your noontime meal or as an accompaniment to the evening dinner, a salad can supply much of your daily vegetable needs.

Don't limit yourself to plain iceberg lettuce day after day. Any vegetable or fruit can be fare for the salad of your dreams; the best salad bars around are those with the most variety.

Go for color with kernels of corn, shavings of carrot, and a spoonful or two of red cabbage. Use last night's leftover vegetables. Add some fresh pears or apples. Try all the different types of lettuce—bibb, romaine, butter, leaf—as well as the traditional iceberg. Mix two or three types together.

Then think about the dressings to top it all off. Ah, but there's the rub. Most commercially prepared salad dressings are prepared with whole eggs, saturated fats, and often a lot of sugar. Either look at the labels carefully before you buy, or start preparing your own. Try some of the new oil-free dressings. They have really improved and are delicious.

Yogurt Dressing

- 1 cup nonfat plain yogurt
- 1 tablespoon fresh lemon or lime juice
- 1 ½ teaspoons fresh basil (½ teaspoon if dry)
- 1 large garlic clove, finely minced
- 1 tablespoon honey

Combine all the ingredients in a storage container and let stand in the refrigerator for at least 2 hours before serving to develop the full flavor.

Nutritional Information per Serving
Serving: 2 tablespoons
Cholesterol: 0.4 milligrams
Protein: 1.34 grams

Carbohydrates: 3.71 grams
Fat: 0.05 grams
Saturated: 0.03 grams
Polyunsaturated: 0.002 grams
Monounsaturated: 0.01 grams
Fiber: 0.005 grams
Sodium: 17.6 milligrams
Calories: 20.2

• •

Honey-Lime Dressing

¼ cup fresh lime juice
⅛ cup honey
¼ teaspoon Dijon mustard

Combine all ingredients and serve cold. Delicious over a salad of romaine and honeydew melon.

Nutritional Information per Serving
Serving: 2 tablespoons
Cholesterol: 0
Protein: 0.04 grams
Carbohydrates: 4.4 grams
Fat: 0.02 grams
   Saturated: 0.001 grams
   Polyunsaturated: 0.002 grams
   Monounsaturated: 0.001 grams
Fiber: 0
Sodium: 2.17 milligrams
Calories: 16.4

Tomato Dressing

1 cup salt-free tomato juice
½ cup peeled and chopped fresh
    tomatoes
1 tablespoon fresh lemon juice
1 tablespoon fresh chopped parsley
1 tablespoon fresh chopped cilantro
Pepper to taste

Combine all ingredients in a storage container and let the mixture stand overnight to fully develop the flavor. This has just a few calories in the whole batch.

Nutritional Information per Serving

Serving: 2 tablespoons
Cholesterol: 0
Protein: 0.32 grams
Carbohydrates: 1.71 grams
Fat: 0.05 grams
  Saturated: 0.007 grams
  Polyunsaturated: 0.02 grams
  Monounsaturated: 0.008 grams
Fiber: 0.56 grams
Sodium: 3.52 milligrams
Calories: 7.25

Thousand Island Dressing

1 cup low-fat mayonnaise
2 tablespoons tomato ketchup
1 tablespoon sweet pickle relish

Combine all ingredients in advance. Store and use as needed over all sorts of salads.

Nutritional Information per Serving

Serving: 2 tablespoons
Cholesterol: 10 milligrams
Protein: 0.05 grams
Carbohydrates: 3.13 grams
Fat: 8 grams
  Saturated: 4.35 grams
  Polyunsaturated: 1.2 grams
  Monounsaturated: 2.45 grams
Fiber: 0
Sodium: 43
Calories: 84.5

Herb Dressing

1 cup nonfat plain yogurt
1 tablespoon fresh lemon juice
1½ teaspoons fresh basil
1½ teaspoons fresh tarragon
1½ teaspoons fresh chervil
1 large clove garlic, minced fine
1 teaspoon ground red pepper (optional)

Combine all ingredients in advance. Store and use as desired over salads. Use 2 tablespoons per serving.

Nutritional Information per Serving

Serving: 2 tablespoons
Cholesterol: 0.5 milligrams
Protein: 1.73 grams
Carbohydrates: 2.65 grams
Fat: 0.11 grams
  Saturated: 0.04 grams
  Polyunsaturated: 0.02 grams
  Monounsaturated: 0.02 grams
Fiber: 0.006 grams
Sodium: 22 milligrams
Calories: 18

DESSERTS TO YOUR HEART'S CONTENT

There's no reason to think that just because you're trying to reduce fats and cholesterol you can never have anything but a piece of fruit for dessert. You'll just have to be a bit more careful than most people, and a bit more creative.

For openers, start looking more selectively for items in the supermarket. Read labels before you buy to avoid not only eggs but also "partially hydrogenated oils" and palm oil and coconut oil, which are just as saturated as animal fats and butter. The more you shop the more you'll realize how many acceptable products there are on the market. And as more and more people become diet and health conscious you can expect even more delicious food alternatives to come along.

Frozen yogurt is an excellent example. Available in a wide variety of flavors, these products are even better tasting than when they were first introduced in the 1970s. And there are new desserts based on yogurt that have practically no fat or cholesterol at all.

Also keep an eye out for shops and restaurants with desserts your heart and waistline will love you for. Such places and products are clearly on the increase as the business world recognizes the pent-up demand. Awhile back I took my children out for the evening and as a special treat decided to get them ice-cream cones. Naturally I expected to watch them eat while I lived with memories of the gooey sundaes I've sworn off. Surprise! As we walked into our local 31 Flavors Ice Cream shop, there was a sign for specially formulated, Special Diet, ice-cream treats with a negligible amount of fat and practically no cholesterol. As I'm writing this, there are four flavors available: my favorite is coffee. I can eat this with no guilt and lots of pleasure. Thanks, Baskin-Robbins. (Get on the bandwagon, Häagen Dazs!)

Angel-food cake is made with egg whites, not

the yolks. Most of those cakes, pies, and cookies, though, are loaded with eggs and butter.

The solution is to start getting into dessert making yourself. Believe me, it's really easy. Before going onto this program myself I never baked a cookie in my life. The recipes I've listed here are simple to follow and practically foolproof. It's fun to make cookies, and if you've got kids, it's a great way to keep them entertained helping you.

Apple-Oatmeal Treats

 4 medium-sized apples
 4 teaspoons cinnamon
 1 tablespoon honey
 1 tablespoon lemon juice
 2 egg whites
 ¼ cup oat-bran cereal
 ¼ cup oatmeal
 ½ cup powdered skim milk (dry, nonfat)

First halve, core, and chop the apples. Put them in a steamer, sprinkle with cinnamon, and steam until tender, usually about 10 minutes. (If you don't have a steamer, try placing a strainer in a pot with about two inches of water and cover.)

Next, combine all the other ingredients. By

the time you're done, the apples will be tender and aromatic from the cinnamon. Put them into a blender and liquefy. Combine all ingredients and plop the batter by teaspoonfuls onto a nonstick cookie sheet (or one sprayed with Baker's Joy).

Bake in a preheated 350°F. oven for 20 minutes. This will make 2 to 3 dozen cookies, depending on how big you make them.

Nutritional Information per Serving
Serving 1 cookie
Cholesterol: 0.17 milligrams
Protein: 0.7 grams
Carbohydrates: 4.41 grams
Fat: 0.17 grams
  Saturated: 0.01 grams
  Polyunsaturated: 0.09 grams
  Monounsaturated: 0.005 grams
Fiber: 0.54 grams
Sodium: 16.2 milligrams
Calories: 21

Traditional Oatmeal Cookies

¾ cup all-purpose flour
¼ teaspoon baking soda
2 teaspoons vanilla
2 ounces vegetable oil
½ cup granulated sugar

½ cup brown sugar
1 container of Egg Beaters egg substitute
    (equal to 2 eggs)
1 ½ cups 1-minute oatmeal
¼ cup chopped walnuts or pecans

Here's a traditional recipe for delicious oatmeal cookies, minus the cholesterol and much of the fat. It comes from the pages of one of my wife's magazines, with a few substitutions that make it fit for the program.

First, sift the flour and baking soda together. Next blend vanilla, oil, and sugars, then add the egg substitute. Finally stir in the flour, oatmeal, and nuts. Preheat your oven to 350°F. and spray a cookie sheet with Pam. Drop the dough onto the sheet with a teaspoon. Bake for 8 minutes.

NOTE Yes, there are sugar and fat in the recipe. But remember that you're making 72 cookies in this batch. A little quick division shows that you can afford to have a cookie or two once in a while without any guilt at all. You can store these cookies in the freezer; one batch will last a long time.

Nutritional Information per Serving

Serving: I cookie
Cholesterol: 0
Protein: 0.63 grams

Carbohydrates: 4.61 grams
Fat: 1.09 grams
  Saturated: 0.116 grams
  Polyunsaturated: 0.61 grams
  Monounsaturated: 0.24 grams
Sodium: 17.5 milligrams
Calories: 29

Untraditional Oatmeal Cookies

2 very ripe bananas
½ cup brown sugar
3 teaspoons vanilla
1 container Egg Beaters egg substitute
    (equal to 2 eggs)
2 cups all-purpose flour
1½ cups 1-minute oatmeal
1 teaspoon baking powder
½ teaspoon baking soda
½ cup evaporated skim milk
½ cup chopped nuts

This is the recipe for those who either don't want to have just one or two cookies or don't want any fat at all. They're almost as tasty as the slightly more sinful traditional variety. These are chewy, tasty little treats you'll enjoy when that urge for a nibble strikes.

First mash the bananas with a fork or blend in a blender to a liquid. Place in a large bowl and mix the sugar, vanilla, and egg substitute with the bananas. Mix together the flour, oatmeal, baking powder, and soda. Alternately add the flour mixture and the milk to the banana mixture, and finally add the nuts.

Preheat the oven to 375°F. and spray a cookie sheet with Pam or Baker's Joy. Plop the batter 1 teaspoonful at a time onto the sheet and bake for 10 minutes, till the cookies are just barely browned at the edges.

Nutritional Information per Serving
Serving: 1 cookie
Cholesterol: 0.28 milligrams
Protein: 1.56 grams
Carbohydrates: 8.78 grams
Fat: 0.61 grams
   Saturated: 0.45 grams
   Polyunsaturated: 0.33 grams
   Monounsaturated: 0.11 grams
Fiber: 0.32 grams
Sodium: 26 milligrams
Calories: 32

Sweet Potato and Apple Cobbler

   2 large apples, cored and cut in 1-inch
      chunks
   2 large sweet potatoes, peeled and cut in
      1-inch chunks
   ½ cup brown sugar

½ cup oat-bran cereal, milled to flour in
    blender or food processor
½ cup 1-minute oatmeal
½ teaspoon cinnamon
⅓ cup unsalted soft margarine

This definitely isn't for someone trying to lose weight. It's got all the delicious calories with none of the cholesterol and little of the fat normally found in such a scrumptious treat. For those of us following a low-fat diet, this is a nice reward.

Mix the chunks of apples and potatoes in a 9-inch pie pan, and sprinkle with 2 tablespoons of the sugar. Mix the remaining sugar, oat bran, oatmeal, and cinnamon in a bowl. Work the margarine in a bit at a time until the mixture is crumbly. Sprinkle the crumbs over the apples and potatoes. Preheat the oven to 350°F. Bake about 50 minutes, or until the potatoes are tender and the topping is browned. Serve when still warm.

For a special treat, beat chilled evaporated skim milk with a teaspoon of vanilla to form a "whipped-cream" topping.

Nutritional Information per Serving
Serving: ⅙ cobbler
Cholesterol: 0
Protein: 1.74 grams
Carbohydrates: 41.2 grams

Fat: 10.3 grams
  Saturated: 1.6 grams
  Polyunsaturated: 4 grams
  Monounsaturated: 3.25 grams
Fiber: 3.61 grams
Sodium: 180 milligrams
Calories: 261

• •

Prune Bars

⅓ cup brown sugar
⅓ cup vegetable oil
¼ cup apple-juice concentrate
1 cup whole-wheat flour
½ cup oat-bran cereal
1 ½ cups oatmeal
1 cup diced prunes
1 cup raisins

Here's a yummy way to get a lot of nutrition into a dessert.

Mix the sugar, oil, and apple juice. Separately mix the dry ingredients. To them, gradually add all other ingredients, mixing just until crumbly. Put the mixture into a 9-inch baking pan sprayed with Pam. Bake in a preheated 375° oven for 20 minutes or until resilient to the touch. *Cut into 12 bars.*

VARIATIONS Let your imagination run wild: For the prunes substitute apricots or other dried fruits, or try other frozen fruit-juice concentrates.

Nutritional Information per Serving
Serving: 1 bar
Cholesterol: 0
Protein: 2.94 grams
Carbohydrates: 43.1 grams
Fat: 6.42 grams
Saturated: 0.74 grams
Polyunsaturated: 3.24 grams
Monounsaturated: 1.37 grams
Fiber: 3.46 grams
Sodium: 77 milligrams
Calories: 235

• •

Pie Crusts

1 cup sifted all-purpose flour
¾ teaspoon salt (optional)
¼ cup light corn syrup
2 tablespoons skim milk

I happen to be a real pie lover, but the crusts can be loaded with lard. Just take a look at the ingredient labels of pre-made pie crusts, or at the recipes found in any cookbook. Here's a recipe for a traditional pie crust without saturated fat.

Preheat the oven to 475°F. Mix the flour

and salt in a bowl. Combine the syrup and milk and add all at once to the flour mixture. Stir with a fork until thoroughly mixed. Shape the mixture into a ball and place it between two squares of wax paper lightly dusted with flour, roll the pastry into a circle large enough to fit a 9-inch pie pan. Spray pan with Baker's Joy. Arrange pastry in the pan. Cut off the edges with a knife and press with a fork. Prick the bottom all over with a fork. Bake about 10 minutes or until golden brown. Cool before adding filling.

Nutritional Information per Serving
Serving: 1/6 pie
Cholesterol: 0.08 milligrams
Protein: 2.34 grams
Carbohydrates: 36.1 grams
Fat: 0.18 grams
Saturated: 0.04 grams
Polyunsaturated: 0
Monounsaturated: 0.002 grams
Fiber: 0.59 grams
Sodium: 186 milligrams
Calories: 158

See also:
BRAN BROWNIES, page 497

FRUIT

While there are a number of low-fat, non-cholesterol desserts you can choose from don't forget to include lots of fresh fruits in your diet. Fruit is packed with vitamins and fiber for a terrific nutrition mix, it is convenient, easy to prepare, and a fast picker-upper. Best of all, fruit is delicious.

A long time ago, when I was still eating rich foods, I took a series of Provincial French cooking lessons. Needless to say, most of the recipes I learned then are off-limits today. But I clearly remember how the chef regarded fruit highly for dessert. As a challenge, I asked how the lowly orange could be made into a culinary treat.

The teacher, Josie, smiled. She peeled a large navel orange, and cut it into sections. Then she put the fruit into a bowl and poured an ounce or two of dark Jamaican rum over it. Sound simple? It's fantastic! Try the same thing with other fruits and liquors. Here are a few to get you started:

- Banana slices and Grand Marnier
- Apple slices and calvados
- Raspberries and chocolate liqueur
- Pineapple and crème de menthe
- Strawberries and Cointreau

- Cherries and rum
- Peaches and brandy

Every nutrition book you pick up, going back years and years, lists the need for two servings of fruit each day as part of the four-food-group approach to eating. What most people don't read, however, is that those two servings are the *minimum*. Try to have three, four, five, even six servings of fruit each day, depending on your calorie needs.

It's really not hard to do. Start your day with one of the shakes listed in this book. That'll give you a banana, let's say, and a serving of fruit juice. Next, have a big glass of fresh fruit juice at midmorning. Then an apple or a pear for lunch. And some fruit for dessert at dinner. That's five servings right off the bat.

Your body will love you for it, and you'll love your body when you see the pounds disappear. Replace the fats and refined sugars in your diet and you can't go wrong.

BOUNTIFUL BREAKFASTS

No question about it, the most artery-clogging American meal is the Big Breakfast. For many years moms prepared those bacon-and-egg meals thinking they were doing their families a favor on Sunday mornings. Even today restaurants tout their breakfast specials, including eggs, bacon, sausage, and pancakes dripping with melted butter. Looking at a typical restaurant menu, in fact, is like looking at a list of forbidden foods. Even the innocent-appearing waffle is prepared with egg yolks.

When eating out, one should limit oneself to such staples as oatmeal or other hot or cold cereals, English muffins with honey instead of butter, and a variety of fruits and juices. But at home some of the ever-popular treats can be prepared in a safe and sane manner. It's a simple matter of substitution for the most part, and such meals also provide an opportunity to get even more oat bran into the diet.

Buttermilk Pancakes

6 egg whites (or egg substitute equal to
    3 eggs)
3 cups 1-percent-fat buttermilk (or
    nonfat milk mixed with Saco
    buttermilk mix)
6 tablespoons vegetable oil
1 cup self-rising flour
2 cups oat-bran cereal
1 tablespoon baking powder
3 tablespoons sugar

This recipe will make a lot of pancakes—enough for your family's breakfast and plenty to store in the freezer for those occasions when you don't have time to cook. The pancakes freeze well. Just pop them into the microwave. Or, if you don't have a microwave oven, let them thaw at room temperature and warm for three minutes in a standard oven at 350°F.

Simply mix the ingredients together and bake on a griddle sprayed with Pam.

Serve the pancakes with fruit compotes, purées, or syrups. Remember that the commercial syrups have a lot of sugar—fresh fruits put through the blender taste even better, without the extra calories.

TIP To make nonfat buttermilk, you can use Saco-brand buttermilk mix. Use 3 tablespoons per cup of nonfat milk.

Nutritional Information per Serving
Serving: 1 pancake
Cholesterol: 2.25 milligrams
Protein: 5.04 grams
Carbohydrates: 22.1 grams
Fat: 8.69 grams
   Saturated: 1.22 grams
   Polyunsaturated: 4.02 grams
   Monounsaturated: 1.8 grams
Fiber: 3.39 grams
Sodium: 230 milligrams
Calories: 196

German Apple Pancakes

FRUIT MIXTURE

1 large green apple, halved, cored, and
    sliced
¼ cup sugar
¼ cup applesauce
⅛ teaspoon nutmeg
½ teaspoon cinnamon

BATTER INGREDIENTS

8 egg whites (or egg substitute equal to
    4 eggs)
1 cup skim milk
1 teaspoon vanilla extract
1 tablespoon vegetable oil
¼ cup self-rising flour
½ cup oat-bran cereal
1 teaspoon baking powder
1 tablespoon sugar
⅛ teaspoon nutmeg

This recipe is incredibly delicious. You'll want to share it with all your friends and relatives on special occasions. These pancakes are just as good as you'd get in a pancake restaurant, without the fat and cholesterol.

Spray an ovenproof glass casserole dish with Pam. Mix the apples, sugar, applesauce, and spices, and spread in the dish. Bake at 425°F.

for 10 minutes to partially cook the apples. In a large bowl, mix liquid ingredients for the batter, then add dry ingredients. Stir only until ingredients are mixed. Then pour the batter over the fruit and bake at 375° for another 20 minutes.

The recipe as stated serves two substantial appetites. Increase ingredients as needed for more people.

Nutritional Information per Serving
Serving: I pancake
Cholesterol: 2 milligrams
Protein: 19.8 grams
Carbohydrates: 76.5 grams
Fat: 9.4 grams
   Saturated: 1.15 grams
   Polyunsaturated: 4.09 grams
   Monounsaturated: 1.72 grams
Fiber: 7.25 grams
Sodium: 604 milligrams
Calories: 476

• •

French Toast

    1 slice sourdough bread (nice and big
        and thick)
    Egg Beaters egg substitute equal to 1 egg
    1 ounce (2 tablespoons) skim milk
    1 dash of vanilla extract, orange extract,
        or almond extract

No cholesterol-conscious person would ever order French toast in a restaurant, but this recipe is both delicious and nutritious. The amount given is for one serving.

Mix the egg substitute, milk, and flavoring in a bowl and dip in the bread to soak up the mixture. Grill on a griddle sprayed with Pam.

Serve with syrup, a fruit mixture, or, for something different, sprinkle with powdered sugar.

Nutritional Information per Serving
Serving: 1 piece, or 1 recipe
Cholesterol: 0.5 milligrams
Protein: 11.90 grams
Carbohydrates: 19.59 grams
Fat: 1.42 grams
  Saturated: 0.24 grams
  Polyunsaturated: 0.01 grams
  Monounsaturated: 0.15 grams
Fiber: 0.55 grams
Sodium: 289 milligrams
Calories: 134

Waffles

4 egg whites (or egg substitute equal to
    2 eggs)
2 cups skim milk (evaporated skim milk
    is even better)

1 cup oat-bran cereal
1 cup self-rising flour
1 teaspoon baking powder
3 tablespoons vegetable oil

If you have a waffle iron, here's a recipe that's sure to please your entire family. The first one always sticks to the iron, so plan accordingly.

Preheat the iron. Mix all ingredients in a container with a spout, and pour onto the waffle iron. Bake each waffle for about 5 minutes or until the steam stops. Enjoy while hot. *Makes 6 large waffles.*

Nutritional Information per Serving
Serving: 1 waffle
Cholesterol: 1.33 milligrams
Protein: 7.35 grams
Carbohydrates: 28 grams
Fat: 8.38 grams
  Saturated: 0.99 grams
  Polyunsaturated: 4.01 grams
  Monounsaturated: 1.69 grams
Fiber: 3.68 grams
Sodium: 357 milligrams
Calories: 229

Hot Oat-Bran Cereal

1 cup water (or any of various fruit juices)
1 cup evaporated skim milk

1 teaspoon honey (or brown sugar or
    molasses)
½ cup oat-bran cereal
¼ cup raisins (or dates, or prunes, or
    dried apricots)

There are many ways to make hot oat-bran cereal by using different combinations of the ingredient options in this recipe. Try a number of combinations and you'll never get tired of it.

Bring water and milk to a boil. Stir in the remaining ingredients and cook gently for 10 minutes.

Nutritional Information per Serving

Serving: 1 cup
Cholesterol: 5.1 milligrams
Protein: 10.7 grams
Carbohydrates: 43.8
Fat: 2.21 grams
   Saturated: 0.18 grams
   Polyunsaturated: 0.03 grams
   Monounsaturated: 0.08 grams
Fiber: 6.23 grams
Sodium: 150 milligrams
Calories: 247

BREAKFAST MEATS

I haven't had a slice of bacon in years. What with the fat, cholesterol, and chemical additives, it's something I can do without. And if you read the ingredient labels, even the bacon substitutes don't sound too healthful. So for a meat side dish at breakfast, you can't beat ham. That may sound surprising, but depending on the brand, a slice of low-fat ham contains only one gram of fat. And when you get a craving for breakfast sausage, these next two recipes fill the bill with ground turkey breast substituting for fat-laden pork. Note that these recipes call for ground turkey breast from your butcher, not packaged ground turkey.

• •

Garlicky Turkey Sausage

1 pound ground turkey breast
¾ teaspoon ground coriander
½ teaspoon salt
½ teaspoon pepper
1 clove garlic, minced fine

Mix all ingredients in a bowl and form into 8 patties. Refrigerate. Spray a skillet with Pam and fry for about 12 minutes.

NOTE These sausages can be frozen either raw or cooked for later use. And you may also enjoy them for lunch with a salad and bread.

Nutritional Information per Serving
Serving: 1 patty
Cholesterol: 47.3 milligrams
Protein: 17.3 grams
Carbohydrates: 0.63 grams
Fat: 0.56 grams
  Saturated: 0.14 grams
  Polyunsaturated: 0.13 grams
  Monounsaturated: 0.18 grams
Fiber: 0.01 grams
Sodium: 152 milligrams
Calories: 80

• •

Favorite Breakfast Sausage

1 pound ground turkey breast
1 packet Butter Buds
¼ teaspoon each cumin, marjoram,
    pepper, oregano, cayenne pepper
½ teaspoon each basil, thyme, sage
⅛ teaspoon each garlic powder, nutmeg,
    ginger
1 tablespoon oat-bran cereal (just
    enough to "bind" the sausage)

This one comes really close to tasting like commercial pork breakfast sausage. Again, you can prepare a large quantity in advance and freeze it either raw or cooked. The flavor comes from the large number of spices and herbs used. Vary the amount of seasonings to match your own preferences. I like mine spicy.

Mix the ground turkey with the seasonings and refrigerate for a few hours. Form patties and bake in a 400°F. oven or fry in a pan sprayed with Pam.

Nutritional Information per Serving

Serving: 1 patty
Cholesterol: 47.3 milligrams
Protein: 17.1 grams
Carbohydrates: 1.1 grams
Fat: 0.6 grams
   Saturated: 0.15 grams
   Polyunsaturated: 0.12 grams
   Monounsaturated: 0.08 grams
Fiber: 0.29 grams
Sodium: 29.9 milligrams
Calories: 83.5

EGGS

Although some cholesterol watchers will eat egg yolks in moderation, I prefer to avoid them entirely. Using either the whites or egg substitutes, I can make omelets, scrambled eggs, or just about anything else—even "sunny side up" style without the sunny side.

APPETIZERS AND
HORS D'OEUVRES

Awhile back I attended a presidential reception at a medical meeting and I was absolutely shocked at the foods served on the buffet table. Here were health professionals filling their plates with fat-laden goodies such as rumaki (chicken liver wrapped with bacon), fried chicken wings, greasy meatballs, and plates of cheese. That's the kind of occasion when you just have to munch on the fresh vegetables, and wait for dinner. But, when you have the opportunity to prepare your own buffet, there's no limit to the treats you can come up with for your guests and yourself. These are just a few examples.

Marinated Scallops

1 pound scallops
Juice of 1 lemon or 2 limes
2 tablespoons vegetable oil
1 onion, sliced thin
2 tablespoons capers
½ tablespoon celery seed
1 teaspoon Worcestershire sauce
2 or 3 drops Tabasco

Marinate the scallops overnight in the remaining ingredients and serve with crackers or toast points.

Nutritional Information per Serving
Serving: 2½ ounces
Cholesterol: 40.2 milligrams
Protein: 17.8 grams
Carbohydrates: 3.67 grams
Fat: 5.69 grams
  Saturated: 0.59 grams
  Polyunsaturated: 2.69 grams
  Monounsaturated: 1.13 grams
Fiber: 0.27 grams
Sodium: 209 milligrams
Calories: 134

• •
Pickled Mushrooms

MARINADE
¼ cup each olive oil, lemon juice, water
1 large garlic clove, minced
¼ teaspoon pepper (white pepper is best)

VEGETABLES
1 pound fresh mushrooms
1 red or green pepper, sliced
Parsley sprigs

Mix the marinade ingredients and pour over the mushrooms and pepper slices. Store in the refrigerator at least 3 hours. Drain and serve with parsley sprigs as garnish.

Nutritional Information per Serving
Serving: 2 ounces mushrooms
Cholesterol: 0
Protein: 1.35 grams
Carbohydrates: 4.63 grams
Fat: 7.04 grams
  Saturated: 1 gram
  Polyunsaturated: 0.69 grams
  Monounsaturated: 4.98 grams
Fiber: 1.19 grams
Sodium: 2.13 milligrams
Calories: 81

• •
Marinated Vegetables

MARINADE
1 cup olive oil
½ cup white wine vinegar
½ cup water
1 teaspoon each sugar, thyme, marjoram, basil, pepper
1 large garlic clove, minced
1 large bay leaf

VEGETABLES
Carrot slices
Zucchini slices
Cherry tomatoes

Broccoli flowerets
Cauliflower
Celery chunks
Baby corn ears
Mushrooms

Mix the marinade, add the vegetables, and store in the refrigerator for several hours. Drain the vegetables thoroughly and place in a bowl to serve.

Nutritional Information per Serving
Serving: ½ teaspoon (not including vegetables)
Cholesterol: 0
Protein: 0.01 grams
Carbohydrates: 0.09 grams
Fat: 1.13 grams
   Saturated: 0.16 grams
   Polyunsaturated: 0.09 grams
   Monounsaturated: 0.83 grams
Fiber: 0
Sodium: 0.02 milligrams
Calories: 10.1

Chicken Teriyaki Sticks

MARINADE
⅔ cup soy sauce
¼ cup sweet sherry
1 tablespoon brown sugar
½ teaspoon freshly grated ginger root

1 large clove garlic, minced
Juice of 1 lemon
1 pound boneless, skinless chicken
    breasts in chunks
Pineapple chunks

Mix together the marinade ingredients. Add the chicken and marinate in the refrigerator overnight. Skewer on bamboo sticks or chopsticks, alternating with chunks of pineapple. Broil about 10 minutes until done. Prepare in individual-sized portions.

Nutritional Information per Serving
Serving: 1 teaspoon sauce and 1/5 pound chicken
Cholesterol: 0
Protein: 0.36 grams
Carbohydrates: 0.79 grams
Fat: 0.003 grams
  Saturated: 0.001 grams
  Polyunsaturated: 0.001 grams
  Monounsaturated: 0
Fiber: 0
Sodium: 227 milligrams
Calories: 4.45

California Sunshine Soup

1 quart bottle Clamato juice
½ cup chopped cucumber
¼ pound tiny cocktail shrimp,

imitation surimi shrimp,
   or crab
½ cup tofu, cut into ½-inch cubes
1 small avocado, cut into cubes
⅓ cup fine-chopped onion
2 tablespoons each olive oil and red wine
   vinegar
1 tablespoon sugar
1 large clove garlic, minced
⅓ teaspoon Tabasco

Serve this chilled super soup in a glass bowl with a ladle and little cups the way you would a punch. Give your guests spoons to scoop up the morsels. It'll be a big hit, especially during warm months.

Preparation is really easy: just mix all the ingredients together in a large container and refrigerate overnight to bring out all the flavors.

Nutritional Information per Serving
Serving: 1 cup (8 ounces)
Cholesterol: 17.1 milligrams
Protein: 5.52 grams
Carbohydrates: 8.28 grams
Fat: 7.37 grams
   Saturated: 0.98 grams
   Polyunsaturated: 0.75 grams
   Monounsaturated: 0.45 grams
Fiber: 19.32 grams

Sodium: 618 milligrams
Calories: 112

● ●
Salmon Spread

1 large (15 ½-ounce) can salmon
½ cup low-fat cottage cheese
2 tablespoons minced onion
1 tablespoon lemon juice
1 teaspoon prepared white horseradish
½ teaspoon salt
¼ teaspoon white pepper

Clean the salmon of all bones and skin (or buy the Hormel boneless and skinless variety). On the other hand, you may wish to mash the bones in with the salmon for the calcium they provide. Place the cottage cheese in a strainer and place under running water to clean off all milk. Pat the cottage-cheese curds dry with a paper towel. Combine all ingredients in a bowl and mash until smooth and creamy. Chill in the serving bowl. Serve with crackers, toast points, or slices of cucumber and other fresh vegetables.

Nutritional Information per Serving
Serving: 2 tablespoons
Cholesterol: 10.9 milligrams

Protein: 6.19 grams
Carbohydrates: 0.46 grams
Fat: 1.66 grams
Saturated: 0.36 grams
Polyunsaturated: 0.65 grams
Monounsaturated: 0.49 grams
Fiber: 0.02 grams
Sodium: 222 milligrams
Calories: 43.3

● ●

Toothpick Meatballs

1 small bottle ketchup
10 ounces grape jelly
Juice of 1 lemon
1 pound ground turkey breast
¼ cup oat-bran cereal

Here's an example of substitution working beautifully. The original recipe called for ground beef, but ground turkey breast actually works better, forming firm meatballs that don't fall off the serving toothpicks. This is a simple yet festive buffet treat.

Mix the ketchup, jelly, and lemon juice in a medium-sized saucepan or flameproof casserole. Heat until bubbling. Meanwhile, mix the turkey with the oat bran, adding the oat bran a little at a time until the mixture is firm enough to form into walnut-sized balls. Drop the balls into the bubbling mixture to cook for about 30 minutes. Serve hot, with toothpicks to spear the meatballs.

This dish is even better when prepared the night before your party and stored overnight in the refrigerator to bring out all the flavors. Reheat at serving time. Don't let the weird combination of flavors fool you—your guests will go wild over this one and they'll be amazed when you give them the recipe.

Nutritional Information per Serving
Serving: 1 ounce
Cholesterol: 23.6 milligrams
Protein: 8.57 grams
Carbohydrates: 23.3 grams
Fat: 0.33 grams
  Saturated: 0.07 grams
  Polyunsaturated: 0.06 grams
  Monounsaturated: 0.04 grams
Fiber: 0.3 grams
Sodium: 253 milligrams
Calories: 129

Hummus (Garbanzo Bean Dip)

⅓ cup sesame tahini
¼ cup lemon juice
5 cloves garlic (minced)
5 drops Tabasco

¼ cup water
½ teaspoon cumin
2 fifteen-ounce cans garbanzo beans
    (chick peas), drained

This dish increases the soluble fiber content of the diet, a good way to control cholesterol levels. It can be served to company or kept in the refrigerator for quick snacks along with wedges of toasted pita bread.

Simply combine all ingredients and blend until smooth. The easiest way to do this is in a food processor. If you do not have one, place ingredients in a large bowl and blend with an electric mixer.

Nutritional Information per Serving

Serving: 2 tablespoons
Cholesterol: 0
Protein: 0.46 grams
Carbohydrates: 1.41 grams
Fat: 0.38 grams
    Saturated: 0.04 grams
    Polyunsaturated: 0.15 grams
    Monounsaturated: 0.07 grams
Fiber: 0.002 grams
Sodium: 6.75 milligrams
Calories: 10.5

ASIAN CUISINE

One of the earliest observations during the study of cholesterol and heart disease was that Asian populations consuming little animal fat and cholesterol had virtually no heart disease. As Asians migrated to the United States, their food habits changed and they began developing the same problems of clogged arteries. Many health authorities therefore recommend leaning heavily toward Asian delicacies. And, since there's so much diversity, it's really easy to have Chinese, Japanese, Thai, and Korean foods frequently.

If you've never done any cooking of this sort, it may at first appear formidable. Yes, you'll have to buy a wok and a few utensils not now in your kitchen. And yes, you'll need some ingredients you don't have. But they're all easy to find in almost any supermarket across the nation.

You'll also want to get a cookbook or two that will show you in a step-by-step manner how to create some fabulous dishes in your own kitchen. There are a number on the market. One I particularly recommend is published by *Consumer Guide*, titled *The Chinese Cooking Class Cookbook*.

Chinese Chicken and Vegetables

  1 cup chicken broth
  1 pound skinless chicken breasts cut as strips
  4 medium carrots cut either as strips or
      circles
  1 small bunch broccoli cut as small
      flowerets
  1 cup bean sprouts
  1 green or red bell pepper cut in strips
  1 can straw mushrooms, drained
  1 tablespoon reduced-sodium soy sauce
  2 tablespoons oyster sauce
  1 tablespoon dry sherry
  1 teaspoon or more ground red pepper
      (cayenne)
  1 tablespoon grated fresh ginger
  2 large cloves garlic, chopped fine

One of the nicest things about Chinese wok cooking is that you can use all the ingredients you love and cut out those you don't. In this recipe, for example, our kids prefer to have only carrots and broccoli along with the chicken. So my wife makes a separate batch that way. She and I prefer a variety of things in ours. And we think we've got the sauce perfected—spicy but not too spicy. To make it even better, we now use only chicken broth in the wok instead of oil to further reduce our fat intake. Mix and match vegetables to your own taste.

Heat 2 ounces of chicken broth in wok. Add chicken strips and stir-fry until tender. Remove chicken and put aside. Add remaining broth to wok, heat, and add vegetables. Cook till tender. Mix sauces and flavorings. Add chicken to wok. Pour in sauce mixture. Stir-fry till entire dish is heated through. Serve with lots of steamed rice.

Nutritional Information per Serving

Serving: 1/2 cup
Cholesterol: 64.3 milligrams
Protein: 26.4 grams
Carbohydrates: 10.6 grams
Fat: 3.28 grams
   Saturated: 0.92 grams
   Polyunsaturated: 0.77 grams
   Monounsaturated: 1.08 grams
Fiber: 2.34 grams
Sodium: 396 milligrams
Calories: 180

When you look at a menu in a Chinese or other Asian restaurant, you'll find that a number of the dishes are strictly vegetables. But these dishes are far from bland and boring. The sauces make them a meal in themselves. Here's a recipe for a vegetable dish we love to have over and over again.

Straw Mushrooms and Baby Corn

1 clove garlic, crushed
½ teaspoon grated fresh ginger
1 tablespoon peanut oil
1 fifteen-ounce can baby corn, drained
2 tablespoons oyster sauce
(essential to bring out the flavor)
4 tablespoons chicken broth
⅛ teaspoon sugar
1 fifteen-ounce can straw mushrooms,
    drained

Make sure you use straw mushrooms, not any other kind. These are found in cans in supermarkets, right next to the cans of baby corn ears. For a complete meal, you can also add some pieces of chicken or fish or scallops.

In a hot wok (375°F. in an electric wok or when a drop of water sizzles), stir-fry the garlic and ginger in the oil for a minute or two. Add the corn, and stir-fry until hot. Add the oyster sauce, chicken broth, and sugar. Stir and toss. When the mixture is hot, add the mushrooms and stir gently until all the food is heated through. *This recipe serves 3 or 4.*

Be sure to make plenty of steaming-hot rice to go along with this and all Asian dishes. You'll be amazed at how much rice you'll want to eat. And don't forget you can enjoy a large quantity of this low-fat, low-cholesterol, and low-calorie food.

Nutritional Information per Serving
Serving: 1 generous cup
Cholesterol: 2.91 milligrams
Protein: 4.94 grams
Carbohydrates: 21.9 grams
Fat: 5.55 grams
  Saturated: 1.27 grams
  Polyunsaturated: 1.68 grams
  Monounsaturated: 2.14 grams
Fiber: 2.92 grams
Sodium: 301 milligrams
Calories: 140

• •

Tori No Sanmi Yaki

3 tablespoons sesame seeds
2 large garlic cloves, crushed
½ small dried red pepper, without seeds
1 teaspoon fresh ginger (¼ teaspoon
    ground ginger)
¼ cup sake (or you can use dry sherry)
⅓ cup soy sauce
¼ cup honey
2 boneless, skinless chicken breasts
1 large green bell pepper, cut in strips
1 tablespoon vegetable oil (peanut oil is best)
6 thin lemon slices without seeds
2 cups hot cooked rice

Here's a Japanese recipe for three-flavored chicken. It's baked, not fried.

Toast the sesame seeds in a little pan for about 5 minutes. Mash the seeds along with the garlic, pepper, and ginger. Add sake, soy sauce, and honey. Coat the chicken breasts with the mixture and place in a glass casserole. Marinate the chicken at least 4 hours, or make it the night before and keep it in the refrigerator. Bake in a 325°F. oven for 15 minutes, turn chicken breasts, bake 10 minutes more. Broil just a few minutes to crisp the chicken. Meanwhile, sauté the green-pepper strips until tender. Arrange chicken, peppers, and lemon slices on a platter. Serve with lots and lots of steaming-hot rice.

Nutritional Information per Serving

Serving: ¹/₆ recipe
Cholesterol: 48.7 milligrams
Protein: 21.8 grams
Carbohydrates: 33.3 grams
Fat: 7 grams
  Saturated: 1.28 grams
  Polyunsaturated: 2.17 grams
  Monounsaturated: 2.6 grams
Fiber: 2.98 grams
Sodium: 868 milligrams
Calories: 301

ITALIAN COOKERY

The same scientists who studied the Asian populations also found that people living in Mediterranean regions such as southern Italy have low rates of heart disease. Again, the cuisine of southern Italy is low in animal fat and cholesterol, and high in carbohydrates. These Italians use a lot of olive oil in their cooking, another monounsaturated fat that's been shown to reduce cholesterol levels while retaining the beneficial HDL levels. Note that we're not talking about northern Italian food, which is rich and fatty.

Italian cookbooks abound, each with variations on pasta and vegetable themes. The sauces are fresh and bubbly and delicious. *Consumer Guide* also publishes *The Italian Cooking Class Cookbook,* another step-by-step approach to cooking, with foolproof instructions to prepare dishes that will look exactly like the color pictures next to each recipe. Remember that any dish that calls for veal can be made just as tender and delicious by substituting turkey breast.

But you don't have to get fancy to enjoy Italian cookery. Sure, you can prepare those multi-ingredient dishes when you have the time and the inclination. But, when it's just a matter of getting some hot food on the table fast, Italian food can come out of cans and jars.

My personal favorite sauce is Newman's Own, which was also noted by the editors of *Consumer Reports*. They also liked the Prego sauce without salt added—an important consideration for those watching their sodium intakes. For a little more variety, try adding some mushrooms, capers, black olives, or what have you to the prepared sauces.

Pasta is the mainstay of Italian cooking. Keep your pantry well stocked with pasta of all shapes and sizes. If you haven't already discovered this, pasta tastes much different when it's thin like vermicelli rather than thick like linguine. Try them all.

Just get the biggest pot you have in the kitchen, fill it halfway with water, bring to a boil, and add the pasta a little at a time so the water keeps boiling. Cook for about 7 or 8 minutes, or until *al dente,* or just a bit chewy to the bite. Meanwhile, heat the sauce to bubbling.

Put together a simple salad with a nice Italian dressing, slice a loaf of bread, and you're ready to sit down and eat within 20 to 30 minutes. A nice glass of Chianti wouldn't hurt.

If you have just a few minutes more, try adding some seafood to the sauce. Nothing fancy; just sauté a quarter of a pound of scallops, for example, and toss them into the sauce. You can do the same, without even cooking, with the imitation crab and lobster products. If sodium is a problem, you may wish to soak the pieces in some lemon water before serving to remove some of the salt.

To get over the pizza craving that's bound to set in when you start reducing the fat and cholesterol in your diet, here's a perfectly satisfying and delicious alternative. Just go to the store and buy the following ingredients:

- Chilled prepared pizza crusts
- Commercially prepared pizza sauce
- Green pepper
- Onion
- Fresh mushrooms
- Tomatoes
- Olives

Preheat your oven to 375°F. while you prepare the toppings. Ladle out the sauce over the crusts and top with sliced pepper, onion, and mushrooms, cut-up tomatoes and olives. Pop the pizza into the oven for 10 minutes or less.

What about the cheese, you say? Well, first of all, the pizza tastes delicious without any cheese at all. But, if you wish, you can pick up one of the "filled" cheeses or an imitation, such as Pizza-Mate. The fat content remains the same, but the cholesterol has been removed along with the saturated fat. You'll get about 6 to 7 grams of fat per ounce of cheese. And it's amazing how just an ounce of cheese adds zip to the pizza.

The crust, by the way, is made without any eggs or animal fat, so you're perfectly safe in enjoying it. Again, if sodium is a problem, you may wish to make your own sauce rather than using the kinds that come out of jars. Just mix some low-sodium tomato sauce with ¼ teaspoon each of Italian seasoning, oregano, and garlic powder. You may also wish to add just a teaspoonful of olive oil to the sauce.

ANOTHER WORD ABOUT BEEF . . .

I want to make it perfectly clear that I do not advocate completely eliminating beef or other red meats from the diet. Yes, the recipes in this book call for chicken, turkey, and seafood. Simply enough, they are much lower in fat per serving size. Make your own comparisons in the charts included in Chapter 4, "Winning by the Numbers." But once in a while you and I will want to enjoy the flavor of a good piece of beef.

When you decide that you'd like to have a beef dish, just follow two simple rules. First, remember that a serving size is 4 ounces un-cooked. If that sounds like a small amount, think of it as a quarter of a pound, as the burger advertisers tell us. Second, select those cuts of meat that are lowest in fat. Happily, at least in my opinion, one of those cuts is filet mignon cut from the tenderloin. And here's one of my favorite beef recipes that's fit for a king.

• •

Beef en Brochette

MARINADE
½ cup red wine
¼ cup vegetable oil
1 teaspoon each Worcestershire sauce and
        sugar
1 tablespoon vinegar
2 tablespoons ketchup
1 clove garlic, minced
½ teaspoon each marjoram and rosemary
1 pound beef tenderloin (filet mignon)
        cut in cubes
16 large fresh mushrooms
2 green bell peppers
2 onions
2 tomatoes

Mix the marinade ingredients together in a large plastic food-storage bag. Cut the meat and vegetables into chunks suitable for skewering. Marinate in the bag for 2 to 3 hours. Skewer the meat and vegetables and broil until the meat is at the doneness you prefer. Serve with wild rice or rice pilaf. They are beautiful on the plate, and delicious and tender.

This recipe serves 4 good-sized appetites. No one ever complains about wanting more meat. It is a good example of how meat need not predominate in the meal.

Nutritional Information per Serving

Serving: 1/4 recipe

1/4 marinade	1/4 pound beef
Cholesterol: 0	111.9 milligrams
Protein: 2.06 grams	34.89 grams
Carbohydrates: 14 grams	0
Fat: 14.2 grams	16.95 grams
Saturated: 1.81 grams	3.88 grams
Polyunsaturated: 8.23 grams	0.44 grams
Monounsaturated: 3.35 grams	5 grams
Fiber: 2.84 grams	0
Sodium: 101 milligrams	66.88 milligrams
Calories: 201	181

In the same way, lean cuts of meat can be used in a variety of recipes that are probably near and dear to you and your family. Soups, stews, casseroles, and other dishes need no more than 4 ounces per person. You'll note that in almost all cases meat is browned first, then other ingredients are added. When you do that, just remember to drain off the fat rather than keeping it in the pan. You really won't miss it at all.

COOKING WITH SEAFOOD

For many reasons, you'll want to start including more seafood in your meal planning. First, of course, fish and shellfish have the least amount of fat of any selection from the meat group. Second, the fat they do contain is particularly useful to those wishing to reduce cholesterol levels. Salmon, especially, is a great source of the alpha-three fatty acids, which have been shown time and again to lower lipid levels. Third, and possibly just as important as any other reason, fish offer an almost incredible variety to choose from in selecting dish after dish. Don't just stick with your favorites, but rather start to experiment with new and exciting types you come across at the seafood counter.

The following recipes happen to be favorites of mine that I've developed over the years. But you'll also want to get at least one good seafood cookbook. The best one, in my opinion, is James Beard's *New Fish Cookery*. He talks about selecting fish, cooking methods, and recipes for just about anything that moves in fresh or salt water. In the meantime, however, give these recipes a try.

But before getting into the recipes, I want to mention the importance of selecting fresh fish. The frozen types just aren't as good. Find a fish seller you can trust and ask his opinion about which fish is best on a particular day. Fish should have a fresh, not fishy aroma. If whole, the eyes should not be sunken and the fins should not be shriveled. Fillets must not have a dried appearance.

● ●
Frozen Fish Fiesta

> 1 medium onion, sliced thin
> 1 cup water
> 2 teaspoons chili powder
> 1 teaspoon ground cumin
> 1 teaspoon oregano
> 1 large bay leaf
> 1 large garlic clove, minced
> 6 stuffed olives, sliced
> 1 pound frozen cod (or other fish)

There are always times when you have to settle for frozen fish, and it's a good idea to have some in the freezer ready for an "emergency." One of the fish that freezes best is cod. Store it in 1-pound pieces in plastic storage bags.

Combine all ingredients except the fish in a saucepan and heat to a bubbling boil. By this time the fish should be partly thawed, enough to cut into 2-inch chunks. Toss in the chunks with the sauce and reheat to boiling, then simmer 20 minutes or less, until fish flakes easily. Serve over noodles for a hearty meal. You'll also want some big chunks of bread to soak up the sauce—this is hearty eating, so go ahead and get primitive.

Nutritional Information per Serving
Serving: ¼ pound fish
Cholesterol: 66 milligrams
Protein: 31.8 grams
Carbohydrates: 3.06 grams
Fat: 7.3 grams
　Saturated: 0.12 grams
　Polyunsaturated: 0.05 grams
　Monounsaturated: 0.01 grams
Fiber: 0.44 grams
Sodium: 168 milligrams
Calories: 217

Pescatori (Italian-Style Shellfish)

1 medium onion
1 tablespoon olive oil
1 large clove garlic, minced
½ teaspoon each oregano, thyme, and
　crushed red pepper

2 medium tomatoes, cut up
1 large green pepper, cut up
8 ounces raw clams
8 ounces raw scallops

In a saucepan place all ingredients except the shellfish, and cook over medium heat for 4 to 5 minutes, until the pieces of onion and green pepper become tender and a saucelike consistency is reached. Then add the shellfish and simmer for just 5 more minutes, no more or the fish will be overcooked. *Serve over pasta for 4.*

Nutritional Information per Serving

Serving: ¼ recipe
Cholesterol: 232.8 milligrams
Protein: 86.18 grams
Carbohydrates: 32.76 grams
Fat: 20.3 grams
   Saturated: 2.88 grams
   Polyunsaturated: 2.34 grams
   Monounsaturated: 10.88 grams
Fiber: 5.86 grams
Sodium: 908 milligrams
Calories: 651

Serving: 1 cup spaghetti
Cholesterol: 0
Protein: 7 grams
Carbohydrates: 39 grams
Fat: 1 gram

Saturated: 0
Polyunsaturated: 0
Monounsaturated: 0
Fiber: 0.91 grams
Sodium: 1 milligram
Calories: 190

• •

Fish Baked in Paper

1 pound fish fillets such as sea bass,
grouper, or snapper
1 cup carrots, sliced into strips
1 small onion
2 teaspoons each dill weed and thyme
leaves (or 1 tablespoon of each fresh)
Freshly ground pepper

Cut 4 circles of parchment paper (not waxed paper) about 15 inches in diameter. Place the fish, cut into equal pieces, on the 4 pieces of paper, and cover with vegetables. Season to taste with herbs and pepper. Fold the paper and crimp to seal. Place on a cookie sheet and bake in a preheated oven at 350°F. for about 12 minutes. *Serves 4, with small boiled potatoes and bread.*

Nutritional Information per Serving
Serving: ¼ pound fish and ¼ recipe
Cholesterol: 66.5 milligrams

Protein: 30.4 grams
Carbohydrates: 4.68 grams
Fat: 6 grams
   Saturated: 0.02 grams
   Polyunsaturated: 0.05 grams
   Monounsaturated: 0.01 grams
Fiber: 1.11 grams
Sodium: 129 milligrams
Calories: 199

• •

Mexican Fish Delight

   1 tablespoon olive oil
   Juice of 1 fresh lime
   1 pound fish fillets, such as snapper
      or sea bass
   Freshly ground pepper
   Chopped parsley
   Chopped black olives
   Chopped tomatoes

Preheat the oven to 450°F. Mix the oil and lime juice together and rub over the fish fillets. Season to taste with pepper. Bake uncovered for 15 minutes without turning. Meanwhile, chop the parsley, black olives, and tomatoes and mix to form a garnish to top the fish with when the fillets come out of the oven.

Serves 4, with vegetarian refried beans, rice,

and warm tortillas. A nice Mexican beer makes the meal a fiesta.

Nutritional Information per Serving
Serving: ¼ pound fish with ¼ sauce
Cholesterol: 66.5 milligrams
Protein: 30.4 grams
Carbohydrates: 4.5 grams
Fat: 11.4 grams
  Saturated: 0.71 grams
  Polyunsaturated: 0.35 grams
  Monounsaturated: 2.5 grams
Fiber: 1.33 grams
Sodium: 182 milligrams
Calories: 242

Polynesian Scallops

½ cup diced green bell pepper (or mix
    with red bell pepper)
1 tablespoon chopped green onion
¼ cup sliced water chestnuts
¼ cup pineapple cubes
1 teaspoon Worcestershire sauce
1 teaspoon wine vinegar
¼ cup pineapple juice
Juice of 1 lime
Cornstarch (optional)
1 pound scallops

Mix all ingredients except the scallops in a flame-proof casserole and heat on the stove top until the vegetables are tender. Thicken, if you wish, with cornstarch, added a bit at a time. Add scallops and mix. Cover the dish and bake in a preheated 350°F. oven for just 5 minutes—more will overcook the delicate scallops. *The recipe serves 4. Try it served with rice and Asian vegetables.*

Nutritional Information per Serving

Serving: ¼ pound scallops, ¼ recipe
Cholesterol: 60.3 milligrams
Protein: 26.7 grams
Carbohydrates: 9.21 grams
Fat: 1.71 grams
  Saturated: 0.01 grams
  Polyunsaturated: 0.05 grams
  Monounsaturated: 0.01 grams
Fiber: 0.34 grams
Sodium: 314 milligrams
Calories: 155

Baked Salmon Loaf

1 one-pound can salmon
½ cup chopped celery
¼ cup chopped onion
¼ pound chopped fresh mushrooms
¼ cup evaporated skim milk
2 egg whites or egg substitute equal to 1 egg

1½ tablespoons dill weed (fresh is best
   if possible)
1 cup breadcrumbs or oat-bran cereal

Mix all ingredients well in a bowl. Spray with Pam a meatloaf pan large enough to accommodate the mixture. Bake in a 375°F. oven for 45 minutes. Cut into slices. *Serves 4 with potatoes and vegetables of your choice.*

While you're at it, you might as well make 2 loaves and freeze one for a future meal when you don't have time to cook.

Nutritional Information per Serving
Serving: ¼ loaf
Cholesterol: 45.9 milligrams
Protein: 27.1 grams
Carbohydrates: 17.4 grams
Fat: 8.82 grams
  Saturated: 1.25 grams
  Polyunsaturated: 2.87 grams
  Monounsaturated: 2.02 grams
Fiber: 5.49 grams
Sodium: 650 milligrams
Calories: 280

Teriyaki Salmon

¼ cup soy sauce
2 tablespoons brown sugar

2 tablespoons grated fresh ginger
1 pound salmon fillets or steaks

Mix the soy sauce, sugar, and ginger together in a plastic food-storage bag. Marinate
the salmon for at least 30 minutes, preferably
1 hour. Broil the salmon in the oven broiler or
over charcoal. Figure 10 minutes per inch of
thickness for broiling time.

Nutritional Information per Serving

Serving: ¼ pound salmon, ¼ recipe
Cholesterol: 68 milligrams
Protein: 26.1 grams
Carbohydrates: 8.81 grams
Fat: 10.6 grams
   Saturated: 1.46 grams
   Polyunsaturated: 3.34 grams
   Monounsaturated: 2.43 grams
Fiber: 0
Sodium: 1032 milligrams
Calories: 239

• •

Salmon Patties

1 one-pound can salmon
4 egg whites or egg substitute equal to 2 eggs
⅔ cup oat-bran cereal
1 medium onion, minced fine
1 tablespoon fine-chopped parsley
1 tablespoon fresh-squeezed lemon juice

Mix all ingredients together and make 8 patties shaped like hamburgers. Spray a non-stick pan with Pam and fry until crisp. I love these best with mashed potatoes, canned corn, and a dash of ketchup—just the way we ate them as children in my family. *Serves 4.*

Nutritional Information per Serving
Serving: 1/4 pound salmon (2 patties)
Cholesterol: 45.3 milligrams
Protein: 28.6 grams
Carbohydrates: 11.2 grams
Fat: 8.02 grams
   Saturated: 1.22 grams
   Polyunsaturated: 2.84 grams
   Monounsaturated: 2.02 grams
Fiber: 3.64 grams
Sodium: 641 milligrams
Calories: 243

• •

Halibut Marengo

2 cups canned whole tomatoes, chopped
1/2 orange, sliced
1/4 cup each mushrooms, celery, green pepper
1/4 teaspoon each thyme and white pepper
2 tablespoons chopped onion
1 pound halibut (this is a nice, firm fish)

Mix all ingredients except fish and bring to a boil in a medium saucepan. Place the fish in a glass baking dish and pour the sauce over. Bake 15 minutes in a 375°F. oven.

Nutritional Information per Serving
Serving: ¼ pound fish, ¼ recipe
Cholesterol: 68 milligrams
Protein: 30.3 grams
Carbohydrates: 8.6 grams
Fat: 8.39 grams
  Saturated: 0.06 grams
  Polyunsaturated: 0.16 grams
  Monounsaturated: 0.05 grams
Fiber: 1.66 grams
Sodium: 355 milligrams
Calories: 233

• •

Tuna- or Salmon-Salad Sandwiches

1 can tuna or salmon
¼ cup fine-chopped apples
6 stuffed green olives, sliced
1 green onion, minced
¼ teaspoon dill weed (or 1 teaspoon fresh)
¼ cup chopped celery
3 drops Tabasco
Juice of ½ lime
Just enough reduced-fat mayonnaise to
      hold it all together

Even people who flat-out don't like fish enjoy these sandwiches. Choose albacore tuna packed in water. Hormel has also brought out salmon without skin or bones, to avoid the problem of cleaning the fish as it comes out of the can. Or just discard the skin and mash the bones. This might sound a bit unusual; most people wouldn't think of including apples in tuna salad, but give it a try. Even my fish-hating wife thinks it's delicious enough to serve for dinner, when we don't want a big meal.

Mix all the ingredients together, refrigerate long enough to cool, and serve on lightly toasted slices of sourdough bread.

Nutritional Information per Serving

Serving: $1/4$ recipe
Cholesterol: 17.4 milligrams
Protein: 12.1 grams
Carbohydrates: 2.7 grams
Fat: 3.61 grams
  Saturated: 0.08 grams
  Polyunsaturated: 0.32 grams
  Monounsaturated: 0.004 grams
Fiber: 0.47 grams
Sodium: 282 milligrams
Calories: 88.8

Seafood Kabobs

  Juice of 2 lemons
  $1/4$ cup white wine

3 large garlic cloves, minced
3 tablespoons fine-chopped parsley
1 tablespoon vegetable oil
2 teaspoons oregano
½ teaspoon white pepper
1 pound scallops or fish chunks or both

Combine all ingredients except fish or scallops to form a marinade. Add scallops or fish and marinate 1 hour. Drain and skewer. Broil 10 minutes in the oven broiler or over charcoal. You may wish to alternate the chunks of fish on a skewer with chunks of green pepper, mushrooms, or other vegetables for variety and color. Baste with the marinade as you're broiling to keep the fish moist.

Nutritional Information per Serving

Serving: ¼ pound scallops
Cholesterol: 60.3 milligrams
Protein: 26.7 grams
Carbohydrates: 6.07 grams
Fat: 5.03 grams
   Saturated: 0.44 grams
   Polyunsaturated: 2.01 grams
   Monounsaturated: 0.82 grams
Fiber: 0.21 grams
Sodium: 303 milligrams
Calories: 175

CHERISHED FAMILY RECIPES

It's important to stress that Life After Cholesterol can go on much as it did before. By all means one should continue to eat similar kinds of foods. It would be practically impossible to expect lifelong success eating nothing but foods foreign to what you're used to.

Maybe people in California can go on day after day eating broiled fish and boiled artichokes. But in Milwaukee and Chicago and all over the country, people have gotten used to many kinds of ethnic foods.

The trick is not to give up such foods, but rather to alter them to eliminate as much fat and cholesterol as possible. Use egg substitutes or whites for yolks. Broth instead of oil for sautéing. Turkey instead of beef or veal. Pam for frying rather than butter or oil. Evaporated skim milk instead of cream. Yogurt instead of sour cream.

Everyone has his or her own family recipes that shouldn't be forgotten. One of the things my mother used to make many years ago when I was growing up in Chicago was called *galumki*, with the "l" pronounced as a "w." It's Polish stuffed cabbage. It calls for eggs and beef in the original recipe, but with a couple of simple substitutions, we have a perfect low-fat, low-cholesterol meal that's hearty and satisfying. The same kinds of substitutions can bring almost any recipe right into line with the prudent approach to eating. Following is Mom's altered recipe.

• •

Galumki (Polish Stuffed Cabbage)

1 head of cabbage, cored
1 ½ pounds ground turkey breast
2 cups cooked rice
1 packet Butter Buds
2 medium onions, chopped
Ground pepper
Egg substitute equal to 1 egg

Boil the cored cabbage head in water sufficient to cover for 10 minutes. Cook turkey in a skillet, stirring until the pinkness is gone. Combine the turkey, rice, Butter Buds, onions, pepper, and egg substitute in a bowl. Cool the cabbage and remove the leaves whole. Divide the mixture and place on cabbage leaves, wrap, and secure with wooden toothpicks. Place in a casserole, cover, and bake in a 325°F. oven for 1 hour.

Other family recipes for similar dishes include sour cream. Instead, use nonfat yogurt sweetened with a bit of sugar and dollop over the stuffed cabbage leaves. You may also wish to baste the stuffed cabbage with some tomato juice while cooking. Mom never did, but other families did so.

Serve with chunks of hearty bread. It's a meal in itself.

Nutritional Information per Serving
Serving: ¼ pound turkey
Cholesterol: 94.3 milligrams
Protein: 36.4 grams
Carbohydrates: 13.80 grams
Fat: 1.27 grams
  Saturated: 0.3 grams
  Polyunsaturated: 0.32 grams
  Monounsaturated: 0.17 grams
Fiber: 3.13 grams
Sodium: 77.3 milligrams
Calories: 219

Notes

Chapter 1. Cholesterol: No More Controversy

1. Schaefer, E. J., et al. "The Effects of Low Cholesterol, High Polyunsaturated Fat, and Low Fat Diets on Plasma Lipid and Lipoprotein Cholesterol Levels in Normal and Hypercholesterolemic Subjects." *American Journal of Clinical Nutrition*, 1981: volume 34, pages 1158–63.

2. Stamler, J. "Diet and Coronary Heart Disease." *Biometrics*, 1982: volume 38 Supplement, pages 95–118.

3. Friedman, M., and Rosenman, R. *Type A Behavior and Your Heart*. A. A. Knopf, New York, 1974.

4. Cooper, R., et al. "Seventh-Day Adventist Adolescents—Life-Style Patterns and Cardiovascular Risk Factors." *Western Journal of Medicine*, 1984: volume 140, number 3, pages 471–77.

5. Caggiula, A. W., et al. "The Multiple Risk Intervention Trial (MRFIT) IV. Intervention on Blood Lipids." *Preventive Medicine*, 1981: volume 10, pages 443–75.

6. Lipid Research Clinics Program. "The Lipid Research Clinics Coronary Primary Prevention Trial Results. II. The Relationship of Reduction in Incidence of Coronary Heart Disease to Cholesterol Lowering." *Journal of the American Medical Association*, 1984: volume 251, number 3, pages 365–74.

7. Pritikin, N., and McGrady, P. M. *The Pritikin Program for Diet and Exercise.* Grosset & Dunlap, New York, 1979.

8. Rifkind, B. M., and Segal, P. "Lipid Research Clinics Reference Values for Hyperlipidemia and Hypolipidemia." *Journal of the American Medical Association,* 1983: volume 250, number 14, pages 1869–72.

9. Stamler, J., et al. "Is Relationship Between Serum Cholesterol and Risk of Premature Death from Coronary Heart Disease Continuous and Graded?" *Journal of the American Medical Association,* 1986: volume 256, pages 2823–28.

10. Uhl, G. S., et al. "Relation Between High Density Lipoprotein Cholesterol and Coronary Artery Disease in Asymptomatic Men." *American Journal of Cardiology,* 1981: volume 48, number 5, pages 903–10.

11. Kannel, W. B., et al. "Is Serum Total Cholesterol an Anachronism?" *Lancet,* 1979: volume 2, pages 243–44.

12. Council on Scientific Affairs. "Dietary and Pharmacologic Therapy for the Lipid Risk Factors." *Journal of the American Medical Association,* 1983: volume 250, number 14, pages 1873–79.

13. *Dietary Guidelines for Americans.* U.S. Department of Agriculture and U.S. Department of Health, Education and Welfare, Washington, D.C., 1980.

14. Oster, P., et al. "Diet and High Density Lipoproteins." *Lipids,* 1981: volume 26, pages 93–97.

15. Brown, W. V., et al. "Treatment of Com-

mon Lipoprotein Disorders." *Progress in Cardio-vascular Diseases,* 1984: volume 27, number 1, pages 1–20.

Chapter 2. Special Considerations for Women, Children, and the Elderly

1. Weidman, W. H., et al. "Nutrient Intake and Serum Cholesterol Level in Normal Children 6 to 16 Years of Age." *Pediatrics,* 1978: volume 61, number 3, pages 354–59.

Chapter 5. Getting the Scoop on Oat Bran

1. Burkitt, D. P., et al. "Effects of Dietary Fibre on Stools and Transit Times, and Its Role in the Causation of Disease." *Lancet,* 1972: volume 2, pages 1408–11.

2. Anderson, J. W., and Chen, W. L. "Plant Fiber: Carbohydrate and Lipid Metabolism." *American Journal of Clinical Nutrition,* 1979: volume 32, pages 346–63.

3. Trowell, H. "Fiber: a Natural Hypocholesterolemic Agent." *American Journal of Clinical Nutrition,* 1972: volume 25, pages 464–65.

4. DeGroot, A. P., et al. "Cholesterol-Lowering Effect of Rolled Oats." *Lancet,* 1963: volume 2, pages 303–304.

5. Fisher, H., and Griminger, P. "Cholesterol-Lowering Effects of Certain Grains and of Oat Fractions in the Chick." *Proceedings of the Society for Experimental Biology and Medicine,* 1967: volume 126, pages 108–111.

6. Anderson, J. W., et al. "Hypolipidemic Ef-

fects of High-Carbohydrate, High-Fiber Diets." *Metabolism,* 1980: volume 29, pages 551–58.

7. Kirby, R. W., et al. "Oat-Bran Intake Selectively Lowers Serum Low-Density Lipoprotein Cholesterol Concentrations of Hypercholesterolemic Men." *American Journal of Clinical Nutrition,* 1981: volume 34, pages 824–28.

8. Anderson, J. W., et al. "Cholesterol-Lowering Properties of Oat Products." In press. Presented at the American Association of Cereal Chemists' annual meeting, 1982.

9. Anderson, J. W., et al. "Hypocholesterolemic Effects of Oat-Bran or Bean Intake for Hypercholesterolemic Men." *American Journal of Clinical Nutrition,* 1984: volume 40, pages 1146–55.

10. Ney, D. M., et al. "Soluble Oat Fiber Tends to Normalize Lipoprotein Composition in Cholesterol-Fed Rats." *Journal of the American Institute of Nutrition,* 1988: volume 118, pages 1455–62.

11. Kinosian, B. P. and Eisenberg, J. M. "Cutting into Cholesterol. Cost-Effective Alternatives for Treating Hypercholesterolemia." *Journal of the American Medical Association,* 1988: volume 259: pages 2249–54.

12. Anderson, J. W., et al. "Mineral and Vitamin Status on High-Fiber Diets: Long-Term Studies of Diabetic Patients." *Diabetes Care,* 1980: volume 3, pages 38–40.

13. Anderson, J. W. "Medical Benefits of High-Fiber Intakes." *The Fiber Factor,* August 1983. Quaker Oats Company, Chicago.

14. *Dietary Guidelines for Americans.* U.S. Department of Agriculture and U.S. Department of Health, Education and Welfare, Washington, D.C., 1980.

15. *The Surgeon General's Report on Nutrition and Health.* 1988. U.S. Department of Health and Human Services, Public Health Service. DHHS (PHS) Publication No. 88–50211.

Chapter 6. The Amazing Story of Niacin

1. Council on Scientific Affairs. "Dietary and Pharmacologic Therapy for the Lipid Risk Factors." *Journal of the American Medical Association,* 1983: volume 250, number 14, pages 1873–79.

2. Hotz, W. "Nicotinic Acid and Its Derivatives: a Short Survey." *Advances in Lipid Research,* 1983: volume 20, pages 195–217.

3. Wahlqvist, M. L. "Effects on Plasma Cholesterol of Nicotinic Acid and Its Analogues (Niacin)." In *Vitamins in Human Biology and Medicine.* CRC Press, Boca Raton, Florida, 1981, pages 81–94.

4. Hunninghake D. B. "Pharmacologic Therapy for the Hyperlipidemic Patient." *American Journal of Medicine,* 1983: volume 74, number 5A, pages 19–22.

5. Paoletti, R, et al. "Influence of Bezafibrate, Fenofibrate, Nicotinic Acid and Etofibrate on Plasma High-Density Lipoprotein Levels." *American Journal of Cardiology,* 1983: volume 52, number 4, pages 21B–27B.

6. Kane, J. P., et al. "Normalization of Low-Density Lipoprotein Levels in Heterozygous Fa-

milial Hypercholesterolemia with a Combined Drug Regimen." *New England Journal of Medicine,* 1981: volume 304, number 5, pages 251–58.

7. Nessim, S. A., et al. "Combined Therapy of Niacin, Colestipol, and Fat-Controlled Diet in Men with Coronary Bypass. Effect on Blood Lipids and Apolipoproteins." *Arteriosclerosis,* 1983: volume 3, number 6, pages 568–73.

8. Kane, J. P., and Malloy, M. J. "Treatment of Hypercholesterolemia." *Medical Clinics of North America,* 1982: volume 66, number 2, pages 573–50.

9. Hoeg, J. M., et al. "An Approach to the Management of Hyperlipoproteinemia." *Journal of the American Medical Association,* 1986: volume 255, number 4, pages 512–21.

10. "U.S. Defines Cholesterol Hazards and Offers Treatment Guidelines." *New York Times,* October 6, 1987, page 1.

11. Blankenhorn, D. H., et al. "Beneficial Effects of Combined Colestipol-Niacin Therapy on Coronary Atherosclerosis and Coronary Venous Bypass Grafts." *Journal of the American Medical Association,* 1987: volume 257, pages 3233–41.

12. Cohen, L. "Successful Treatment of Hypercholesterolemia with a Combination of Probucol and Niacin." Presented at the Annual Meeting of the Federation of American Societies for Experimental Biology, April, 1985.

13. *Family Practice News.* Volume 16, number 2, page 65, 1986.

14. Luria, M. "Effect of Low-Dose Niacin in High-Density Lipoprotein Cholesterol and Total

Cholesterol/High-Density Lipoprotein Choles-terol Ratio." *Archives of Internal Medicine,* 1988: volume 148, pages 2493–95.

15. The Coronary Drug Project Research Group. "Clofibrate and Niacin in Coronary Heart Disease (the Coronary Drug Project)." *Journal of the American Medical Association,* 1975: volume 231, pages 360–81.

16. Mevacor advertisement. Merck, Sharp & Dohme. *Journal of the American Medical Association,* 1987: volume 258, pages 1884 A–H.

Index